Ron Schuren
6/6/88.

LINEAR GROWTH RETARDATION IN LESS DEVELOPED COUNTRIES

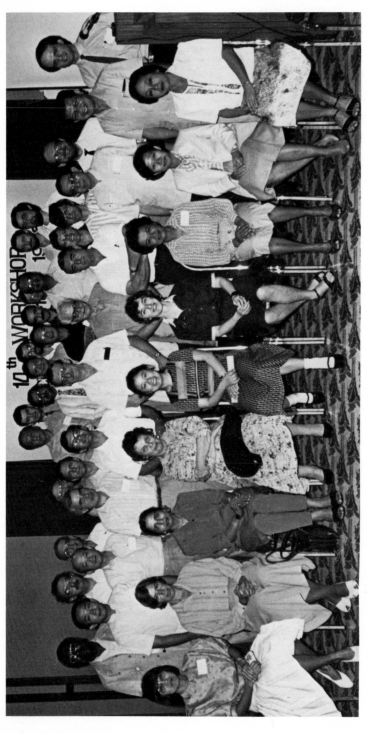

Linear Growth Retardation in Developing Countries, Fourteenth Nestlé Nutrition Workshop, Cha-am, Thailand, March 11–13th, 1986

Conference Participants *(from left to right):* First row—K. Sriwatanakul, M. Colombo, P. Kaur, B. Tanner, M. Yang, B. Golden, O. Thanangkul, P. Kuncharanussorn, K. Karijadi. Second row—D. Nnanyelugo, K. Tontisirin, T. -Y. Huang, R. Rappaport, D. P. Davies, R. Martorell, G. B. Spurr, J. C. Waterlow, P. R. Guesry, A. Tomkins, Ph. Goyens, A. Valyasevi, M. Golden, S. Saowakontha, D. Nabarro. Third row— W. Keller, M. Hernandez Rodriguez, J. M. Tanner, W. Gandawidjaja, D. Milner, D. Mukherjee, W. Chatranon, W. Van Lerberghe, Syarikat Tarigan, M. T. Lahrech, D. R. Fraser, S. Daili, J. Ehrlich, A. Jacob.

Linear Growth Retardation in Less Developed Countries

Editor

John C. Waterlow, M.D., F.R.S.

Emeritus Professor of Human Nutrition
London School of Hygiene and Tropical Medicine
University of London
London, England

Nestlé Nutrition
Workshop Series
Volume 14

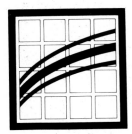

NESTLÉ NUTRITION, VEVEY

RAVEN PRESS ■ NEW YORK

Nestec Ltd., Avenue Nestlé, 1800 Vevey, Switzerland
Raven Press, Ltd., 1185 Avenue of the Americas, New York, New York 10036

Made in the United States of America

Library of Cataloging-in-Publication Data

Linear growth retardation in less developed countries.

(Nestlé Nutrition workshop series ; v. 14)
Based on papers presented at the 14th Nestlé Nutrition workshop, held in Cha-am, Thailand, Mar. 11–13th, 1986.
Includes bibliographies and index.
1. Malnutrition in children—Developing countries—Congresses. 2. Children—Developing countries—Growth—Congresses. 3. Children—Developing countries—Constitution—Congresses. 4. Stature, Short—Developing countries—Congresses. I. Waterlow, J. C. (John Conrad) II. Nestlé Nutrition S.A. III. Series. [DNLM: 1. Body Height—in infancy & childhood—congresses. 2. Developing Countries—congresses. 3. Growth Disorders—etiology—congresses. 4. Growth Disorders—in infancy & childhood—congresses. W1 NE228 v.14 / QZ 45 1986] RJ399.M26L56 1988 618.92 87-32216
ISBN 0-88167-378-1 (Raven Press)

The material contained in this volume was submitted as previously unpublished material, except in the instances in which credit has been given to the source from which some of the illustrative material was derived.

Great care has been taken to maintain the accuracy of the information contained in the volume. However, neither Nestec nor Raven Press can be held responsible for errors or for any consequences arising from the use of the information contained herein.

9 8 7 6 5 4 3 2 1

Preface

In many Third World countries, 30% or more of children under 5 years may be diagnosed as malnourished solely on the basis of a low height or length for age by comparison with international standards. For brevity this deficit in linear growth is often referred to as stunting, a term that was introduced because it is purely descriptive. What right have we to diagnose this growth deficit as malnutrition? There is grave danger of a circular argument. It is probably true that nutritional deficiency in general leads to impairment of linear growth; it is certainly not true that all such impairment is caused by malnutrition, although there may perhaps be a common final metabolic or endocrine pathway. If one asks, "How do we know that malnutrition causes this growth deficit in the Third World?" the only answer in the present state of knowledge is that the existence of the deficit defines the presence of malnutrition.

This is clearly a most unsatisfactory situation, particularly because the problem is not a trivial one. Stunting is not only very prevalent, but it has important social implications, since it is widely regarded as an index of poverty. At the biological level, some look on stunting as a useful adaptation that enhances the chances of survival; others emphasize the physical and psychological handicaps that may be associated, directly or indirectly, with stunting.

It seems that the only way to make progress in this situation is to withdraw from concepts that cannot be defined, such as malnutrition and poverty, and to look objectively at the facts that we do have: the epidemiology and natural history of the process; the biological mechanisms that determine growth failure, because in the end there must be a metabolic cause; the environmental factors that set the process going; and the handicaps, if any, associated with it or even caused by it.

The question has important implications for policy. Are these large numbers of children malnourished in any meaningful way? I myself do not think it is enough simply to say that stunting is an index of poverty and that this requires a holistic approach. This may be true, but it is not particularly helpful. A useful approach may be that if we regard stunting as an indicator, it is difficult to develop a rational policy, even a policy to do nothing, unless we know more about what the indicator really means. Such knowledge should help in using limited resources more effectively.

This position is an article of faith, and I do not expect everyone to agree with it. Nevertheless, I do believe that the Workshop may have contributed to a better definition of the problem and hence may stimulate further research and discussion.

JOHN C. WATERLOW

v

Acknowledgments

As the initiator of the Fourteenth Nestlé Nutrition Workshop, I wish to record my gratitude to Nestlé for its generous and imaginative support, and in particular to Dr. P. Guesry, who made that support possible. We are greatly indebted to M. P. Guinand and his colleagues who were responsible for the arrangements in Thailand; to Dr. P. Goyens for his assistance in editing the discussions, and to Mrs. Jennifer Bohn-Pink who surmounted the difficulties of transcribing them.

Foreword

The idea of this workshop, *Linear Growth Retardation in Less Developed Countries,* came from the need to get a better understanding of a condition that, though extremely common, has been studied very little from a scientific point of view.

What could be more appropriate than a Nestlé Nutrition Workshop bringing together research scientists and practicing pediatricians in a forum for discussion of the subject in depth? Many aspects of "nutritional stunting" were extensively discussed, with contributions from epidemiologists, auxologists, nutritionists, endocrinologists, and pediatricians.

More questions were raised than can be answered, but progress was made in defining the extent of the problem, its implications for pediatricians, and the needs for further research.

PIERRE R. GUESRY, M.D.
Vice President
NESTEC Ltd.
Avenue Nestlé 55
1800 Vevey, Switzerland

Contents

Contributors

I. de Andraca
Unidad de Neuropsicologia
Instituto de Nutrición y Tecnologia de los
Alimentos (INTA)
Universidad de Chile
Casilla 15138
Santiago 11, Chile

Claudia Cassels
Department of International Community
Health
Liverpool School of Tropical Medicine
Pembroke Place
Liverpool L3 5QA, England

*Marta Colombo
Unidad de Neuropsicologica
Instituto de Nutrición y Tecnologia de los
Alimentos (INTA)
Universidad de Chile
Casilla 15138
Santiago 11, Chile

Ricardo Castillo
Department of Pediatrics
Stanford Medical School
Stanford, California 94305

*D. P. Davies
Department of Paediatrics
Prince of Wales Hospital
The Chinese University of Hong Kong
Shatín, New Territories, Hong Kong

*D. R. Fraser
Department of Animal Husbandry
University of Sydney
New South Wales 2006, Australia

Michael H. N. Golden
Tropical Metabolism Research Unit
University of the West Indies
Kingston 7, Jamaica

*C. Gopalan
The Nutrition Foundation of India
B - 37 Gulhomar Park
New Delhi 110049, India

M. J. R. Healy
London School of Hygiene and Tropical
Medicine
Keppel Street
London WC1E 7HT, England

Peter Howard
Institute of Medical Research
Papua New Guinea

*W. Keller
Nutrition, World Health Organization
Geneva, Switzerland

I. López
Unidad de Neuropsicologia
Instituto de Nutrición y Tecnologia de los
Alimentos (INTA)
Universidad de Chile
Casilla 15138
Santiago 11, Chile

*Reynaldo Martorell
Food Research Institute
Stanford University
Stanford, California 94305

---

*Workshop participants.

Fernando Mendoza
Department of Pediatrics
Stanford Medical School
Stanford, California 94305

*R. D. G. Milner
Department of Paediatrics
Children's Hospital
Sheffield S10 2TH, England

*David Nabarro
Department of International Community
  Health
Liverpool School of Tropical Medicine
Pembroke Place
Liverpool L3 5QA, England

Nigel Padfield
East Street Health Centre
Thame, Oxford, England

Mahesh Pant
International Irrigation Management
  Institute
Kathmandu, Nepal

*R. Rappaport
Research Unit on Developmental Biology
  and Growth
INSERM U. 30
Hôpital des Enfants-Malades
149 rue de Sèvres
Paris 15ème, France

*G. B. Spurr
Research Service
Zablocki
Veterans Administration Medical Center
Milwaukee, Wisconsin 53295

*J. M. Tanner
Institute of Child Health
University of London
Guilford Street 30
London WC1N 1EH, England

*Andrew Tomkins
Department of Human Nutrition and
  Department of Clinical Tropical
  Medicine
London School of Hygiene and Tropical
  Medicine
Keppel Street
London WC1E 7HT, England

*W. Van Lerberghe
ENOV-URESP, Unit for Research and
  Training in Public Health
Institute for Tropical Medicine
Nationale Straat 155
B-2000 Antwerp, Belgium

*John C. Waterlow
London School of Hygiene and Tropical
  Medicine
Keppel Street
London WC1E 7HT, England

Alet Wijga
KHARDEP Impact Studies of the Kosi
  Hill Area Rural Development
  Programme
Dhankuta, Nepal

*Min Yang
Department of Health Statistics
West China University of Medical
  Sciences
South Ren-min Road
Chengdu, Sichuan, People's Republic
  of China

F. Y. Zumrawi
P.O. Box 20P3
Khartoum, Sudan

Invited Attendees

H. A. Aponso/*Peradeniya, Sri Lanka*
Wirapong Chatranon/*Bangkok, Thailand*
Syamsir Daili/*Padang, Indonesia*
John Erlich/*Alice Springs, Australia*
Winadi Gandawidjaja/*Jakarta, Indonesia*
Barbara E. Golden/*Kingston, Jamaica*
Teh-Yang Huang/*Taipei, Taiwan*
Albert Jacob/*Agadir, Morocco*
Koesriatoen Karijadi/*Surabaya, Indonesia*
Pyar Kaur/*Kedah, Malaysia*
Pawadee Kuncharanussorn/*Bangkok, Thailand*
M. T. Lahrech/*Rabat, Morocco*

Dilip Mukherjee/*Calcutta, India*
Dickson Nnanyelugo/*Nsukka, Nigeria*
K. Ramanchandran/*New Delhi, India*
Manuel Hernandez Rodriguez/*Madrid, Spain*
Sastri Saowakontha/*Khon Kaen, Thailand*
Kitima Sriwatanakul/*Bangkok, Thailand*
Bernice Tanner/*London, U.K.*
Syarikat Tarigan/*Medan, Indonesia*
Ousa Thanangkul/*Chiang Mai, Thailand*
Kraisid Tontsirin/*Bangkok, Thailand*
Aree Valyasevi/*Bangkok, Thailand*
Komol Wongsrisart/*Bangkok, Thailand*

Nestlé Participants

Pierre R. Guesry
Vice President
Nestec, Switzerland

Philippe Goyens
Nestec, Switzerland

Steve R. Allen
Eastreco, Singapore

Nestlé Nutrition Workshop Series

LINEAR GROWTH RETARDATION
IN LESS DEVELOPED COUNTRIES

Linear Growth Retardation in Less Developed Countries, edited by John C. Waterlow. Nestlé Nutrition Workshop Series, Vol. 14. Nestec Ltd., Vevey/Raven Press, Ltd., New York © 1988.

Observations on the Natural History of Stunting

J. C. Waterlow

London School of Hygiene and Tropical Medicine, London WC1E 7HT, England

The reason for organizing this workshop is very simple. If we use a low weight for age as the basis for the anthropometric diagnosis of malnutrition, then in many countries some four-fifths of the children considered to be malnourished are simply small in size, with normal weight for height (Table 1). However, it is remarkable that there has been no systematic attempt to tackle the question: Is it meaningful or realistic to call these small children malnourished? To establish a valid definition, we must avoid a circular argument: nutritional status is assessed by measurement of body size; therefore, a small child is malnourished.

The question posed above is of great public health importance, and attempts to answer it will bring us into difficult territory. It may be useful to divide the question into two parts. First, does smallness imply any impairment of health or functional capacity? More precisely, what are the relationships between body size and different functions after interfering factors have been removed (if, indeed, they can be removed)? Here we are dealing with the *mal* in malnutrition. The second part of the question is whether the effects are caused primarily by nutritional factors and, if they are, by what mechanism? The chapters in this volume are addressed to different aspects of these two questions. These in turn encompass a third question: Does stunting represent a situation that calls for action in countries where resources are scarce, and, if so, what kind of action?

TABLE 1. *Prevalence of malnutrition (percentage) in preschool children according to different criteria[a]*

Criterion of malnutrition	Nepal	Sri Lanka	Vietnam refugees
Wasted, stunted, or wasted and stunted	56.2	37.1	65.7
Wasted or wasted and stunted (excluding children who are stunted only)	7.3	6.6	10.8

[a]Cut-off points: wasted, <80% of reference median; Stunted, <90% of reference median.

1

I introduced the term stunting some 10 years ago (1,2) to describe what one actually sees: a deficit in attained length or height of children compared with international standards. It is not a very pleasant-sounding word, and it is difficult to translate into other languages, but at least it is concise and objective. Moreover, it is very convenient that in English we can distinguish between stunting, which is a process and could be regarded as a velocity term, and stunted, which in Tanner's terminology is a distance term. One cannot make this distinction with the word "short." Moreover, "stunted" conveys the impression that the child does not have to be short, that something has gone wrong. However, it is not justified to take the further step of equating stunting with chronic malnutrition, because that begs all the questions raised above.

NATURAL HISTORY OF STUNTING

By natural history I mean the evolution of stunting in time as opposed to its geographical prevalence, which is described elsewhere in this volume by Keller. I concern myself with two particular questions: When does stunting begin in the populations with which we are concerned? What are the possibilities for catch-up? Obviously, there are many other matters that are relevant to the natural history, but they are discussed in other chapters.

At the beginning there is the problem that stunting or growth retardation are comparative terms—stunting in relation to what? At the present time there does not exist an adequate reference for height velocity. In Tanner's original standards (3), the intervals are too long for detailed study of growth velocity during the first 2 years of life, which I believe to be the critical period.

The findings presented in Figs. 1 and 2 are derived from various studies in developing and developed countries. Wherever possible I have chosen longitudinal or semilongitudinal studies. Even when children have been measured longitudinally, the published results usually give only average heights at different ages. Differences between heights at different ages thus represent average increments rather than velocities; they give no information about the standard deviations (SD) or centiles of growth velocity, so that no judgment can be made about the range of so-called normality. Moreover, the process of putting together different sets of figures and making comparisons involves many sources of variability and error. In some studies the sexes are not separated; it is often not possible to be certain about the accuracy of the ages; some of the data are clearly not of good quality; in some Third World countries there may be seasonal effects that were not allowed for; different authors use different age intervals, e.g., 4-week periods, months, decimal years. Social class may vary; some studies are urban, others rural. The numbers of children also vary greatly, both between and within studies. When overall averages have been calculated, no attempt has been made to weight them for numbers. Finally, I make no claim to have taken into account all results that may be available in the literature; there are many studies reported in local journals that are not so easily accessible. Even among the four sets of values from industrialized countries, there are not inconsiderable differences among the average increments.

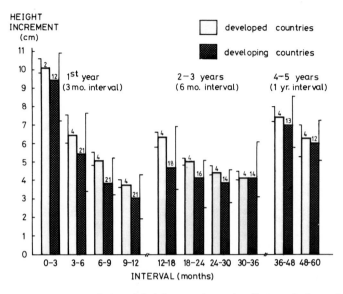

FIG. 1. Average increments in length/height over 3 months (first year), 6 months (second and third years), and 1 year (fourth and fifth years) in children from developing (*filled bars*) and developed (*open bars*) countries. The bars represent the range of variation between studies, not between individuals. Numbers above the columns indicate the number of studies. Sources of data for developing countries (boys or mixed sexes): Australian aborigines (4), China (5), Egypt (6), Gambia (7), Gaza Strip (8), Guatemala (9,10), India (11–14), Jamaica (15), Jordan (16), Kenya (17), Malaysia (18), Nigeria (19,20), Papua–New Guinea (21), Philippines (22), Senegal (23), Thailand (24), Zaire (25); for developed countries (boys): Netherlands (26), UK (3), USA (27,28).

My aim is simply to take a preliminary look to see whether patterns or trends emerge that are worth a more detailed examination.

When Does Stunting Begin in Third World Children?

The results in Fig. 1 for increments over 3-month periods seem to confirm the suggestion made 10 years ago (2) that linear growth begins to fall off in the second 3 months of life if not earlier. The average increments remain low, at about 80% of reference, until at least the end of the second year, and then there is a suggestion that they pick up.

The young infant is of particular interest. Figure 2 is an attempt to find out whether the deficit starts even before 3 months. The results in this figure are not very satisfactory, since I found only 11 studies with monthly measurements of length, and it is likely that over such short intervals differences are not very accurate. At this age there are also likely to be large variations between ethnic groups in feeding practices, seasonal effects, and so on. By comparison with the industrialized countries, there is some evidence of faltering after the third month but not before that.

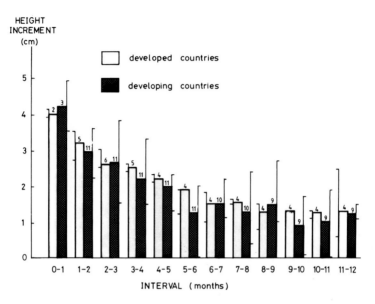

FIG. 2. Average monthly increments in length during the first year of life in children from developing (*dark bars*) and developed (*light bars*) countries. The *bars* represent the range of variation between studies. Numbers above the columns indicate the number of studies. Sources of data for developing countries (boys or mixed sexes): Australian aborigines (4), China (5), Eskimos (29), India (13,14), Kenya (17), Nigeria (19), Pakistan (30), Papua–New Guinea (21), Philippines (22), Zaire (23); for developed countries (boys): Australia (see 24), Netherlands (26), UK (31), USA (28,32,33).

Is the Comparison Between Third World and Industrialized Countries Appropriate?

Conclusions drawn about faltering may be criticized on the grounds that the so-called standards of developed countries are inappropriate. The major questions about genetic and environmental influences on growth are discussed elsewhere in this volume by Davies and Martorell et al., but there are two other points that should be taken into account.

The first is the influence of breast feeding. The NCHS reference, its predecessor, the Harvard standards, and possibly both Tanner's standards and the Dutch ones reflect the growth of infants who were probably mainly formula fed, because these were compiled before the recrudescence of breast feeding in industrialized countries. In the words of Whitehead and Paul (34):

> It is perhaps not unreasonable . . . to suggest that now infant feeding practices have changed so markedly we might consider the systematic collection of data for the reconstruction of new growth centile charts. Surely we should not just assume that what was happening to the growth of children 20 to 50 years ago, when the majority of children were fed on what we now realize were inappropriately constituted and administered formulae, coupled with the early administration of solids, is the rational anthropometric target to aim for at the present time.

Whitehead and Paul's figures seem to show some falling off in attained length in boys at about 9 months and in girls at about 6 months (34). It is puzzling that most of these infants had been exclusively breast fed for not more than 4 to 6 months, so that the faltering seems to begin and to be maintained after supplements were introduced.

Table 2 shows results of three comparisons in developed countries between formula-fed and exclusively breast-fed infants. The increments between 0 and 3 months were the same with both types of feeding; after 3 months they were consistently less in the exclusively breast-fed babies and close to those of the developing countries shown in Fig. 1. If the average growth curve in those countries is close to that of breast-fed babies, is it fair to use the word "faltering" with its connotation of something undesirable? That is not a question that can be taken up in this chapter, which is concerned with data rather than with interpretations.

A second problem is that in developing countries there is a high proportion of infants with low weight at birth. Could the "bad start" that these children have cause the falling off in average increments during the first year? A great deal of work has been done in developed countries on the growth of premature and small-for-date infants. The impression is that at least the prematures usually show greater than normal incremental growth (e.g., 37).

Table 3 shows comparisons made in India and Guatemala of growth in length of low-birth-weight and normal-birth-weight infants. In this table I have excluded the extremes of low birth weight since we are not concerned here with frankly pathological states. Except in the study of Bhargava et al. (11), most of the low-birth-weight children were probably small for gestational age. There seems, within this range, to be no consistent difference in growth in length related to low birth weight. Therefore, I conclude that the falling off shown in Fig. 1 is not caused by dilution of the samples by infants of low birth weight. However, more evidence on this point is needed.

TABLE 2. *Comparison of increments in length during the first year of life in exclusively breast-fed and formula-fed infants in industrialized countries with average increments in Third World countries*[a]

Age interval (months)	Increment (cm)		
	Formula-fed	Breast-fed	Third World
0–3	9.6	9.5 (3)	9.5
3–6	6.2	5.8 (3)	5.5
6–9	4.6	3.95 (2)	3.9
9–12	4.1	3.6 (1)	3.1

[a]Numbers of studies in parenthesis. Breast- and formula-fed data from Owen et al. (35), Evans (31), Salmenperä et al. (36). Third World data from Fig. 1.

TABLE 3. *Increments in length of low-birth-weight and normal-birth-weight infants*

Age interval (months)	India[a] Mean birth wt. (kg)		India[b] Birth wt. (kg)		Guatemala[c] Birth wt. (kg)	
	1.8 ± 0.2	3.0 ± 0.3	2.0–2.5	2.5–3.0	2.0	3.0
0–3	9.1	10.7	8.7	8.9	8.7	8.4
3–6	7.4	6.2	5.5	5.4	5.5	4.8
6–9	4.8	3.3	3.5	3.8	3.7	3.9
9–12	3.4	4.2	3.4	3.3	3.3	2.2
Total, first year	24.7	24.4	21.1	21.4	21.2	19.3
Length at birth (cm)	44.6	49.3	47.9	49.3	41.6	49.3

[a]Data of Datta Banik et al. (38) for mixed AGA and SGA infants.
[b]Data of Bhargava et al. (11) for AGA infants.
[c]Date of Mata (9) for mixed AGA and SGA infants.

How Long Does It Take to Become "Significantly" Stunted?

The calculations that follow are all in terms of increments, and for this purpose the NCHS reference (27) is used rather than the "mixed" reference of Fig. 1. A child whose increments from month to month are less than those of the NCHS median is described as having an incremental deficit; his increments will be expressed as a percentage of the reference median increments. The calculations also assume, for the sake of simplicity, that a child has the same incremental deficit throughout the first 3 years of life. Obviously this is not true, but one has to start with some simplifying assumptions.

Figure 3 shows the attained length at different ages, expressed as a percentage of NCHS reference median, of children whose average increments were 80%, 65%, and 50% of the reference increments. From Tanner's velocity data (3), these deficits correspond very roughly to -1, -2, and -3 SD. The figure also shows a line for 90% of NCHS median length, which is commonly taken as a cut-off point for a child to be classified as stunted. It is obvious that the smaller the incremental deficit, the longer it takes for a child to cross the cut-off line. It follows that in a population of children with varying degrees of incremental deficit, the number that cross the line will increase with time. In this model, the prevalence and distribution of stunting remain constant, but the prevalence of stunted children increases. For this reason it seems quite unjustified to draw the conclusion, as some have done, that "chronic malnutrition" is a more serious problem in older than in younger preschool children.

The argument implies that what matters from a physiological point of view is not a deficit in attained length or height but a deficit in increment, i.e., in rate of growth. If that is correct, it follows that it is unsound to use a cut-off point for attained length that is the same over the whole age range. If we are going to use cut-off points at all, and they are sometimes necessary for public health purposes,

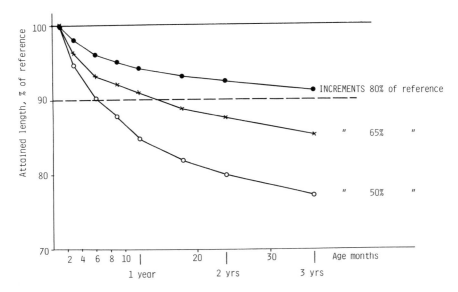

FIG. 3. Effect of deficits in incremental growth on attained length, expressed as percentage of reference (NCHS) length for age (boys). *Solid circles, crosses,* and *open circles* represent length when increments are 80%, 65%, and 50%, respectively, of reference increments. *Dashed line,* 90% of reference attained length.

it would be more logical to put the cut-off point at each age as the length representing the result of a given deficit in incremental growth, say, 65% of the reference median increment. This value might be chosen as a cutoff because it corresponds roughly to −2 SD of standard velocity. When we have more data on the SD of increments, we can, if we want to, choose a more appropriate cut-off point. The result of this approach is shown by line B in Fig. 4; this line could be called the "incremental cutoff." Line A represents the conventional cutoff of 90% of reference median attained length. It is apparent that line B will lead to more children being classified as stunted at younger ages and fewer at older ages. I believe that from the public health point of view this would present a much more realistic picture. It would be very simple to prepare charts of attained length that show this new cut-off line; it would be more difficult to explain how it was derived.

VARIABILITY OF LINEAR GROWTH

It is common to regard growth in length as much less variable than growth in weight. This is probably wrong: it is the measurement that is more difficult. Tanner's velocity data show a coefficient of variation during the first 3 years of life of about 16% (3). I presume that this represents between-subject variation. Fomon and his colleagues have recently been analyzing their data on the growth of infants

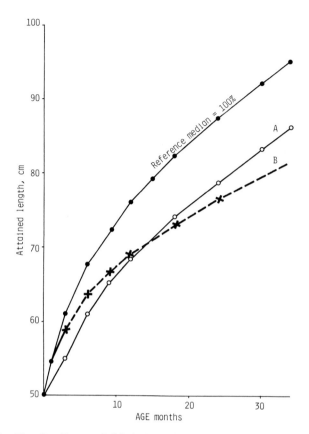

FIG. 4. Attained length with age. *Solid circles,* references (NCHS) median, boys; *open circles,* curve **A,** 90% of reference median (the conventional cut-off point for stunting); *crosses,* curve **B,** attained length when increments are 65% of the reference increments.

up to about 4 months. Measurements were made at intervals of 2 to 4 weeks. As one might expect, the growth from one period to another is more variable in some children than in others. Fomon should be able to tell us the range between subjects of within-subject variability. This will be very important information.

In Third World countries there are marked seasonal variations of growth in length or height, which can be shown very clearly over periods as short as 2 months. They are documented in this volume by Nabarro et al. and by Tomkins, so I need not discuss them further here except to conclude that the rate of growth in height as well as in weight is quite sensitive to environmental factors.

CATCH-UP

The term "catch-up" is somewhat ambiguous. It is obviously necessary to distinguish between catch-up in attained height, so that final height is within normal limits for sex and age, and catch-up in the rate of growth. There is also a problem in assessing the extent of catch-up in rate, because the observed increment over any period can be compared with the expected increment either in children who start at the same age or in children who start at the same height. Either method seems to have its logic.

The possibility for catch-up in attained height is limited by the maturation of the ossification centers, which seems in general to be less retarded than linear growth (39). There is a large literature on catch-up growth, but much of it is concerned with rather older children than those considered here and with the effects of making good hormonal deficits, e.g., of thyroid and growth hormones, as discussed in this volume by Rappaport. However, if the rate of growth in height is indeed responsive to environmental, including nutritional, factors, one would expect catch-up growth to occur whenever nutritional conditions become favorable. There is impressive evidence that this can indeed happen. As one example, Prader and co-workers (40) have shown remarkable gains in height when treatment is instituted in previously untreated children with celiac disease. These children were, of course, living in a good and clean environment, but the findings illustrate what is physiologically possible in young children.

Further evidence of the rapid responsiveness of linear growth is provided not only by the seasonal changes mentioned above but also by the catch-up that can occur during a relatively short period of treatment of malnourished children in hospital (Golden, *this volume*).

Table 4 summarizes the results of three long-term studies in which children who had been severely malnourished were reexamined after several years. In the Peruvian study (43), a small group (A) of malnourished children, after discharge from hospital, were brought up in the homes of well-to-do foster parents. These were

TABLE 4. *Later catch-up growth of children malnourished in infancy*

	Height as percentage of standard (NCHS, boys)	
South Africa (41)		
Admission to hospital	86.6 (35)[a]	
Follow-up, 5 years	87.4 (77)	
Follow-up, 10 years	90.1 (78)	
Jamaica (42)		
Admission to hospital	92.8 (56)	
Follow-up, 2–8 years	101.1 (56)	
Peru (43)	Group A[b]	Group B[c]
Admission to hospital	86.1 (8)	86.0 (8)
Discharge from hospital	91.2 (8)	90.1 (8)
Follow-up, 6–10 years	97.9 (8)	89.7 (8)

[a]Numbers of children in parentheses.
[b]Taken by well-to-do foster parents.
[c]Returned to impoverished homes.

compared with a group (B) of children matched for age and sex who, on discharge from hospital, returned to their own poor families.

One can conclude from the Jamaican study (42) and from the Peruvian group A that even after severe retardation, virtually complete restoration of normal height is possible, at least up to the age of about 10 years. The failure of catch-up shown by the South African children (41) and by the Peruvian group B is presumably the result of continuing deprivation.

The question then arises whether even in these children eventual catch-up would be possible as a result of delayed maturation and prolongation of the pubertal growth spurt. Only one study has gone on long enough to address this question, that of Satyanarayana and co-workers in India (44). They separated 5-year-old children into different groups according to their height and reexamined them at intervals up to the age of 20. The initial deficit of the shortest group was 15.5 cm; they were still 10 cm shorter at 20 years, but between the ages of 5 and 20 the increment was greater in the initially shorter children and equal to that of American boys over the same age interval. Thus, although a serious deficit was established by the age of 5, it did not prevent these children from growing at a normal rate thereafter. But why could they not grow at a faster rate than normal and so catch up in attained height? Was the limiting factor food intake or infection or heavy manual work? Or was growth during this phase of life controlled by genetic factors, small adults producing small children, who in turn became small adults? In the society in which this study was done, there is evidence that smallness may be a disadvantage when it comes to earning capacity, so that perhaps people are particularly poor because they are small rather than the other way around.

These questions provide an introduction to the chapters that follow by Martorell et al. and Davies.

CONCLUSION

In the early years of life, growth in length is very sensitive to nutritional and other environmental influences. In developing countries the growth rate often falls off within a few months of birth but tends to return to normal after the age of 3 years. This leaves the children with a deficit in attained height and body size compared with their better-off peers. Is it acceptable to regard this as an adaptation? (for discussion see refs. 45, 46). If conditions are favorable, young children may achieve remarkable degrees of catch-up in linear growth, so the physiological capacity is preserved but only seldom expressed. We do not know the extent to which short stature in adults in developing countries is determined by deficits in early life. Is it possible that genetic differences in height become established at the time of the pubertal growth spurt?

REFERENCES

1. Waterlow JC. Note on the assessment and classification of protein–energy malnutrition in children. *Lancet* 1973;2:87–9.

2. Waterlow JC, Rutishauser IHE. Malnutrition in man. In: Cravioto J, Hambraeus, L, Vahlquist B, eds. *Early malnutrition and mental development.* Swedish Nutrition Foundation Symposia XII. Stockholm: Almqvist and Wiksell, 1974:13–26.

3. Tanner JM, Whitehouse RH, Takaishi M. Standards from birth to maturity for height, weight, height velocity and weight velocity. British children, 1965, part II. *Arch Dis Child* 1966;41:613–35.

4. Kettle ES. Weight and height curves for Australian aboriginal infants and children. *Med J Aust* 1966;53:972–7.

5. Su T-F, Liang CJ. Growth and development of Chinese infants of Hunan province. *Chin Med J* 1940;58:104–12.

6. Abbasy AS. *Growth and development of the Egyptian child, birth to five years.* Alexandria: University of Alexandria, Department of Paediatrics, 1972.

7. McGregor IA, Rahman AK, Thompson B, Billewicz WZ, Thomson AM. The growth of young children in a Gambian village. *Trans R Soc Trop Med Hyg* 1968;62:341–52.

8. Guinema AHI. Protein–calorie malnutrition in young refugee children in the Gaza Strip. *Environ Child Health* 1977;23:38–57.

9. Mata LJ. *The children of Santa Maria Cauqué: a prospective field study of health and growth.* Cambridge, MA: MIT Press, 1978.

10. Yarbrough C, Habicht J-P, Malina RM, Lechtig A, Klein RE. Length and weight in rural Guatemalan Ladino children, birth to seven years of age. *Am J Phys Anthropol* 1975;42:439–48.

11. Bhargava SK, Kumari S, Choudhary P, Ghosh S, Butani R, Bhargava V. Longitudinal study of linear physical growth in preterm infants from birth to six years. *Indian J Med Res* 1983;78:74–7.

12. Datta Banik ND, Krishna R, Mane SIS, Raj L. Longitudinal growth pattern of children during pre-school age and its relationship with different socio-economic classes. *Indian J Pediatr* 1970;37:438–47.

13. Jha SJ. A longitudinal study in infants belonging to a sweeper community in Bombay city. *Pediatr Clin India* 1969;1:49–56.

14. Mukherjee DK, Sethna NJ, Mahdavan R. Height, weight, height velocity and weight velocity of Bengali Hindu children from birth to 18 months. *Indian J Pediatr* 1970;37:429–37.

15. Standard KL, Desai P, Miall WE. A longitudinal study of child growth in a rural community in Jamaica. *J Biosoc Sci* 1969;1:153–76.

16. Hijazi SS. *Child growth and nutrition in Jordan.* Amman: Royal Scientific Society Press, 1977.

17. Oomen HAPC, Blankhart DM, Mannetje W't. Growth pattern of pre-school children. In: Van Ginneken JK, Multer AS, eds. *Maternal and child health in rural Kenya.* London: Croom Helm, 1984:183–96.

18. Millis J. Growth of pre-school Malay infants in Singapore. *Med J Malaysia* 1957;12:416–21.

19. Ecoma EE. Observations on the growth of children in the Nsukka Division, Eastern Nigeria. *J Trop Pediatr* 1959;5:59–63.

20. Morley DC, Woodland M, Martin WJ, Allen I. Heights and weights of West African village children from birth to the age of five. *West Afr Med J* 1968;17:8–13.

21. Bailey KV. Growth of Chimbu infants in the New Guinea Highlands. *J Trop Pediatr* 1964;10:3–15.

22. Fernandez TL, Guthrie GM, Ruiz-Lambo NR. *A study on the problems of weaning and the maintenance of lactation in Cebu, Philippines.* Report to Nestlé Nutrition Research Grant Programme. Cebu, Philippines: Cebu Institute of Medicine, Department of Preventive and Social Medicine, July 1982–June 1985.

23. Massé G, Moreigne F, Sénécal J. Poids et tailles d'enfants dakarois pendant les quatre premières années de la vie. *Bull Soc Med Afr Noire Langue Fr* 1961;6:661–72.

24. Bailey SM, Gershoft SN, McGandy RB, et al. A longitudinal study of growth and maturation in rural Thailand. *Hum Biol* 1984;56:539–58.

25. Van Lerberghe W. Weight, height and arm circumference in 0 to 5 year old children from Kasongo (Zaire). *Ecology Food Nutr* 1982;12:19–28.

26. Van Wieringen JC. *Secular changes of growth: 1964–1966 height and weight surveys in the Netherlands in historical perspective.* Leiden, Netherlands: Institute for Preventive Medicine TNO, 1972.

27. Hamill PVV. *NCHS growth curves for children, birth to 18 years.* Hyattsville, MD: National Center for Health Statistics, 1977; DHEW publication no. (PHS) 78-1650.

28. Stuart HC, Stevenson SS. Physical growth and development. In: Nelson WE, ed. *Textbook of pediatrics.* Philadelphia: WB Saunders, 1959:12.

29. Heller CA, Scott EM, Hammers LM. Height, weight and growth of Alaskan Eskimos. *Am J Dis Child* 1967;113:338–44.
30. Ahmad MS, Kazmi SI, Mubarak MM. Height, weight and arm circumference norms of rural children (a community study). *Pakistan J Med Res* 1984;23:29–38.
31. Evans TJ. Growth and milk intake of normal infants. *Arch Dis Child* 1978;53:749–51.
32. Fomon SJ. *Infant nutrition.* 2nd ed. Philadelphia: WB Saunders, 1974:118–51.
33. Thompson H. Data on the growth of children during the first year after birth. *Hum Biol* 1951;23:75–92.
34. Whitehead RG, Paul AA. Growth charts and the assessment of infant feeding practices in the Western world and in developing countries. *Early Hum Dev* 1984;9:187–207.
35. Owen GM, Garry PJ, Hooper EM. Feeding and growth of infants. *Nutr Res* 1984;4:727–31.
36. Salmenperä L, Perheentupa J, Siimes MA. Exclusively breast fed healthy infants grow slower than reference infants. *Pediatr Res* 1985;19:307–12.
37. Cruise MO. A longitudinal study of the growth of low birth weight infants. *Pediatrics* 1973;51:620–8.
38. Datta Banik ND, Krishna R, Mane SIS, Raj L. A longtudinal study on physical growth of children of different birth weight groups from birth to 5 years. *Indian J Pediatr* 1970;37:95–101.
39. Martorell R, Yarbrough C, Klein RE, Lechtig A. Malnutrition, body size and skeletal maturation; interrelationships and implications for catch-up growth. *Hum Biol* 1979;51:371–89.
40. Prader A. Catch-up growth. *Postgrad Med J* 1978;54[suppl]:133–43.
41. Keet MP, Moodie DD, Wittmann W, Hansen JDL. Kwashiorkor: a prospective ten-year follow-up study. *S Afr Med J* 1971:45:1427–49.
42. Garrow JS, Pyke MC. The long-term prognosis of severe infantile malnutrition. *Lancet* 1967;1:1–4.
43. Graham GG, Adrianzen TB. Late "catch-up" growth after severe infantile malnutrition. *Johns Hopkins Med J* 1972;131:204–11.
44. Satyanarayana K, Prasanna Krishna T, Narasinga Rao BS. Effect of early childhood undernutrition and child labour on growth and adult nutritional status of rural Indian boys around Hyderabad. *Hum Nutr Clin Nutr* 1986;40C:131–40.
45. Gopalan C. "Small is healthy?" For the poor, not for the rich! *Bull Nutr Found India* 1983:Oct.
46. Waterlow JC. Mechanisms of adaptation to low protein and energy intakes. *Annu Rev Nutr* 1986;6:495–526.

DISCUSSION

Dr. Davies: You referred, Dr. Waterlow, to the faster growth of bottle-fed versus breast-fed babies. One of the problems in making these comparisons is that we are often comparing one population with another, and often at a different time. What we need to do is to compare breast- and bottle-fed babies within the same time period. If this were done we would obtain a far more accurate comparison between bottle-fed and breast-fed babies. We are currently studying the growth of South Chinese babies born in Hong Kong and in Canton using similar methodology. These babies share a similar population genotype. Hong Kong is now largely a bottle-fed population; very few are breast fed. In South China most babies are still breast fed. Yet the pattern of linear growth and weight gain over the first 6 months of life is almost identical in Hong Kong and Canton.

Dr. Barbara Golden: I suggest that ethnicity may affect length more than weight for length, and therefore the standards may be more variable between communities. Thai community standards, for example, will be more different from the NCHS standards than the Jamaican ones.

Dr. Guesry: Is it true that static measurements of final height will depend much more on ethnicity than velocity measurements?

Dr. Van Lerberghe: I do not have any concrete evidence on that, but it seems to me that errors of age and errors arising from ethnic differences, which are so important in the analysis of static measurements (attained length), probably become much less important when we analyze velocity measurements, certainly as far as their implication and clinical significance are concerned.

Dr. Waterlow: The question of ethnic differences will be fully covered in the chapters by Drs. Davies and Martorell et al., so I think that we could leave that for the moment.

Dr. Martorell: Yes, we will indeed be focusing on ethnic differences in growth. It should be underscored that most of us are interested in this issue because we use growth data to assess nutritional status. We would like to evaluate children using appropriate reference data. It is also important that we concentrate, where possible, on longitudinal data and not on attained status. Growth monitoring in young children is a useful tool for selecting children at risk of poor health. A key question is whether the functional implications of growth retardation vary by age. I believe this is the case and that the earlier the retardation, the more likely that it will be associated with poor nutritional outcomes.

Dr. Guesry: I would like to return to the question of the faster growth of formula-fed compared with exclusively breast-fed babies. I am prepared to accept that the faster weight gain may be considered deleterious, although adult obesity does not seem to be related to infant obesity. However, I can hardly imagine how faster growth in length could be deleterious.

Dr. Waterlow: I do not know whether it may be deleterious. I was simply trying to present facts. For example, in Owen's study (1) in the United States, the gain in length of exclusively breast-fed infants in the first 3 months of life was 98% of the reference, and in the second 3 months it was 88% of the reference. The NCHS reference is, of course, based largely on data from formula-fed infants.

Dr. Guesry: It has been said that excessive protein intake early in life could induce excessive insulin release, which could be responsible for faster growth, at least in length, and later on could induce diabetes. Dr. Rappaport, could you comment on this?

Dr. Rappaport: I have no specific comment on insulin. A high protein intake will also stimulate the production of growth factors.

Dr. Milner: This workshop is concerned with stunting in the Third World, and later we shall be considering whether a low food intake can produce a deficiency of growth factors. In Western countries, when growth hormone deficiency has been diagnosed, it takes several years' treatment to produce catch-up in height.

Dr. Waterlow: I wonder whether clinical data of this kind in older children are relevant to our problem.

Dr. Nabarro: Our main concern is with the growth of children in developing countries. We need to be careful when applying the results of clinical experience in Western countries. However, this experience may help us to identify the questions to be solved. We should not apply the experiences from one environment to another without the necessary supporting data.

Dr. Rappaport: I agree that the growth hormone model may not be the most appropriate model in the present context. We discuss this in later chapters. I hope also that during this meeting we will be able to elaborate more on the question of catch-up growth. In this connection I would like to return to the earlier discussion on breast feeding and growth. Dr. Waterlow, did you not say that between 1 and 2 years of age, infants have the same pattern of growth whether they have been breast fed or artificially fed? That would imply that there is catch-up growth during the second semester of life.

Dr. Waterlow: I did not mean to imply anything so positive. The studies that I am familiar with, comparing breast-fed and formula-fed babies, have usually not gone on long enough to answer the question. If Dr. Davies' study will continue into the second year, it should be possible to answer Professor Rappaport's question.

Dr. Davies: The intention is to continue the study for 5 years.

Dr. Milner: As a clinician I have serious reservations about whether measuring length in the first to second year of life is practical.

Dr. Aponso: As regards the feasibility of linear growth measurements in infancy: yes, these measurements can be carried out for any specific research project. For instance, we are currently conducting a research project on linear growth in babies and preschool children in collaboration with the London Institute of Child Health. It would, however, be almost impossible for a busy practicing physician to look at linear growth as a measure of growth and development in infancy. In fact, what is the importance of linear growth during the first 6 months of life in Third World countires? Is it all that important?

Dr. Waterlow: I am not proposing that these measurements be done by busy clinicians. I am thinking of research, surveys, and child welfare clinics. Admittedly, it takes three people to measure the length of a young child accurately, but if it does turn out that these measurements are important for public health, not just for clinical pediatrics, then we should try to make them.

Dr. Guesry: An additional problem is that when assessing "faltering" in linear growth, we need to know the exact age of the infant, which is not the case when we assess wasting, because then we relate body weight to height.

Dr. Milner: Age is indeed critical for the assessment of growth retardation, because the "normal" velocity is much higher from 3 to 9 months, for example, than from 15 to 21 months.

Dr. Waterlow: Indeed, a small difference in age will have a very big effect in the first 6 months. That is why we need velocity standards covering shorter intervals than the 3-month intervals of Tanner's standards. I hope that this Workshop will conclude that monthly increments in length are important. I should also like to stress again the variability of monthly increments. This is another subject on which we need more information.

Dr. Golden: Length measures the growth of the whole skeleton. Do we need something more?

Dr. Waterlow: I know that there are ethnic differences in the relative lengths of different parts of the skeleton, e.g., trunk and limbs (2). I do not know whether these differences exist in infants and, if they do, whether they are large enough to interfere with using linear growth to assess nutritional state.

Dr. Davies: It is also a mistake to presume that all babies keep within the same centile channel in the early months after birth. This is a period of very considerable growth shift, both upward and downward. In individual infants this sometimes makes the interpretation of an apparent faltering difficult. In some instances, and this obviously applies far more to children in the developed world, apparent faltering could well be physiological.

Dr. Tomkins: The attained weights and heights of children in relation to the reference may vary considerably in different periods of the year. A child's length may be satisfactory at one moment but may not be so 3 months later. This makes the interpretation of longitudinal data very difficult.

Dr. Waterlow: I accept Dr. Davies' point that it is unrealistic to suppose that a child will grow along the same channel for 2 or 3 years. I agree with Dr. Tomkins that, as he, Dr. Nabarro, and others have shown, linear growth, as well as weight gain, is quite sensitive to environmental influences. Unfortunately, it is difficult to make use of this sensitivity because of the variability in the rate of linear growth even in "normal" children. One of the problems in the data that I had access to was that they told us nothing about the variability among different children. As I have said, we need much more information on this before we can plan how to make the best use of data on length velocity.

Dr. Kraisid: Does one observe differences in growth velocity between infants receiving milk-based and non-milk-based supplementary food? When milk-based supplementary foods such as cow's milk are given, growth velocity may not falter as it does in children receiving non-milk-based supplements.

Dr. Waterlow: I cannot answer that question. The data that I presented are derived from over 20 studies conducted in various countries. Most of them say little about the feeding pattern, so I doubt if it will be possible to answer your question. However, I would draw your attention to a study by Fomon and co-workers (3) in which they showed that babies fed on a skim-milk mixture, which is high in protein but low in energy, grew as well in height but less well in weight as children on a normal formula.

Dr. Ousa: We have had the opportunity to study the growth pattern of children from low socioeconomic classes and with a background of poor sanitation. The growth velocity of children with low birth weight is quite good when they are breast fed because the amount of breast milk may be adequate for these small babies. However, in those with high birth weight, the growth velocity fell off sooner. We have difficulty in analyzing the weight-for-length data of our children under 1 year because they are much below the growth pattern of the developed countries. I think that the international standards may not be appropriate and that a local reference should be used.

A related question is whether the duration of pregnancy and of intrauterine growth retardation have any influence on subsequent stunting.

Dr. Waterlow: With regard to your first point, I am glad to hear what you say. I mentioned in my chapter evidence for catch-up by low-birth-weight babies (provided that they survive); I tried to argue that because of this catch-up, dilution of the sample by large numbers of low-birth-weight babies could not account for the apparent falling off in growth rate after the first 3 months of life. I think that your second point, the applicability of an international reference, would be best discussed after Dr. Keller's chapter.

Dr. Martorell: We need to distinguish between the two types of low-birth-weight infants: those with low weight for length at birth and those with adequate weight for length. In an investigation carried out in 200 Guatemalan children, we found that postnatal growth and development patterns were very different for these two groups (4). Low-birth-weight infants with low weight for length experienced catch-up growth in weight during the first few months because of increased fat deposition. Overall, the low-birth-weight infants with adequate weight for length remained lighter and shorter and had smaller head circumferences at 3 years of age. These infants also performed poorly on developmental tests. These effects, we believe, reflect differences in the timing and duration of the nutritional insult. Our hypothesis is that newborns with low weight for length are affected late in pregnancy, whereas infants who are small but symmetrical (i.e., adequate weight for length) are affected earlier in pregnancy and for a longer period of time. One might consider these situations to be equivalent to acute and chronic intrauterine growth retardation, respectively.

Dr. Guesry: Dr. Martorell, is it also related to prematurity and intrauterine growth retardation?

Dr. Martorell: Prematurity is a very important determinant of postnatal growth and development. However, I neglected to say that in the study I just cited, we considered only term low-birth-weight infants.

Dr. Valyasevi: I hope that one result of this Workshop will be to provide indicators of when preventive measures are necessary.

Dr. Waterlow: That raises the key question that we have not yet tackled. If we accept that deficits in linear growth do occur, what is their significance?

Dr. Guesry: How long does a child need to be stunting before he becomes stunted?

Dr. Golden: Referring to Fig. 4 of the chapter, the time that it takes to cross line B has to be taken into consideration.

Dr. Waterlow: Yes, indeed. The question is: How much does it matter to have been subjected to a process of linear growth deficit (stunting) for 3 years compared to 6 months. If we want to use cut-off points, which are sometimes useful for public health purposes, line B would represent the continuation of a process and might be a more physiological cutoff than the conventional line A.

Dr. Guesry: Could one of the practical conclusions from this session be a suggestion to modify the way of assessing stunting, thus leading to intervention, as requested by Professor Aree Valyasevi earlier. Has anyone a comment on the practicability of changing the cut-off points for the assessment of stunting?

Dr. Nabarro: I think that we should, at this stage, make recommendations on how the length growth of individual children should be charted and what should be considered the desirable rate of length increment. In the 3 days of this Workshop, we have to answer some basic questions first and then think about practical implications later. The important questions to be asked are (a) What is happening? and (b) Does it matter?

Dr. Waterlow: We may have some idea about the first question, but we have virtually none about the second. What are the physiological implications of growing at two-thirds of the normal velocity for the first 6 months of life compared to the second year of life? Or suppose a child grows at 65% of the standard rate for 6 months and then gets better, whereas another child grows at 80% of the standard rate for 2 years. I would like to know whether they will be in the same physiological state when they are at the same point for attained height.

Dr. Milner: The one who suffered growth retardation longer will be more disadvantaged.

Dr. Waterlow: Even if the retardation is mild? I wonder. The effect may depend not only on the degree of deficit and how rapidly it is established but also on when it occurs, according to Dobbing's concept of vulnerable periods.

I hope that other chapters may throw more light on these questions. The objective of this session was to raise them.

REFERENCES

1. Owen GM, Garry PJ, Hooper EM. Feeding and growth of infants. *Nutr Res* 1984;4:727–31.
2. Eveleth PB, Tanner JM. *Worldwide variation in human growth*. Cambridge: Cambridge University Press, 1976.
3. Fomon SJ, Filer LJ, Ziegler EE, Bergmann KE, Bergmann RL. Skim milk in infant feeding. *Acta Paediatr Scand* 1977;66:17–30.
4. Villar J, Smeriglio V, Martorell R, Brown CH, Klein RE. Heterogeneous growth and mental development of intrauterine growth retarded infants during the first three years of life. *Pediatrics* 1984;74:783–91.

Linear Growth Retardation in Less Developed Countries, edited by John C. Waterlow. Nestlé Nutrition Workshop Series, Vol. 14. Nestec Ltd., Vevey/Raven Press, Ltd., New York © 1988.

The Epidemiology of Stunting

W. Keller

Nutrition, World Health Organization, Geneva, Switzerland

The process of growth inhibition in children (stunting) leads to "stunted growth." Stunted growth implies the existence of inhibiting factors without which growth would have continued unabated according to the genetically determined growth potential of the individual.

The degree to which growth is stunted can be assessed by comparing attained growth with the growth that would have been achieved without environmental inhibition. This theoretical value, which corresponds to the genetic potential for growth, is not known for any given population or individual. However, reasonable assumptions can be made. Although worldwide there is large variation in human growth, the growth patterns in affluent countries are in general very similar, and average growth curves are close to each other. In affluent or "elite" groups of poor countries, the growth of children is much closer to the patterns of affluent but ethnically different populations than to the growth pattern of poor but ethnically similar groups. This observation had led to the hypothesis that (a) the average growth potential of young children is similar in different ethnic groups and that (b) with some exceptions observed differences between and among groups arise from environmental influences. Thus, one genetically determined average growth curve should be applicable to all or most populations. This assumption of an equal growth potential for different populations, i.e., a common standard, makes possible geographic comparisons of growth patterns and of possible environmental influences.

REFERENCE POPULATION

Since it is impossible to develop a true standard of growth potential, instead it is customary to use cross-sectional data of presumably healthy, well-nourished populations from industrialized countries. For several reasons, these are no real standards: (a) the nature of an equal growth potential is hypothetical; (b) a secular trend continues even in the wealthy populations; and (c) even generally healthy, well-nourished populations suffer an unknown degree of morbidity and malnutrition. It is therefore preferable to talk about reference populations rather than standards. A widely used reference population is one developed by the U.S. National

Center for Health Statistics and the U.S. Centers for Disease Control (1). It is recommended by the WHO for national and international comparisons of growth data (2).

Geographical Distribution

By comparing different growth data with the reference population and by applying as cutoff a defined point along the distribution of the reference values, one can obtain comparable prevalence values for stunting.

Growth data of preschool children from different parts of the world have been collected over a number of years and processed using as cutoff the mean of the NCHS reference population minus two standard deviations (3). The increasing prevalence with age and the geographical distribution of prevalences are shown in Fig. 1 and in Tables 1–3 for the first 3 years of life. Although the quality and validity of the data sets vary considerably so that conclusions about individual countries cannot be drawn directly, certain general trends may be noted. The highest prevalences are found in a belt reaching from the horn of Africa over the Indian subcontinent to the Philippines and Papua–New Guinea. It includes a variety of ethnic and "racial" identities as well as areas with very high and with very low population densities.

Age Distribution

A second phenomenon that the data illustrate is the general increase in prevalence with age. Below 1 year of age, prevalences of stunting below 10% are common (Table 1), and those more than 40% are rare. Between 2 and 3 years (Table

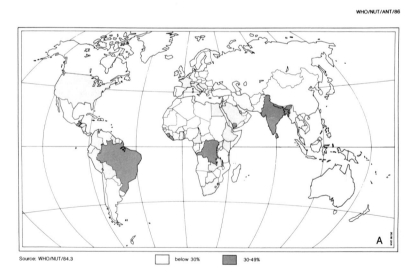

WHO/NUT/ANT/86

Source: WHO/NUT/84.3   below 30%   30-49%

FIG. 1. Geographical distribution of stunting in children at ages less than 1 **(A)**, 1 **(B)**, and 2 years **(C)**.

WHO/NUT/ANT/86

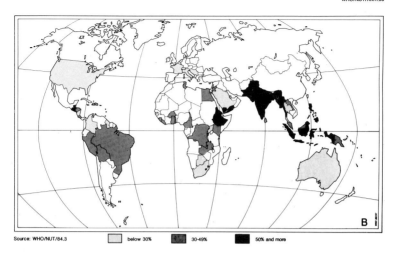

Source: WHO/NUT/84.3   □ below 30%   ▨ 30-49%   ■ 50% and more

WHO/NUT/ANT/86

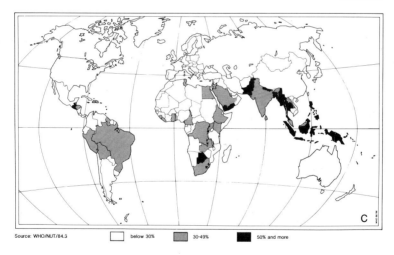

Source: WHO/NUT/84.3   □ below 30%   ▨ 30-49%   ■ 50% and more

FIG. 1.   (continued). B and C.

TABLE 1. *Prevalence (%) of stunting before 1 year of age: countries by WHO region*

Region	Percentage stunting (%)								
	0	10	20	30	40	50	60	70	80
Africa	Botswana Burundi Ghana S. Africa Uganda	Rwanda Togo	Cameroon Kenya Burkina Faso Zambia	Sierra Leone Zaire	Liberia	Lesotho			
Americas	Bolivia Colombia Jamaica	Barbados Belize Costa Rica Dominica Guyana Haiti Honduras Nicaragua St. Vincent	Panama	Brazil Salvador Guatemala					
Eastern Mediterranean	Saudi Arabia	UNRWA	Yemen D.R. Egypt Iran Jordan Tunisia	Yemen A.R.					
Southeast Asia		Burma Thailand	Indonesia	India Sri Lanka	Bangladesh Nepal				
Western Pacific	Papua–New Guinea Singapore	Laos Solomon Is. W. Samoa	Malaysia Philippines						
Europe	France Italy	Yugoslavia							

TABLE 2. *Prevalence (%) of stunting at 1 year of age: countries by WHO region*

Region	Percentage stunting (%)								
	0	10	20	30	40	50	60	70	80
Africa			Botswana S. Africa Uganda	Burundi Cameroon Ghana Kenya Sierra Leone Togo Burkina Faso	Liberia Zaire Zambia	Lesotho Rwanda			
Americas	Barbados	Dominica Jamaica	Colombia Guyana	Belize Bolivia	Brazil Dominican Republic		Salvador	Guatemala	
			Nicaragua St. Vincent	Costa Rica Haiti Honduras Panama					
Eastern Mediterranean			Saudi Arabia	Jordan UNRWA	Egypt Tunisia	Yemen D.R. Pakistan	Yemen A.R.		
Southeast Asia			Thailand		Sri Lanka	Burma India	Indonesia	Nepal	Bangladesh
Western Pacific		Singapore	W. Samoa	Malaysia Solomon Is.	Laos Papua–new Guinea		Philippines		
Europe	France Italy		Yugoslavia						

3), most prevalences are between 20% and 70%, and in no developing country except Singapore is there a stunting prevalence of less than 10%.

National prevalences can be used to make an approximate estimate of world-wide stunting in order to obtain an idea of the size of the phenomenon. A weighted estimate of stunted children in developing countries (excluding China and the countries of temperate climate in South America) gave a prevalence of about 40% in children under 5 and a total of about 125 million (Table 4). However, figures of this kind should be used with caution; not only is the data base unreliable, but the definition of stunting is quite arbitrary. The distribution of heights is continuous and near normal, and although the transformation into a dichotomous variable may be justified for practical reasons, the resulting prevalence figures depend mainly on the choice of the cut-off values.

Socioeconomic Factors

Stunting is a nonspecific response to a number of specific noxious agents. In the individual case it may be possible to identify a specific cause that prevents a child from thriving. At the population level this is usually impossible. It has been shown that growth is usually retarded under less than optimal living conditions. Differences in growth persist between social classes even when standards of living and of health are high (4,5). Nonspecific socioeconomic indicators such as income, housing, and possessions are usually inversely related to stunting, but the associations are weak since the indicators themselves are not the causes. The addition of more specific indicators can sometimes sharpen an apparent but weak relationship. An example is given in Fig. 2 from a study in Southern India (6). The proportion of stunted children decreases with increasing income. This effect is enhanced if electricity and sanitation are available; it is only slight if this is not the case. In the poorest group, the availability of electricity or sanitation makes no difference.

TABLE 4. *Estimated prevalence and number of cases of wasted and stunted preschool children in developing countries, by region[a]*

	Asia without China		Africa		The Americas		Total	
	Percentage	Millions	Percentage	Millions	Percentage	Millions	Percentage	Millions
Wasted[b]	16	33	7	4	4	2	12	39
Stunted[b]	40	81	35	24	43	20	39	125

[a]Date from WHO, 1983.
[b]Percentage of children 0–4 years old below the mean minus 2 standard deviations of the NCHS reference (1).

TABLE 3. Prevalence (%) of stunting at 2 years of age: countries by WHO region

Percentage stunting (%)

Region	0	10	20	30	40	50	60	70	80	90
Africa			Burkina Faso	Burundi Ghana Kenya Sierra Leone S. Africa Togo Zambia	Cameroon Liberia Uganda Zaire	Botswana Lesotho	Rwanda			
Americas		Barbados Dominica Jamaica Nicaragua	Colombia Costa Rica Panama	Belize Brazil Dominican Republic Guyana St. Vincent	Bolivia Haiti Honduras	Salvador Guatemala				
Eastern Mediterranean			UNRWA	Jordan Saudia Arabia	Egypt Tunizia	Pakistan	Yemen D.R. Yemen A.R.			
Southeast Asia					India Sri Lanka	Thailand	Burma Nepal	Indonesia		Bangladesh
Western Pacific	Singapore		Solomon Is. W. Samoa		Laos Malaysia	Papua–New Guinea	Philippines			
Europe	France Italy	Yugoslavia								

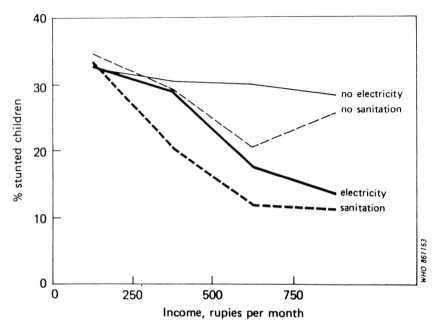

FIG. 2. Stunting at different levels of income in families with and without electricity and sanitation (Kerala) (From Scott and Mathew, ref. 6).

One can speculate on the possible effects of electricity and sanitation on the way of life in the various income groups. The figure says nothing about this or about the causes of stunting.

MALNUTRITION

At present the two commonly recognized and documented causes of stunting are malnutrition or insufficient food intake and continued or repeated infections, especially of the gastrointestinal tract. A reduction in height, or stunting, has been seen as evidence of past malnutrition in contrast to low weight for height, which indicates acute malnutrition (7). This view is probably partly based on clinical observations from children recovering from malnutrition. It has been shown repeatedly (8,9) that in children recovering from severe malnutrition body weight increases rapidly but linear growth resumes only when body weight has returned to normal; rehabilitated children are thus stunted. Similar observations have been made during recovery from measles (10) as well as among populations with seasonal fluctuations in growth, where the velocity of length growth recovers several months after the velocity of weight growth has again attained its higher value (D.

Nabarro et al., *this volume*). Such observations together with the well-known association between stunting and poverty have led to the view of stunting as a sign of past or chronic malnutrition.

INFECTION

Similarly, there are indirect epidemiological indications of a causal relationship between infections and stunting as well as direct ones from case studies. Associations of unfavorable socioeconomic conditions with stunting have already been mentioned. Indicators of housing, sanitation, etc. are often much more strongly associated with stunting than with wasting (11). An example is given in Fig. 3, which shows the proportions of stunted and wasted children in urban and rural populations in a number of countries. One of the differences between urban and rural habitats is the greater exposure to infections in the former.

Evidence for a direct influence of diarrheal infections on linear growth is given

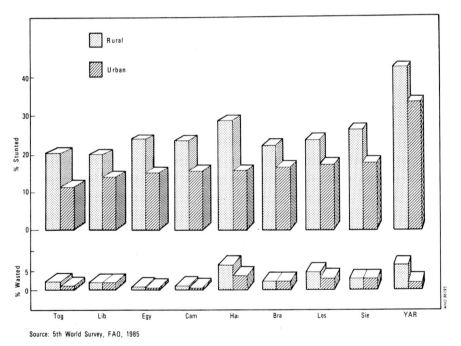

Source: 5th World Survey, FAO, 1985

FIG. 3. Percentages of stunted and of wasted children in the age groups 0–5 years by rural and urban areas in selected countries. Abbreviations: Tog, Togo; Lib, Liberia; Egy, Egypt; Cam, Cameroon; Hai, Haiti; Bra, Brazil; Les, Lesotho; Sie, Sierra Leone; YAR, Yemen Arab Republic.

by Mata, who recently published a number of growth charts of individual children (12). Practically each diarrhea incident is followed by a complete standstill of linear growth, which sometimes lasts for several months. After the first months of life the difference between attained height and reference height increases with each infectious incident. Since one can assume that each attack of diarrhea leads to an acute weight loss (or wasting) that is soon recovered, there is a direct analogy to the observations made during recovery from malnutrition.

Thus, there is evidence that both protein–energy malnutrition and repeated diarrheal infections can lead to stunted growth. Both are interrelated, and both are associated with poverty; their effects cannot easily be separated. However, other observations may disprove the easy assumption that malnutrition and infections constitute the main cause of stunting. Whereas stunting often starts after the first few months of life and continues for several years, the age-dependent incidence of clinical malnutrition (kwashiorkor) in many countries shows a sharp increase in the second year of life (13), a phenomenon that corresponds closely to a similar peak seen in the age-related incidence of wasting (3). Since these peaks in wasting and in clinical malnutrition do not correspond with prevalence curves of stunting, a common causal mechanism for protein–energy malnutrition and stunting seems improbable.

Further doubts are raised by observations that in malnourished as well as well-nourished child populations, weight for height and height for age are not correlated (11; R. Martorell, *this volume*). This makes it unlikely that growth in height and soft tissue mass are determined by the same environmental factors.

SECULAR TRENDS IN STUNTING AND WASTING

To some extent, and in a more dynamic way, the effects of socioeconomic changes on child growth may be studied by examining a number of consecutive surveys.

In Colombia, national nutrition surveys were conducted in 1965–1966 and again in 1977–1980. During this period, important socioeconomic improvements had taken place on a national scale. The lowest income group, which in 1965–1966 included almost 40% of the population, was reduced to 12% in 1977. Infant mortality fell from over 90 per 1,000 to 59 per 1,000 in 1980, preschool mortality from 15 to fewer than seven per 1,000. There were improvements in literacy and primary school attendance. The supply of piped water in homes increased from 44% to 60%, and toilet facilities from 42% to 53%. The distribution curves of weight for height in preschool children (Fig. 4) show that in 1965–1966 there was little wasting, and in 1977–1980 there was no change; in fact, the two curves were almost identical. In contrast, the distribution of heights for age, which indicated a considerable degree of stunting in 1965, had shifted to the right by 1977–1980.

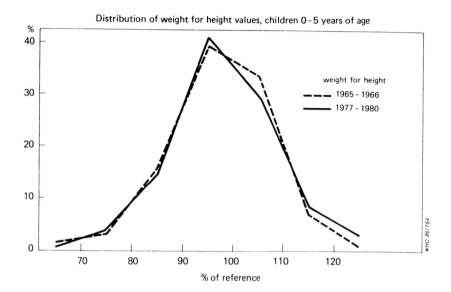

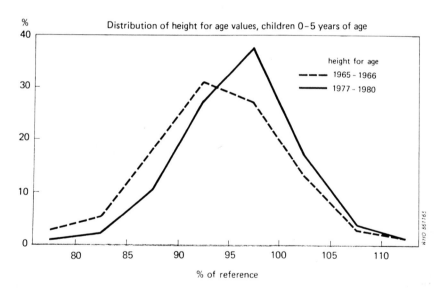

FIG. 4. National nutrition surveys showing changes in weight-for-height and height-for-age distributions in Colombia for 1965–1966 and 1977–1980.

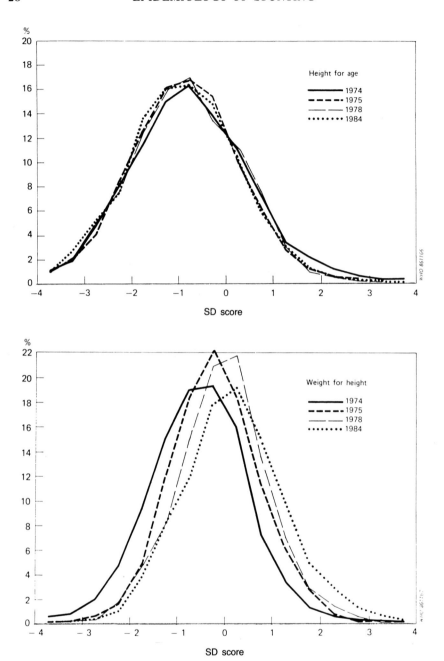

FIG. 5. Changes in height-for-age and weight-for-height distributions among Palestinian refugees for 1974–1984.

Thus, the general improvement in income and hygiene was associated with a reduction in stunting, but there was no change in the already low level of wasting.

The Colombian data seem to correspond well to the model concept that catch-up growth in stature sets in once abnormal weight for height has been established. A recent report from Cuba (14) describes what is presumably the next step, a situation in which stunting has virtually disappeared and a trend toward obesity is visible. But observations from other parts of the world show different behavior of growth in height and weight.

Between 1974 and 1984 the United Nations Relief and Works Agency for Palestinian Refugees (UNRWA) carried out four surveys on the nutritional status of children under their care. During the decade there had been major improvements in sanitation, water supply, and literacy (15) as well as impressive reductions in morbidity, especially from diarrheal diseases (16). As shown in Fig. 5, wasting had practically disappeared by 1978, and in 1984 the distribution curve of weight for height had shifted to the right of that of the reference population, indicating the onset of obesity. There was, however, no improvement in stunting: the successive distribution curves of height for age remained unchanged. In this population, both malnutrition and infection appear to be unlikely causes of stunting. A converse observation can be made in a data set from rural Bangladesh, where a nutrition survey was carried out in 1975–1976 (17) and was repeated in 1980–1981 (18). As Fig. 6 shows, by 1980–1981 there was no improvement in wasting, but there was definitely less stunting at all ages. Unfortunately, no data on socioeconomic change were available.

Observations made as part of a longitudinal study in Kerala, India (6), to which we have already referred (Fig. 2), show yet another pattern. Between 1981 and 1984 there appears to have been a continual improvement in height but also in weight for height, as shown in Fig. 7. During this period a number of changes in the standard of living were observed (6). Although there seems to have been little change in overall income, improvements were recorded in food consumption, particularly rice and milk, and in housing, safe water supply, sanitation, electricity supply, and selected household possessions. It is remarkable that on the whole both stunting and wasting improved, though without reaching normal values.

CAUSES OF STUNTING

These examples of change in populations show no consistent relationship between change in stunting and change in wasting, nor are there consistent associations to changes in specific environmental factors. From the type of evidence examined here, it is impossible to identify one causal factor that could be responsible for the widespread inhibition of growth. The associations between static observations, for example, stunted growth and sanitation, are much too weak to allow

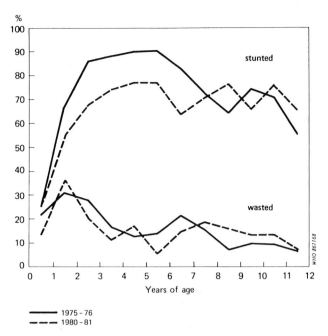

FIG. 6. Changes in the prevalences of stunted and wasted children in rural Bangladesh for 1975–1976 and 1980–1981.

this kind of inference. The measured variables are only proxies for unknown causes. There is possibly no single cause that is responsible for all stunting worldwide; rather, various combinations of unfavorable dietary habits and other conditions that occur in different populations elicit the nonspecific response of growth retardation. In the clinical setting and the laboratory, growth inhibition has been found to be one of the signs of deficiencies in most essential nutrients, but in free-living human populations lack of information has so far restricted epidemiological comparisons almost exclusively to dietary energy.

The complex causality and the varying combinations of causative and contributing factors in different populations probably make it impossible to identify a common cause of stunting applicable to all populations by using this kind of statistical comparison. Especially favorable circumstances may be necessary to distinguish the different dietary and socioeconomic factors in a population. An example is a recent study from Holland that compares dietary intake and growth in children on conventional and several "alternative" diets (19). Only the most extreme (macrobiotic) dietary group showed a major degree of stunting, with over 50% of children below the 10th percentile of the reference. In all dietary groups the children's parents had had higher (university level) education; dietary energy and protein sup-

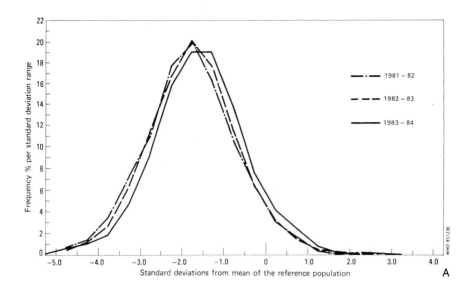

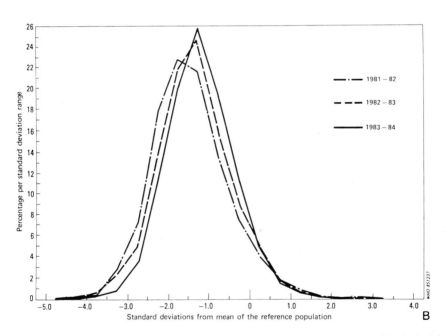

FIG. 7. Changes in height-for-age **(A)** and weight-for-height **(B)** distributions in Kerala (India) for 1981–1982 and 1983–1984.

plies were adequate for all groups, and weights for heights were normal. There were, however, major differences in the composition of their diets. Table 5 shows that there were major differences in the energy contributed by the main food groups and that the pattern for the stunted group was similar to that of the national food balance sheet pattern of a country with a stunted child population. In terms of nutrients, the diet of the stunted group was deficient in calcium, vitamin D, riboflavin, and probably iron. Although the study appears to have considerably narrowed down the possible causative factors for this particular group of children, the question remains open to what extent the result would be applicable to other stunted groups and, if so, whether it would be useful in prevention, and whether specific preventive measures would be considered necessary.

Generally, our knowledge regarding the extent and distribution of stunting is growing, but we are far from understanding its etiology. It is uncertain whether stunted growth is accompanied by functional impairment. Even if this is not the case, stunting must be seen as an indication of adverse living conditions, and a stunted child population calls for exploration into the underlying causes of its growth inhibition.

SUMMARY

Data on the prevalence of growth retardation relative to North American children are presented from 58 countries. The geographical distribution shows a con-

TABLE 5. *Proportions of dietary energy supplied by major food groups (%)*

| Food group | Dutch children (19) | | India: National Food Balance Sheet 1981 (20) |
	Conventional diet	Macrobiotic diet	
Milk and milk products	31	2	3
Cereals and pulses	16	63	72
Vegetables	5	7	2
Fruit and fruit juices	10	9	1
Oils and fats	7	4	7
Sweets and sugar	17	6	9
Meat, fish, poultry	8	1	1

centration of high prevalence figures in a belt from the horn of Africa through southeast Asia. Stunted growth usually becomes evident after the first year of life. There are clear associations with poverty and poor levels of living. No single causative factor can be identified as being generally responsible. Although a multi-causal etiology appears probable, the possible causative role of micronutrients has not yet been sufficiently explored.

REFERENCES

1. United States Public Health Service, Health Resources Administration. *NCHS growth charts.* Rockville, MD: National Center for Health Statistics, 1976; publication no (HRA) 76-1120; (suppl 25):3.
2. World Health Organization. *Development of indicators for monitoring progress towards health for all by the year 2000.* Geneva: World Health Organization, 1981.
3. Keller W, Fillmore CM. Prevalence of protein–energy malnutrition. *World Health Stat Q* 1983;36:129–67.
4. Eveleth PB, Tanner JM. *Worldwide variation in human growth.* Cambridge: Cambridge University Press, 1976.
5. Jones Y, Nesheim MC, Habicht J-P. Influences in child growth associated with poverty in the 1970s: an examination of HANES I and HANES II, cross-sectional US national surveys. *Am J Clin Nutr* 1985;42:714–24.
6. Scott W, Mathew NT. *A development monitoring service at the local level. Vol III. Monitoring change in Kerala: the first five years.* Geneva: United Nations Research Institute for Social Development, 1985.
7. FAO/WHO. *Joint FAO/WHO Expert Committee on Nutrition Eighth Report.* WHO Tech Rep Ser 477. Geneva: WHO, 1971.
8. Ashworth A. Growth rates in children recovering from protein–calorie malnutrition. *Br J Nutr* 1969;23:835–45.
9. Geniès JL, Ricour C. Croissance de rattrapage chez l'enfant en nutrition artificielle. *Arch Fr Pediatr* 1982;39:745–8.
10. Duggan MB, Milner RDG. Measles, energy balance and childhood growth. *Proc Nutr Soc* 1986;45:35A.
11. Keller W. Choice of indicators of nutritional status. In: Schürch B, ed. *Evaluation of nutrition education in third world communities.* Bern: Hans Huber, 1983:101–13 (Nestlé Foundation Publication Series; vol 3).
12. Mata L. Environmental factors affecting nutrition and growth. In: Gracey M, Falkner F, eds. *Nutritional needs and assessment of normal growth.* New York: Raven Press, 1985:165–82 (Nestlé Nutrition Workshop Series; vol 7).
13. Waterlow JC, Vergara A. *Protein malnutrition in Brazil.* Rome: FAO, 1956 (FAO Nutritional Studies; no. 14).
14. Ramos Palmero RM, Estrada Borges O. La malnutrición por excesso en nitros asistentes a tres circulos infantiles de Sancti Spiritus. *Rev Cubana Pediatr* 1985;57:293–302.
15. Jabra A. *Nutrition survey among Palestine refugees in Jordan, West Bank and Gaza.* April–May 1984 (UNRWA Document).
16. United Nations Relief and Works Agency for Palestine. *Refugees in the Near East.* Annual Report of the Director of Health. Vienna: UNRWA, 1985.
17. Institute of Nutrition and Food Science, University of Dhaka. *Nutrition Survey of Rural Bangladesh 1975–76.*
18. Institute of Nutrition and Food Science, University of Dhaka. *Nutrition Survey of Rural Bangladesh 1980–81.*
19. van Staveren WA, Dhuyvetter JHM, Bons A, Zeelen M, Hautvast JGAJ. Food consumption and

height/weight status of Dutch preschool children on alternative diets. *J Am Diet Assoc* 1985;85:1579–84.

20. FAO. *Food Balance Sheets 1979–81 average*. Rome: FAO, 1984.

DISCUSSION

Dr. Waterlow: You have raised a number of very important points. I would like to defer discussion of the points you suggested about causality—infection and nutrient factors—until after some of the later chapters.

Topics that I would like to see discussed at this stage, on which really only the WHO can give us information, are these:

1. Geographical distribution.

2. The changes in time of the prevalence of stunting in different areas.

3. Although this Workshop is really concerned with linear growth, the question of the correlation or absence of correlation between stunting and wasting ought to be considered and perhaps disposed of; we ought to be quite clear in our minds about this because, as Dr. Keller pointed out, this has obvious implications for causality.

4. Any comment on the data from the FAO balance sheets would be very relevant at this particular point, because Dr. Keller is probably the person who is most familiar with these data and their limitations.

5. Finally, the prevalence charts of the WHO are, I believe, based on cut-off points, Z scores, or -2 SD (Fig. 1). I wonder whether this is the best way of presenting the data, and whether a way of expressing the data that shows the whole population distribution might not be better. I would like to ask whether the WHO, with all its statistical expertise, could consider ways of expressing prevalences that do not depend on artbitrary cut-off points but could represent the whole curve. Is this possible? Dr. Keller's data illustrate the value of attempting to do something like that.

Dr. Tomkins: I am worried about the quality of the data that are used for making epidemiological generalizations and particularly about the effect of age. Population distributions can vary enormously with respect to age within the first 2 years of life. However, people still talk about stunted children over 2-year age ranges. It would be useful to have some guidance on the optimal age ranges for analysis. In your Bangladesh data (Fig. 6), you showed prevalence at 1-year intervals, and in your original paper in 1977 (1), you recommended 6-month intervals. What is the optimum?

Dr. Keller: On the world maps (Fig. 1), age groups of 1 year have been used for practical reasons. Many investigations do not start at birth but at 3 or 6 months. With narrower age groups, especially during the first year of life, one finds differences in the onset of stunting. In some populations stunting is present at birth; in others it becomes apparent during the first year or later. If one wants to study the onset of stunting in a population, age groups of 6 months, 3 months, or less should be used, at least during the first year of life. After that, changes are usually minor, and age groups of 1 year would seem sufficient. The choice of age groups depends very much on the purpose of the study.

Dr. Davies: My concern about your data is that you are using a ubiquitous standard, the NCHS standard, to assess the prevalence of stunting. If you are dealing with populations in which the tendency to be smaller is perhaps more genetic, then you will exaggerate the prevalence of stunting. Of some concern to me is your assumption that all children have the same potential to grow in the same way. I am particularly interested in Southeastern Asia, where I believe in general children are smaller for genetic reasons. You are therefore going to exaggerate the prevalence of stunting in this part of the world, and this will have considerable public health implications.

Dr. Keller: I think that for most populations the growth potential of young children is very similar, but there are exceptions. In Africa, the pygmies are almost certainly genetically small, and other groups in Central Africa are genetically tall. As far as Southeast Asia is concerned, I don't think one can generalize. The Indian populations, for example, are not ethnically uniform at all; but there are a number of examples from India of upper social groups growing to the same height as Europeans or North Americans.

Dr. Waterlow: At the beginning, Dr. Keller specifically said that he is using the NCHS as a reference and not as a standard, so that what we have at the moment is geographical prevalences of a certain degree below the reference. The interpretation of the differences as genetic or environmental will come up during the discussion, but the map shows facts.

Dr. Nabarro: I would like to comment on Tables 1 to 3. I note that the prevalence of stunting before 1 year of age (Table 1) in Southeast Asia and the Western Pacific countries is roughly what would be expected, given the economic conditions of those countries. In Table 3 there is a much greater prevalence of stunting at 2 years in the Southeast Asians.

Does the distribution of countries with a high prevalence of stunting under 1 year parallel the distribution of countries with a high infant mortality rate?

Dr. Keller: There is a correlation with infant mortality rate, but it is not particularly close. Mean infant mortality rates for the countries shown in Table 1 rise with increasing prevalence of stunting, but there is a wide range of individual values, especially for prevalences below 30% (Table 6). At 1 and 2 years of age, the association is no longer visible.

TABLE 6. *Percentage prevalence of stunting before 1 year of age and infant mortality rates in the countries shown in Table 1 (except Europe)[a]*

	Percentage stunted					
	0–9	10–19	20–29	30–39	40–49	50–59
Infant mortality	11	18	29	38	112	110
rates	16	21	50	44	133	
	53	23	63	66	144	
	79	35	82	71		
	92	51	85	107		
	94	82	87	118		
	98	85	101	154		
	98	94	101	200		
	103	108	113			
	124	110	117			
	137	113	138			
		122	149			
Mean	82	72	93	100	130	

[a]Adapted from World Statistics in brief (2).

Dr. Aponso: When we look at the geographical distribution, it seems to me that the shaded areas are also areas where the population is bursting at the seams. I don't know whether you have purposely left out the implications of large and small families, birth spacing, age of the mother, and whether they show any correlations with what we have been talking about. I think that most of us are aware of the role of maternal malnutrition on fetal outcome and on the growth of the baby during the first year, but I would like to know more about the recent work that has been done on the role of paternal malnutrition on fetal outcome.

Dr. Waterlow: You said "on fetal outcome." I suggest that this question should be addressed later on after the chapters on this subject. The important point you raised in relation to geographical distribution is "population density." The very interesting point that you made about "populations bursting at the seams," of course, raises many questions about social factors.

Dr. Keller: These are very difficult questions. We do have estimates of population density, but the interpretation of these data is sometimes very difficult. In Switzerland, for example, the population density for the whole country is quite low, but large parts of the country are mountainous and uninhabited; thus, the population density in the plains is high. At present it is impossible to produce data that could be used for such a comparison. As far as the nutritional status of the mother is concerned, there is insufficient information regarding rates of low birth weight to make this comparison. The distribution of low birth weight is not very similar to the distribution of stunting. At least in Southeast Asia, I think that both nutritional status and stunting are in some way related to poverty.

Dr. Waterlow: I am still trying to elicit facts rather than explanations, and you just said something almost in passing that I thought was very interesting: that the distribution of stunting and the distribution of low birth weight are different according to the WHO criteria. If you had to draw a map of the distribution of low birth weight, it would not correspond with these maps of the distribution of stunting. Is that correct?

Dr. Keller: Yes, that is correct.

Dr. Waterlow: That is an extremely important point, even though types of low birth weight, as Dr. Martorell has pointed out, differ. That is a point that is relevant to the chapters that address endocrine and fetal factors.

May I comment on the very interesting data you presented about changes with time in the same populations, though not of course in the same individuals? Several examples you gave showed a decrease in the prevalence of stunting with no change in the prevalence of wasting. It is precisely the opposite of what I naively would have expected. Would anyone like to question Dr. Keller further on this matter?

Dr. Nabarro: Were the studies of wasting and stunting undertaken at the same time of year?

Dr. Keller: I realize that this is an important question, but unfortunately I cannot answer it. I have shown a graph (Fig. 6) in which the curve of wasted children changes with age, although this is not the case for stunting. Of course, it is possible that there are seasonal differences and that there is sometimes less stunting than when the findings were reported. But the same applies to wasting.

Dr. Nabarro: One study in Bangladesh has shown that in a rural community the highest prevalence of wasting in children is observed a few months before the peak prevalence of stunting (3).

Dr. Waterlow: This really brings us to another point you made that is extremely important: the lack of correlation between wasting and stunting. If I understood correctly, there is no correlation within a population, within a collection of individuals; between countries there may be a correlation—where there is a lot of wasting, there tends to be a lot of stunting. Dr. Martorell mentions it also in his chapter. From our point of view, I think this is very important because we have to recognize very clearly that it is useless to talk about acute and chronic malnutrition, wasting, and stunting if they are different things that are not correlated. One of the advantages of having the WHO represented here is that we are able to get a global view.

Dr. Martorell: Stunting and wasting could be elements of the same process and yet appear not to be related under certain circumstances. Think of stunting (as measured by low height for age) as the cumulative result of many, many events that disrupt growth rates in length and cause wasting. Wasting (as measured by low weight for height), on the other hand, is more like a snapshot in that it is more related to recent disruptive events. After such an event, and if conditions are appropriate, weight for height may go back to normal, but catch-up in height may not be possible. Thus, I am not surprised that Dr. Keller does not find significant correlations between stunting (a long-term measure) and wasting (a short-term measure).

Monthly serial data from Bangladesh show that stunting and wasting are related when appropriate measures are used (3). Specifically, Brown and colleagues used monthly serial data to show that growth velocities in length were related to the prevalence of wasting. In other words, when wasting occurs, growth velocities in length (i.e., the mechanism leading to stunting) are reduced.

Dr. Waterlow: So simple correlation or absence of correlations could both possibly be misleading.

Dr. Mukherjee: As Dr. Nabarro pointed out, there are seasonal differences between wasting and stunting, but if stunting is a long-term effect whereas wasting is an acute effect, one naturally wonders if the wasting comes first and stunting later.

Dr. Keller: What we analyzed is not the correlation between stunting and wasting but that between height for age and weight for height. In the populations studied, the correlation coefficients were close to zero irrespective of the presence or absence of wasting and stunting in the population. Moreover, multiple regressions of weight for height and height for age over weight for age had measures of determination (R^2) between 0.95 and 0.98 and slope values very similar to each other (4).

Dr.Waterlow: Would you accept the proposition that wasting and stunting are different processes that may often occur together but do not necessarily occur together? That is a question that I would like to see clarified.

Dr. Keller: In populations there is no doubt that wasting and stunting very often occur together, but that does not mean that they necessarily occur together in individuals. I do not really see any good evidence for a common etiology in general, but there is no doubt, I think, that wasting also leads to a cessation of growth in length. That does not mean that it is the main cause of stunting.

Dr. Waterlow: I think you have answered my question.

Dr. Goyens: We are sometimes able to say that a wasted child is not stunted, but does the sensitivity of our measurements enable us to say that a child is not "stunting," that the "stunting process" is not going on, and that that child will not be considered "stunted" a few months later? Thus, if wasting and stunting occur together in a population, should we not be cautious before deciding that they do not occur together in individuals unless we look very carefully at short-term increments in length?

Dr. Keller: It takes longer to find the results of stunting because the measurement error is relatively large. By the calculation of increments or velocities, the measurement error is multiplied. I don't think that that would be a solution.

Dr. Golden: In support of there being different processes, I think that a number of supplementation studies have shown that you get differential changes in wasting and stunting with supplementation. Malcolm in New Guinea (5) found that children supplemented with milk powder grew in length, yet their arm circumference and skinfold thickness were less than in those given a high-energy supplement. I think that, as in many diseases, the therapeutic test is an efficient way of discriminating causal factors.

Dr. Keller: I fully agree with your comment. However, milk powder is a very complex substance, and we don't know what actually causes what.

Dr. Nabarro: When investigating factors that are associated with the presence or absence of wasting or stunting, we need to select our methods with care. Longitudinal studies of associations between different factors and the velocity of children's weight or height gain are needed. The age groups of the children studied should be clearly defined and as narrow as possible, as already mentioned.

Dr. Keller: All I can do is compare data that are available, and these data at present are exclusively cross sectional. What I wanted to show was only how far one can go using such data. I agree with you that you cannot draw a definite conclusion regarding causality.

Dr. Van Lerberghe: Still, if internationally we can only compare cross-sectional data, it might be useful to compare them on a distribution basis rather than on a cut-off basis. Part of the problem of the lack of correlation that we find is because we are thinking in terms of "below a certain curve" instead of thinking in terms of distribution. I realize that it is more difficult to analyze distributions, and I think more work has to be done in that direction.

Dr. Keller: I think there is a misunderstanding. The correlations are not calculated between prevalences; they are actually calculated from individual data in the population.

Dr. Waterlow: This really brings us back to the starting point of the discussion—the method of expressing data. I think it has been a useful discussion, even though inconclusive. Questions of causality and the roles of malnutrition and infection are taken up again in later chapters (Tomkins, *this volume;* Golden, *this volume*).

REFERENCES

1. Waterlow, JC, Buzina R, Keller W, Lane JM, Nichaman MZ, Tanner JM. The presentation and use of height and weight data for comparing the nutritional studies of groups of children under the age of 10 years. *Bull WHO* 1977;55:489–98.
2. *World statistics in brief. United Nations statistical pocketbook.* 9th ed. New York: United Nations, 1985.
3. Brown KH, Black RE, Becker S. Seasonal changes in nutritional status and the prevalance of malnutrition in a longitudinal study of young children in rural Bangladesh. *Am J Clin Nutr* 1982;36:303–13.

4. Keller W. Choice of indicators of nutritional status. In: Schürch B, ed. *Evaluation of nutrition education in third world communities*. Bern: Hans Huber, 1983:101–13 (Nestlé Foundation Publication Series; vol 3).
5. Malcolm LA. Growth retardation in a New Guinea boarding school and in response to supplementary feeding. *Br J Nutr* 1970;24:297–305.

Linear Growth Retardation in Less Developed Countries, edited by John C. Waterlow. Nestlé Nutrition Workshop Series, Vol. 14. Nestec Ltd., Vevey/Raven Press, Ltd., New York © 1988.

The Use of Short-Term Increments in Length to Monitor Growth in Infancy

*M. J. R. Healy, †Min Yang, ‡J. M. Tanner, and §F. Y. Zumrawi

*London School of Hygiene and Tropical Medicine, London WC1E 7HT, England; ‡Institute of Child Health, London University, London WC1N 1EH, England; and §Department of Home Science, University of Khartoum, Khartoum, Sudan. †Present address: Department of Health Statistics, West China University of Medical Sciences, Chengdu, Sichuan, China

We consider how length measurements taken every 4 or every 8 weeks in infancy may be used to detect slowing down of growth as a result of nutritional or other causes. Mixed longitudinal data from 427 children from the Sudan are presented. Using a simple model, we show that measurements at the shorter interval are quicker to detect growth deficiency, though at the cost of a substantial increase in the false alarm rate.

The possibility of detecting growth deficiency in infants and small children depends on the ability to make and interpret serial (longitudinal) measurements of simple indicators of growth such as length and weight. Since any deficiency should be detected and put right with the minimum delay, frequent measurements are desirable. The interpretation of such measurements in practical situations requires reference to some form of standardizing data, preferably taken from children whose health status is known. Such data are surprisingly scarce and are mostly derived from Western population groups, so that their relevance to Third World conditions is open to question.

This chapter represents a first attempt at the analysis of a large data set from the Sudan. It presents some factual findings on the growth of Sudanese children and draws some methodological conclusions to aid those collecting similar data elsewhere. Our analyses must be regarded as strictly preliminary; there are many aspects of the data that we have not yet attempted to investigate.

THE DATA SET

The data provide mixed longitudinal measurements of supine length for a total of 229 boys and 198 girls. The measurements were taken at 4-week intervals during the first year of life. The children lived in typical Third World conditions in the neighborhood of Khartoum; they were unselected so far as nutrition was concerned. Rather extensive information on illnesses were recorded, but we have not been able so far to make use of this information.

DATA ANALYSIS

The data were scrutinized, and a number of coding and keyboarding errors were detected and corrected. A very small number of lengths that gave rise to negative 4-week length increments of more than 2 cm were rejected as being measurement or recording mistakes. There are almost certainly a few more erroneous readings present in the data analyzed.

Our analyses concentrate on the growth increments at 4-week and 8-week intervals. The numbers of children available at each age are shown in Table 1. The dates of measurement were recorded, and the observed increments have been adjusted proportionately to intervals of exactly 4 or 8 weeks.

The distributions of the increments were first examined by inspecting histograms and normal plots of the data (1). They were distinctly skewed to the right, with apparently a slight shortage of negative increments at the 4-week intervals. Specimen histograms are shown in Fig. 1. Biologically, a real decrease in length is unlikely even over this short period, but measurement errors would be expected to give rise to some negative increments when the true growth in length was small. It is likely that these have been eliminated by a measurer who knew the result of the previous measurement. In addition, the histograms of the actual increments, before adjustment to exact 4- or 8-week intervals, show a heavy preponderance of increments that are exact centimeters or half-centimeters (Fig. 2). This occurs because most of the original measurements were recorded as exact centimeters or half-centimeters. It makes a detailed study of the statistical properties of the data quite difficult.

Table 2 shows the means and standard deviations of the Sudan data, and in Figs.3 and 4 these are compared with several series from the literature (2–6). The mean velocities are somewhat lower than those in Western communities, espe-

TABLE 1. *Numbers of available cases*

	4-week increments					8-week increments		
Weeks	Boys	Girls	Weeks	Boys	Girls	Weeks	Boys	Girls
1–4	178	154	25–28	176	156	1–8	164	141
5–8	171	151	29–32	176	149	9–16	164	129
9–12	164	133	33–36	142	123	17–24	172	149
13–16	176	141	37–40	128	109	25–32	165	146
17–20	177	150	41–44	130	109	33–40	144	116
21–24	176	155	45–48	122	101	41–48	119	102

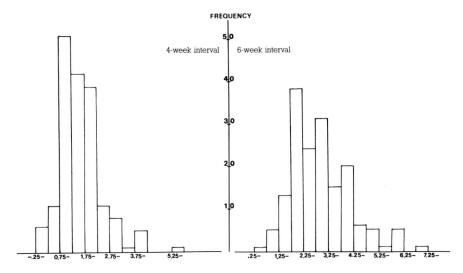

FIG. 1. Histograms of length increments for males at around 6 months of age, 4-week and 8-week intervals.

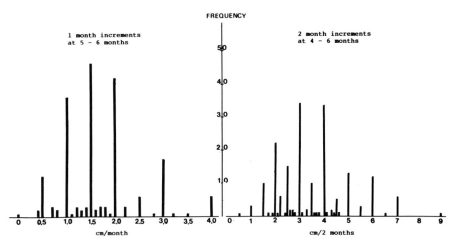

FIG. 2. Histograms of length increments for males as recorded, before adjustment to exact intervals.

TABLE 2. *Means and standard deviations of length increments (cm)*

	4-week increments					8-week increments		
Weeks	Mean	SD	Weeks	Mean	SD	Weeks	Mean	SD
				Boys				
1–4	3.44	1.52	25–28	1.58	0.85	1–8	6.30	1.85
5–8	2.93	1.27	29–32	1.37	0.65	9–16	4.94	1.70
9–12	2.59	1.51	33–36	1.32	0.63	17–24	3.46	1.46
13–16	2.34	1.15	37–40	1.29	0.71	25–32	2.91	1.18
17–20	1.80	1.00	41–44	1.22	0.53	26–40	2.57	0.95
21–24	1.67	0.82	45–48	1.14	0.55	27–48	2.32	0.83

TABLE 2. *Means and standard deviations of length increments (cm)* (continued)

	4-week increments						8-week increments		
Weeks	Mean	SD	Weeks	Mean	SD		Weeks	Mean	SD
				Girls					
1–4	3.41	1.54	25–28	1.42	0.65		1–8	6.20	2.02
5–8	2.80	1.29	29–32	1.39	0.64		9–16	4.51	1.79
9–12	2.32	1.08	33–36	1.28	0.68		17–24	3.61	1.40
13–16	2.23	1.28	37–40	1.29	0.64		25–32	2.81	1.11
17–20	1.96	1.02	41–44	1.15	0.49		33–40	2.55	1.02
21–24	1.64	0.89	45–48	1.11	0.50		41–48	2.27	0.76

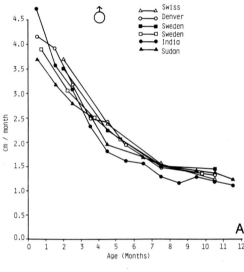

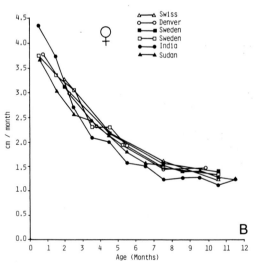

FIG. 3. Means of Sudanese and other growth increment data (from refs. 2–6).

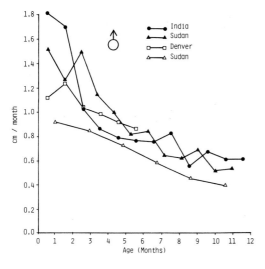

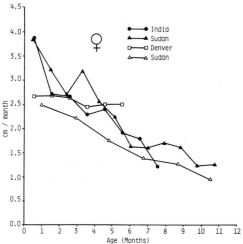

FIG. 4. Standard deviations of Sudanese and other growth increment data (from refs. 2 and 4).

cially during the first 6 months. The 4-week standard deviations are only a little higher than those reported in the Denver series and comparable with those in the Indian series. The standard deviations at the 8-week interval are smaller than those for the 4-week interval by around 30%, which is about what would be expected if successive increments were uncorrelated.

INCREMENT CENTILES

Increment centiles for 4-week and 8-week intervals are shown in Figs. 5 and 6, respectively. The nonnormality of the increment distributions made it necessary to

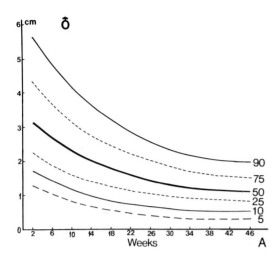

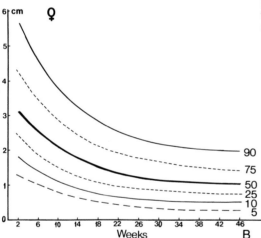

FIG. 5. Increment centiles for 4-week intervals. **A:** Males. **B:** Females.

obtain the centiles by counting inward from the tails. These centiles were quite irregular because of the grouping of the data. They were smoothed by fitting to them the first derivative of the Jenss–Bayley curve in the form

$$y = a + b \exp(ct)$$

but to obtain consistency it was necessary to smooth the coefficients of these curves by plotting them against the normal equivalent deviates of the corresponding percentages. This worked quite well for the 8-week increments, but at the shorter interval some additional manual smoothing was needed. The curves are constructed so that the user plots the increment being examined at the center of the age interval and not (as in some increment standards) at the end of the interval.

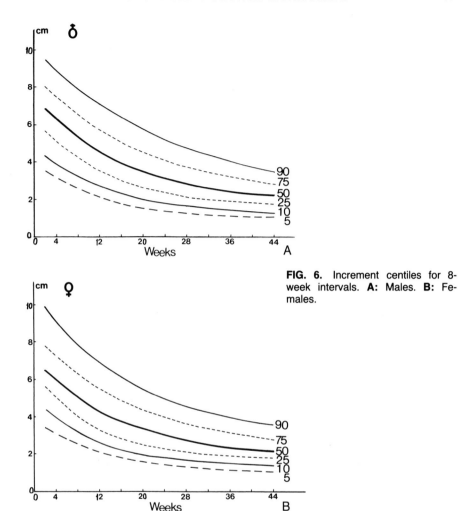

FIG. 6. Increment centiles for 8-week intervals. **A:** Males. **B:** Females.

USING AN INCREMENT STANDARD FOR SCREENING

In practice, a child will be measured at regular intervals, and the growth increments will be compared with the standard centiles. The question arises of how the comparison should be interpreted. There is a close analogy with the situation of industrial quality control when measurements on the output of a production process are being monitored. If a single measurement is extreme, this can be interpreted as meaning that the process is "out of control"—in our context, that the child is growing badly and that intervention is indicated. This procedure may, however, be slow at picking up relatively minor but long-lasting deficits. It is therefore advisable to fix not only an "action limit" at, say, the fifth centile but also a "warning limit'' much closer to the median value. If a growth increment is below the warning limit, the child's record is marked, and the next recorded increment is scrutinized. If this too lies below the warning limit, the two successive signals are taken to indicate abnormality, and intervention is initiated. A possible warning limit is the 25th centile; the chance of a false positive, a normal child with two successive increments below this centile, is approximately $0.25^2 = 6.25\%$. The process is illustrated in Fig. 7.

In a growth context, a scheme like this is wholly inappropriate for distance or length-attained data because of the high correlation between successive measurements—a child who is small on one occasion of measurement is almost certain to be small at the next. However, it is well fitted for judging increments, for which the correlations between one measurement and the next are quite low (see Table 3). When the interval between occasions is fairly short, the contribution of measurement errors to the increment will be appreciable, and a single too-small increment may merely reflect a negative measurement error on the second measurement occasion. This too-small increment, however, will automatically tend to be balanced by a too-high increment over the next interval for precisely the same reason. Successive small increments, on the other hand, even if not individually extreme, are more likely to indicate a genuine slowing down of growth.

The performance of a growth increment standard used in this way must be assessed by examining its ability to pick up cases of deficient growth without raising too many false alarms. These are slight extensions of the usual concepts of sensitivity and specificity. The specificity is, at least in principle, controlled by the use of centile limits. If we take an intervention limit at the fifth centile, we should get a false alarm rate of 5% at each measurement occasion. The sensitivity, though, is more complicated, since both the magnitude and the temporal pattern of the growth deficiency must be taken into account. Take as an example a child who starts by growing normally but whose velocity abruptly changes at a particular

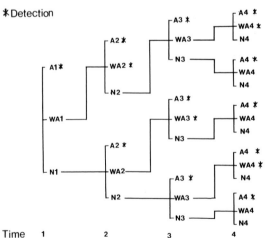

FIG. 7. Scheme showing detection of growth deficiencies using action and warning limits at the fifth and 25th centiles, respectively.

TABLE 3. *Intercorrelations of successive length increments*

Weeks	Boys	Girls
4-week intervals		
1–4 vs. 5–8	− 0.01	+ 0.01
5–8 vs. 9–12	− 0.05	+ 0.03
9–12 vs. 13–16	− 0.08	+ 0.06
13–16 vs. 17–20	+ 0.11	+ 0.03
17–20 vs. 21–24	+ 0.33	+ 0.10
21–24 vs. 25–28	+ 0.30	+ 0.33
25–28 vs. 29–32	+ 0.31	+ 0.48
29–32 vs. 33–36	+ 0.17	+ 0.30
33–36 vs. 37–40	+ 0.07	+ 0.19
37–40 vs. 41–44	+ 0.10	+ 0.15
41–44 vs. 45–48	+ 0.23	+ 0.26
8-week intervals		
1–8 vs. 9–16	− 0.26	− 0.14
9–16 vs. 17–24	+ 0.07	+ 0.16
17–24 vs. 25–32	+ 0.34	+ 0.33
25–32 vs. 33–40	+ 0.21	+ 0.40
33–40 vs. 41–48	+ 0.24	+ 0.36

time to a lower value and remains low. If this occurs shortly before a measurement occasion, the resulting increment will be only slightly less than its expected value and is unlikely to be detected. If the slowing down occurs just after the previous measurement occasion, the increment will be more severely reduced and is more likely to be picked up.

An important question is the optimal interval between measurement occasions. The problem is that with a short interval the amount of growth will be small compared to the variability from measuring errors and other causes. A small deficit in an already small amount is thus unlikely to be detectable. On the other hand, if a longer interval is used, a slowing down in growth may have been present for some time before a measurement occasion occurs to make its detection possible. With some simplifying assumptions, we can get an idea of the probability of detection of a given growth deficit using different intervals between measurement occasions. The method is described in the Appendix.

Table 4 shows some results. The means and standard deviations were taken to be those for 2 months of age, and the action and warning limits were taken at the fifth and 25th centiles. The table shows the average length of time it takes to detect a growth failure, measured from the moment it begins, under the systems of 4-weekly and 8-weekly monitoring. The degree of growth failure is given by the coefficient α, the proportion of the normal growth velocity to which the subject has dropped. When $\alpha = 0$, growth failure is catastrophic and total; when $\alpha = 1.0$, no growth failure occurs, and the cases "detected" are false alarms. It

TABLE 4. *Proportion of growth-deficient children picked up 1–4 weeks after the start of the slowing of growth by monitoring at 4-week and 8-week intervals*[a]

Slowing	Interval	Proportion detected by			
		1 week	2 weeks	3 weeks	4 weeks
$\alpha = 0.00$	A	0.11	1.00	1.00	1.00
	B		0.49		1.00
$\alpha = 0.25$	A	0.14	0.76	1.00	1.00
	B		0.32		0.95
$\alpha = 0.50$	A	0.08	0.43	0.71	0.83
	B		0.14		0.60
$\alpha = 0.75$	A	0.06	0.22	0.35	0.45
	B		0.08		0.20
$\alpha = 1.00$	A	0.05	0.14	0.21	0.29
	B		0.05		0.14

[a]A, 4-week intervals; B, 8-week intervals; α is the proportion of the normal velocity. Thus, slowing may be complete ($\alpha = 0$) or partial ($\alpha = 0.25, 0.50, 0.75$). The row for $\alpha = 1$ shows the proportion of false alarms.

is important to bear in mind that the probabilities in Table 4 are only indicative of the true state of affairs. The underlying model is inevitably oversimplified, and in particular the assumption of normality in the calculations is not really justified. The conclusions are nonetheless fairly clear. A given growth deficit will be picked up a good deal more quickly by the shorter measurement interval, but this advantage is paid for at the cost of a substantial increase in the false alarm rate, that is, the proportion of subjects apparently abnormal who actually do not warrant intervention. A computer program for calculating the probabilities is in preparation, and this would enable other screening rules and situations to be examined.

Finally, we must emphasize that the centile standards we have presented are to be considered as a model only and should not be used uncritically without further examination. The children studied were living in poor Third World conditions and certainly included many with a degree of undernutrition. We need to examine the situation in a well-nourished Western group and also to differentiate between those Sudan children who were moderately well and those who were not. In this chapter we are concerned primarily with methods rather than results.

ACKNOWLEDGMENTS

We are grateful to Prof. J. Waterlow for suggesting this study and to Ms. H. Diamond for help in preparing the data for analysis. This study was supported by a grant from WHO.

REFERENCES

1. Healy MJR. The disciplining of medical data. *Br Med Bull* 1964;24:210–4.
2. Bhalla AK, Kaul S, Kumar V. Longitudinal growth in crown–heel length and weight of Punjabi infants in Chandigarh, India. *Ann Hum Biol* 1986;3:421–3.

3. Heirli E. Longitudinae Wachstumsstudie. *Helv Paediatr Acta* 1960;15:311–35.
4. McCammon RW. *Human growth and development.* Springfield, IL: Charles C. Thomas, 1970:152–3.
5. Karlberg P, Taranger J. Physical growth from birth to 16 years and longitudinal outcome of the study during the same age period. *Acta Paediatr Scand* [suppl] 1976;258:7–76.
6. Persson LA. Infant feeding and growth—a longitudinal study in three Swedish communities. *Ann Hum Biol* 1985;12:41–52.

APPENDIX: PROBABILITIES OF DETECTING A SLOWING IN GROWTH

We suppose that a screening system is set up as suggested in the chapter. Measurements are taken at equally spaced times labeled 0, 1, 2, . . ., and the successive increments are calculated and compared with both action and warning limits. If $\bar{v}_t$, s_t, are the mean and standard deviation for the increments in the interval $(t, t + 1)$, these limits are taken to be of the form $A_t = \bar{v}_t - k_A s_t$, $W_t = \bar{v}_t - k_W s_t$ where k_A, k_W might be taken to be 1.645 and 0.674 to correspond to the fifth and 25th centiles.

Suppose that a child is observed at time 0 growing normally with velocity v and that this velocity changes at time δ $(0 < \delta < 1)$ to a lower value αv. The increment over the $(0,1)$ interval will be $[\delta + \alpha(1 - \delta)] v = \lambda v$, and a collection of such children will have velocities in this interval with mean $\lambda \bar{v}_1$ and SD λs_1.

If one of these children has a velocity low enough to fall below the action limit A_1, immediate action will be recommended; we say that the slowing in growth has been detected. Otherwise, suppose that the velocity in the $(1,2)$ interval is taken at random from a distribution with mean $\alpha \bar{v}_2$ and SD αs_2, independently of that in the preceding interval. The velocities in subsequent intervals are determined in the same way.

We can now calculate the probabilities of detection at times 1, 2, . . . as functions of α and δ. At each time there are three possibilities: the child's velocity can fall below the action limit, between the action and warning limits, or above the warning limit. Call these events A, WA, and N. If normal distributions are assumed, the probabilities at time 1 are

$$pA1 = \Phi\{[(1 - \lambda)\bar{v}_1 - K_A s_1]/\lambda s_1\}$$

$$pWA1 = \Phi\{[(1 - \lambda)\bar{v}_1 - K_W s_1]/\lambda s_1\} - pA1$$

$$pN1 = 1 - pA1 - pWA1$$

where Φ denotes the normal integral. The first of these gives immediately the probability of detection at time 1.

Detection will occur at time 2 if WA1 is followed by WA2 or if WA1 or N1 is followed by A2. The probability is thus more complicated but can be calculated in essentially the same manner. The probabilities of the three events at time 2 are given by formulas like those for time 1 with α replacing λ. Subsequent times introduce still further complications (see Fig. 7 in the text), but the method of calculating the probabilities is unchanged.

It remains to get rid of the unknown quantity δ, the position in the $(0,1)$ interval at which the slowing in velocity occurs. This can be done by assuming that the position is equally likely to be at any point in the interval and averaging the results for values of δ between 0 and 1.

DISCUSSION

Dr. Waterlow: I should like to make a couple of comments about this study. First, I think it is appropriate to say that it was supported by the Nestlé Research Grant Programme. Dr. Zumrawi was working with a very small field team. She was dealing with a very deprived population: mud houses, crowded together, dust and flies everywhere. In the course of the survey, a lot of information was collected regarding morbidity, socioeconomic status, and so on, which of course will be analyzed separately. The first point is that I am amazed and delighted that under those conditions it seems to have been possible, in spite of some defects, to collect data that are usable by experts such as J. M. Tanner, auxologist, and M. J. R. Healy, statistician. It is very satisfactory that there have been some discussions concerning the problem of collecting data, and particularly length data, at short intervals in Third World countries, because this gives for the first time a statistical basis for understanding what we observe. A second point is that the original objective of the study was to relate growth, and particularly in this case growth in weight, to the duration of breast feeding and the introduction of supplementary feeding; also to investigate whether there is a relationship between the length of exclusive breast feeding and the beginning of faltering. I believe that when we turn to the analysis of the weight data, the approach that you have used for height will answer this problem. So I am extremely grateful to Dr. Tanner for the trouble taken for this analysis, because it is going to become a pattern for several other studies in India and Jordan, where similar data have been collected. I would finally agree, Dr. Tanner, although you were asked to try to produce a velocity reference at short intervals, I perfectly appreciate that the brief had to be modified, but the result is possibly even more useful from the point of view of Third World problems.

Dr. Tomkins: You were rather critical about this set of data because of the bunching.[1] How different were the other studies of which you showed slides with regard to bunching? How relevant to the other sets of data were your serious criticisms of this set of data? Secondly, could you give us some indication on how to avoid bunching when taking monthly measurements such as these?

Dr. Tanner: I cannot really answer your first question because I have not got the raw data for these studies. You do not get bunching in longitudinal studies in the developed world such as the Denver study. As for the second question, bunching should really not occur if you measure in millimeters, and there is absolutely no reason not to do so. If you know it is difficult to measure an infant of 6 months, and it certainly is, it does not help to do a coarse measurement. With regard to weight, we did not have to smooth the parameters after we had smoothed the centiles because there was no bunching in weight. As a further answer to your second question, there are perfectly good field techniques for measuring the length of infants with apparatus constructed by UNICEF and others.

Dr. Ramanchandran: Dr. Tanner, your paper projects a simple methodology that could find easy application in different situations, but there are a few points on which I would

---

[1]Bunching: the tendency for values to include many whole numbers and few intermediate ones.

like to seek some information. You showed the curves of height velocities and standard deviations of height velocities to satisfy us that the data were of reasonably good quality and that we could use it. But was an attempt made to study the growth pattern and the variability in the growth pattern of this set of data just by putting them on a graph to see if this could be considered as a reasonably homogeneous group that could be used for deriving reference values?

Dr. Tanner: We looked at all the distributions by plotting them against normal deviates in the regular way. We got these data 6 weeks ago, so we have not yet fitted curves to individuals. We will do this later.

Dr. Ramanchandran: That will directly tell us whether we are dealing with a reasonably homogeneous group. For example, if you find some abnormalities in terms of variability and in terms of the growth itself, you would have to look at the data carefully to possibly eliminate some of these observations.

Dr. Tanner: Absolutely, and this leads me to the next thing we will be doing with Dr. Zumrawi. These data include a number of ''undernourished'' children and a number of ''not undernourished'' children; in the curve fitting, differences will presumably begin to appear. The important thing about this study is that because of her 2-weekly visits Dr. Zumrawi obtained very good morbidity data, although as Dr. Van Lerberghe said, these may introduce a serious bias.

Dr. Ramanchandran: How many measurements do you have on the average on each child in this set of data?

Dr. Tanner: The average would have been 20, the maximum 26.

Dr. Milner: I want to comment on a study that was carried out among older children between the ages of 5 and 10 in 1985, in whom the velocity of growth is much slower than in those that we have been hearing about here. It was a study to evaluate the use of kinemometry, and the children were measured at 4-week intervals by conventional auxology for 6 months. We have a group of some 26 children. Each child was measured absolutely blind on each occasion by two observers; so for one child there would be seven measurements of height at 4-week intervals. Using all the information for one observer and one child, we could calculate a height velocity over 6 months, in other words, the best fit of these seven points to a straight line. Then we cut off month by month to see what was the smallest time increment at which we could get an estimate that had a reasonable correlation with the overall rate over 6 months. It came down to 8 weeks but only if we took the average of the two velocities by the two independent observers. When we were working out the best package to try to get a reasonable estimate of what the height velocity would be over a 6-month period, we found that the best buy was to have a measurement by two observers independently at 0 and 8 weeks (1). That may have some practical application in other environments also.

Dr. Tanner: That is very interesting, but the last thing you said surprises me. You took pairs of measurements?

Dr. Milner: That's right; you have measurements at 0 and 8 weeks by observer A and observer B, working independently; take A8 minus A0 to get that change and B8 minus B0 to get that change. The average of those two explains 80% variance of the growth over 0 to 6 months of that child.

Dr. Tanner: Presumably you explain more and more the longer you continue.

Dr. Milner: Yes. We were surprised that we could use as short a time interval as 8 weeks.

Dr. Tanner: What time of the year was this?

Dr. Milner: Spring through autumn.

Dr. Tanner: This is another problem. You remember the data in the literature on seasonal effect from Marshall (2), who also has 1-month intervals.

Dr. Mukherjee: We have conducted a longitudinal study of growth from birth to 3.5 years, using 14-day intervals (3). You said that we should use 4-week intervals instead of 8-week intervals. Could you comment further on this?

Dr. Tanner: Yes. For the system to work most efficiently, 4 weeks is better than 8, but of course it costs more. We were surprised, but when the statistics are done properly it comes out that in spite of all the unreliability, you still obtain diagnosis faster at 4 weeks.

Dr. Davies: A major dilemma in setting up studies to establish normal standards is the number of children that should be included. I wonder if you could give some general guidance. If you are using precise methods and properly trained personnel, how many children of each sex would you recommend as being a minimum to construct meaningful standards?

Dr. Tanner: A cohort of 250 of either sex, which is not too bad for 1 year.

Dr. Waterlow: You say that successive increments were not correlated. I don't understand how you can get reasonably smooth growth curves unless a period of low growth is followed by a period of better growth.

Dr. Tanner: You mean the increments should be negatively correlated?

Dr. Waterlow: Yes, I would have thought so.

Dr. Tanner: In fact, in these data they are very slightly positively correlated, but the coefficients are less than 0.2. In distance curves, you get very high correlations all the way through, but that is not true in velocity curves. This is the whole point of the exercise. You couldn't do this for distance curves. In a way, that comes back to the point I was making before. I appreciate that anybody can have difficulties with velocity curves, because I do all the time.

Dr. Nabarro: Will the computer programs that have been developed by Professor Healy make it possible to look at the effect of reducing the imprecision in measurements of length on the sensitivity and specificity with which deviations can be detected? If we are attempting to detect growth faltering, we need some idea of the potential for improving sensitivity through training initiatives that concentrate on increasing the precision of measurement. I suspect that considerable increases in sensitivity could result from a small investment in technical training.

Dr. Tanner: I am absolutely delighted to hear you, because I feel so too, but there are a lot of people working in the Third World who do not agree. To answer your question, this particular computer program probably doesn't do that, but you could certainly go through the exercise of generating unbunched and reliable data and see how not having to smooth out the parameters increases the precision.

Dr. Nabarro: I would like to inject a word of caution about the 5% ''action limit'' and the 25% ''warning limit,'' and I am sure that you will agree with this. Can we make absolutely certain that when the final paper appears in the proceedings you emphasize that the choice of cutoffs must be based on some functional criteria. We should make sure that our cutoffs have meaning in terms of risk.

Dr. Tanner: Absolutely. That is why Healy developed the computer program, so that the man in the field could pick his cutoffs. The fifth centile limit is taken purely because the NCHS has got 5 at the bottom and everybody has heard of the NCHS; 25 is out of a hat.

Dr. Rappaport: How does seasonal variation eventually interfere in this type of study, and what is the difference between developed and developing counties?

Dr. Tanner: I think that is a real problem, and it is presumably worse over shorter intervals than over longer ones. About the seasonal effect in developed countries: in the temperate zones, whether north or south, children grow faster in height in the spring and less rapidly in the fall. That is rather well known for primary school children aged 5 to 10. I don't know of any data on babies since those of Bransby (4) in Britain before the war (see also ref. 5). This therefore has to be studied. That is why I think this exercise should be going on somewhere in a developed country as a kind of yardstick, or maybe it is best to consider the developed countries as an extreme. Presumably there are as many seasonal effects in developing countries as there are countries. It depends on the culture, the food situation, differences between the sexes, and so on.

REFERENCES

1. Wales JKH, Milner RDG. Knemometry in assessment of linear growth. *Arch Dis Child* 1987;63:166–71.
2. Marshall WA. Evaluation of growth rate in height over periods of less than a year. *Arch Dis Child* 1971;46:414–20.
3. Mukherjee DK, Sethna NJ, Madhavan R. Height, weight, height velocity and weight velocity of Bengali Hindu children from birth to 18 months. *Indian J Pediatr* 1970;37:429–37.
4. Bransby ER. The seasonal growth of children. *Med Officer* 1945;73:149–51,157–9,165–8.
5. Tanner JM. *Growth at adolescence*. 2nd ed. Oxford: Blackwell Scientific Publications, 1962:110–1.

Linear Growth Retardation in Less Developed Countries, edited by John C. Waterlow. Nestlé Nutrition Workshop Series, Vol. 14. Nestec Ltd., Vevey/Raven Press, Ltd., New York © 1988.

Poverty and Stature in Children

*Reynaldo Martorell, †Fernando Mendoza, and †Ricardo Castillo

Food Research Institute, Stanford University, and †Department of Pediatrics, Stanford Medical School, Stanford, California 94305

The variation in stature among the people of the world is evident to us all. Throughout the years, numerous hypotheses have been advanced to explain differences in stature among populations. Some researchers have postulated that the differences are genetically determined, being the result of adaptations over time to particular climatic or environmental conditions. Other researchers have attributed large explanatory roles to the effects of poverty, namely, malnutrition and infection.

Most investigators would agree that both genetic and environmental factors explain population differences in stature. What remains an issue is the relative importance of genetic and environmental factors at different stages of economic development. In studying the relative importance of genetic and environmental factors, young children must be considered separately from adolescents and adults, for very different answers may be obtained for each group. For example, growth potential may be similar in prepubescent children from around the world, yet adult size may vary because of genetically determined differences in the timing and/or intensity of the adolescent growth spurt.

The main purpose of this chapter is to argue that population differences in stature in young children from around the world are more a reflection of poverty than genetics. This is so because much of the Third World is wretchedly poor. Under these conditions, the explanatory role that can be ascribed to genetics is minor. Conversely, as economic development takes place, the effects of poverty on stature diminish, and genetic explanations acquire greater prominence.

There are four lines of evidence that may be examined with regard to the relative importance of genetic and environmental determinants of stature (Table 1). Although this is not an exhaustive list, a wealth of data exists for all selected approaches. First, secular trends in stature in industrialized nations may be considered, and in this situation, the general assumptions are that genetic endowment remains unchanged while environment changes, generally from poor to better. Second, the stature of socioeconomic groups belonging to the same ancestry group may be examined. In making these comparisons, researchers usually assume that genetic endowment is unrelated to poverty and interpret differences that may be

TABLE 1. *Some approaches for understanding the relative importance of genetic and environmental factors as causes for population differences in stature*

Type of data	Assumption
1. Secular trends in stature in industrialized nations	1. Genetic endowment is constant; hence, trends reflect stature at different stages of economic development
2. Stature of groups classified by poverty indicators in specific populations	2. Genetic endowment is unrelated to poverty; hence, differences among groups reflect the effects of poverty
3. Stature of populations of varying ancestry living in adequate socioeconomic conditions	3. Well-to-do environments allow for the expression of genetic potential; hence, the differences among groups are a reflection of genetic causes
4. Epidemiological and experimental studies of the effects of diet and infection	4. Direct assessment of effects are possible through appropriate study designs and data analysis

found in stature as reflections of poverty. Third, the statures of children of different ancestry or ethnic origin who are growing up under adequate environments may be compared to each other. To the extent that well-to-do environments allow for the expression of genetic potential, differences observed among groups can be said to reflect genetic factors.

In this chapter, we emphasize the three lines of evidence mentioned above. Other chapters in this volume deal with a fourth area, namely, the effects of infection and diet on linear growth. These chapters complement the present one because they provide information on the mechanisms through which poverty affects stature and adds to the persuasiveness of the data reviewed here.

SECULAR TRENDS IN STATURE

There are now considerable data from Europe, North America, and Japan documenting that children and adults are taller today than in the past. The differences observed are larger for children than for adults because maturity has been affected as well. Menarche is reached 2 to 4 years earlier; final adult size is also reached earlier, by 17 to 18 years of age instead of during the mid-20s (1).

To illustrate the magnitude of these changes, data from 19th-century British children who worked in factories are plotted on National Center for Health Statistics (NCHS) curves in Fig. 1. These curves are widely used as reference data (2). The 19th-century data are from Tanner (1) and were collected in 1833 as part of government surveys of the conditions of working children. These data are illustrative of some of the poorest, most deprived sectors of British society in the 19th century. There are several important points. First, the children are very small by modern standards, as mean values are below the NCHS fifth percentile. Secondly, the sample examined was already small at 9 years of age; in fact, its position rela-

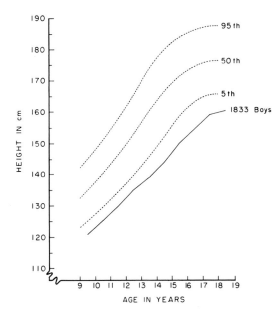

FIG. 1. Mean heights of children working in the Manchester–Stockport area in 1983 (*solid line*) compared to the NCHS percentiles (*dashed lines*).

tive to the NCHS curves remains unchanged throughout the age range studied. This suggests that the principal factors limiting growth operated in the first few years of life. Finally, the 1833 British children had heights similar to those that we see today in the poorest areas of developing countries like India and Guatemala.

There are two general types of explanations for secular changes. The genetic hypothesis argues that the breakdown of small, isolated breeding populations as a result of increased social and geographic mobility produced the phenomenon of heterosis or hybrid vigor; increased stature is one of its manifestations. This hypothesis has not received much support in the literature because hybrid vigor, even in rapidly evolving multiracial societies such as Hawaii, does not appear to exist in humans, certainly not to the extent observed in animals (3,4). This leaves environmental explanations the most favored. No one can deny that dramatic changes have taken place in industrialized countries with respect to environmental sanitation, rates of infection, and food consumption. It is also evident that life for the poor in 19th-century Europe had many of the same adverse features that characterize life for the poor in developing countries today. It is for this reason, we believe, that the size of yesterday's British children is like that of today's children from developing countries.

POVERTY AND STATURE

There are many studies in the literature that show that within particular societies, stature is associated with indicators of wealth such as land, income, and occupation. Some examples are necessary here to show that the magnitude of the differences associated with socioeconomic levels is very large.

Honduras Study

One example comes from Honduras, one of the poorest countries in the western hemisphere. As part of a larger investigation, about 1,000 children less than 7 years of age, in an area largely devoted to subsistence agriculture, were measured between December, 1981 and March, 1982 (5). Standard techniques were used to measure length, weight, head circumference, arm circumference, and triceps and subscapular skinfolds. Subroutines available from the Centers for Disease Control (CDC) were used to generate z scores; these subroutines use NCHS data as reference. We also collected data on simple measures of wealth including characteristics of the home and possession of tools, work animals, appliances, and machines. One of the simplest yet most informative indicators that resulted from these data is the house score (Table 2). Three items make up the score: the presence of a separate kitchen counts as one point; a separate bedroom also gets one point; and a floor other than a dirt one also counts one point. Consequently, the house score can range from 0, which would be a one-room hut with a dirt floor, to 3, a score corresponding to a larger home with a wooden or cement floor.

The first column of numbers in Table 3 shows the simple correlations between the house score and a number of anthropometric variables. The house score was most highly related to z-scores in height and weight and least associated with the weight-for-height z scores. In this sample, height z scores and weight-for-height z scores were unrelated ($r = 0.02$; $n = 985$). Other socioeconomic indicators were also related to the anthropometric variables, but, as might have been expected, a great deal of the variance explained by the socioeconomic indicators was shared and not unique. This is suggested by the multiple correlations that are shown in the second and third columns of numbers. These involve, respectively, the house score and three other socioeconomic scores in column 2 and the house score and six other scores in column 3. Very little additional variance is explained by including more socioeconomic variables in the case of height and weight z scores. In contrast, the correlations involving the arm variables do increase as more socioeconomic variables are considered. With the single exception of weight-for-height z scores, these simple indicators of wealth have multiple correlations of around 0.26 and thus account for a little less than 7% of the variance.

A population taller than the NCHS reference population would have an average z score that is positive. A population similar to the NCHS reference data would have an average z score of 0. Growth-retarded populations would have negative z scores. The statistical and biological strength of the relationship between the house score and the z scores for height is clear as shown in Fig. 2. Honduran children

TABLE 2. *House score components*

Separate Kitchen	No = 0	Yes = 1
Separate Bedroom	No = 0	Yes = 1
Type of Floor	Dirt = 0	Other = 1

TABLE 3. *Correlations between indicators of socioeconomic status and anthropometric variables (n = 940)*

	House	House and 3 other scores[a]	House and 6 other scores[b]
Height *z* score	0.245[c]	0.241[c]	0.258[c]
Weight *z* score	0.215[c]	0.221[c]	0.233[c]
Weight/height *z* score	0.048	0.094	0.111
Arm muscle area	0.106[d]	0.175[c]	0.247[c]
Arm fat area	0.098[d]	0.166[c]	0.259[c]
Arm circumference	0.120[c]	0.199[c]	0.292[c]

[a]House *and* appliances and machines, agricultural tools and work animals, type of iron.
[b]House *and* appliances and machines, agricultural tools and work animals, type of iron, type of house lighting, other house characteristics, field workers' impression of the house.
[c]$p < 0.001$.
[d]$p < 0.01$.

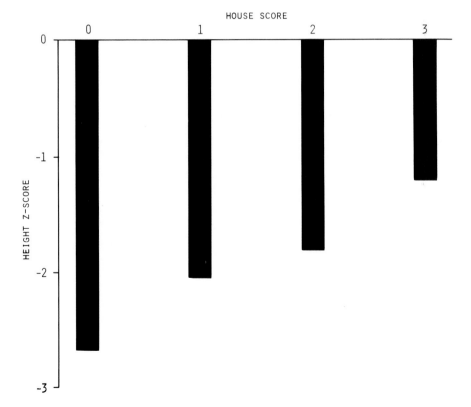

FIG. 2. Relationship between quality of the house and height *z* scores in preschool children from rural Honduras, ($n = 940$, $p < 0.001$).

are very retarded because they have very negative z scores. The z scores for height were -2.68 for a house score of 0, -2.05 for a house score of 1, -1.82 for a house score of 2, and -1.21 for a house score of 3 ($p < 0.008$). Adjusting for age, sex, and locality by analysis of covariance had little effect on the results.

These data from Honduras show that measures of stunting but not wasting are closely related to socioeconomic status and point out that the magnitude of this association is large. It is possible that, in a mestizo society such as Honduras, the proportion of Spanish/Indian ancestry varies with socioeconomic status and therefore that the differences we find among groups might be equally said to reflect ancestry. We do not consider this a credible explanation because the Honduran sample is composed of only rural children and because the variations in socioeconomic status are subtle and not marked as when one compares children from the elite urban classes and the rural poor.

Social Class and Stunting in a Number of Countries

Martorell (6) compared the heights of 7-year-old children of high and low socioeconomic class children from a number of countries. Figure 3 summarizes this work, which incorporates data from Brazil (7), Costa Rica (8), Guatemala (9–11), Jamaican black children (12,13), Nigeria (14,15), India (16), and Hong Kong (17). The NCHS percentiles and the corresponding z scores are shown on the right to facilitate comparison.

Two aspects are clear. First, there are large differences associated with social class, with some countries such as India and Guatemala showing a greater differential than others such as Brazil and Costa Rica. The simplest explanation for these consistent differences is that they reflect the consequences of poverty. However, we know that in some countries, the elite groups may differ somewhat in ancestry from the very poor. Guatemala is a good example. The very poor have a greater degree of Indian admixture than the elite classes. Could the differences we see here result from genetics and not poverty? We do not think this is a likely explanation because it would have to operate in the same direction in every situation, an unlikely event. The second aspect that Fig. 3 makes clear is that differences among high-socioeconomic samples are not that large, as most groups have means that are near the 50th percentile of the NCHS curves.

COMPARISONS OF WELL-TO-DO CHILDREN FROM AROUND THE WORLD

A closer examination of this last issue is presented in Fig. 4, which shows the mean heights of samples of 7-year-old children from industrialized countries and from the highest socioeconomic groups of developing countries. The European studies are those carried out in Czechoslovakia (18), Germany (19), Switzerland (H. Budliger and A. Prader, *unpublished data*), and England (20) under the coor-

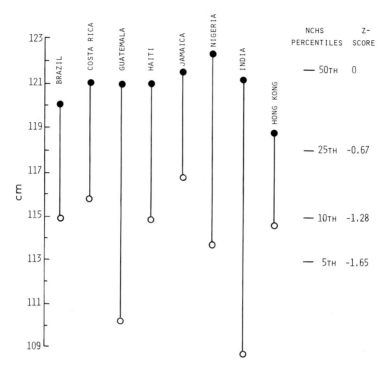

FIG. 3. Mean heights of 7-year-old boys of high (●) and low (○) socioeconomic status. (Adapted from Martorell, ref. 6.)

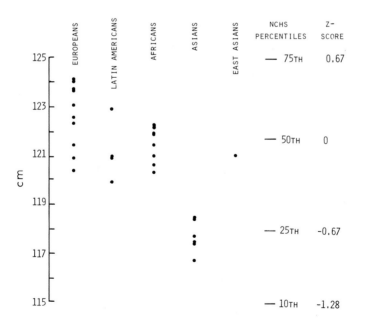

FIG. 4. Mean heights of samples of well-off 7-year-old boys of various ethnic origins. (Adapted from Martorell, ref. 6).

dination of the International Children's Center. These European data, as well as most of those for other areas, are conveniently summarized in tabular form in the work of Eveleth and Tanner (14). The North American data come from major longitudinal studies at Berkeley (21), Boston (22), Cleveland (23), Denver (24), Iowa (25), and Ohio (26). The studies selected from Latin America, as well as those from other developing countries, are those carried out among the countries' elites and represent Brazil (7), Guatemala (9,10), Costa Rica (8), and Puerto Rico (27). The children of African origin are represented by samples from Nigeria (14,15), Haiti (28), Jamaica (12,13), and five studies of black children from the United States (29–34). The Asian group includes samples from Taiwan (35), Hong Kong (17), Jamaica (12,13), Japan (14), and the United States (36,37). The Indian sample is from Hyderabad (16). Presumably, growth and development of children in the samples just cited are not limited by malnutrition and disease but are instead a reflection of genetic differences. This assumption may be incorrect because cultural differences produce dissimilar infant-feeding and child-rearing practices. The importance of this consideration is illustrated by studies of the growth of bottle-fed and breast-fed infants in middle-class families from the United States. Although not enormous, differences of the order of 10 or more percentile points for length in favor of bottle-fed infants have been reported (38).

A second issue to consider in interpreting Fig. 4 is whether the growth of the elite classes is still free from the growth-retarding effects of poverty on previous generations. Small maternal body size, it is known, influences the growth of the next generation. It is said that the secular trend has run out of steam in the United States. It is said also that the new generation of Japanese is the tallest ever and that the secular trend has slowed down considerably (36,39). These findings suggest that at least for some of the groups in Fig. 4, the phenomenon of secular trends should not be a major disturbing element.

In spite of the above caveats, the message in Fig. 4 is simple and clear. With the exception of the group designated as ''Asians,'' the mean heights of samples of diverse ethnic origins center around the 50th percentile. For Asians, the central tendency is near the 25th percentile, equivalent to -0.67 standard deviations below the median. In absolute terms, Asian children are shorter than the NCHS 50th percentile by about 3.5 cm. The data on Asians refer to samples of Japanese and Chinese origin living in Asia as well as in the Americas.

There are obviously many gaps in Fig. 4. For example, the Latin American samples do not include groups of American Indian ancestry. The reason is that, to our knowledge, there are no American Indian populations of well-to-do status, a sad reality. Though other data about Chinese children growing up in London (40) and Korean children in Japan (41) corroborate these findings, data from many other Asian countries are not reviewed. There are also no samples of well-to-do children from New Guinea, and many other exceptions as well. As we fill in the picture, we may discover well-to-do populations with similar or even smaller heights than the Japanese and Chinese. Until we do, the maximal difference in stature at ages 5 to 7 that can be ascribed to genetics is of the order of 3.5 cm. Poverty, on the other hand, can result in populations 12 cm (or more) shorter.

POVERTY AND GROWTH IN THE UNITED STATES

We have advanced the hypothesis that as economic development takes place, the role of genetic factors as explanations for population differences in stature increases. We have used cross-sectional data derived from two surveys carried out by the United States National Center for Health Statistics, HANES I and HANES II, to test this hypothesis. In Fig. 5, height z scores are presented for three age groups: 1 to 5, 6 to 11, and 12 to 17 years. Three ethnic groups are represented: Blacks, Europeans of non-Hispanic origin, and Hispanics, a group of Spanish/American ancestry. The data are presented for three poverty levels defined in terms of an index that relates income to the cost of living and adjusts the results by family size, 1 being the definition of poverty often used by the government.

Data for children 1 to 5 years old are given in the first panel of Fig. 5. Poverty is related to size in all groups, but the differences are small. For instance, the 25th percentile is equivalent to a z score of -0.67, and only one group approaches this level. Blacks are taller than Europeans and Hispanics at early ages. This is well known, and, in fact, Garn and Clark (42) have argued for separate growth standards for blacks, a plea that has gone unanswered because the differences are perceived as too small to consider. Another important point to emphasize is that

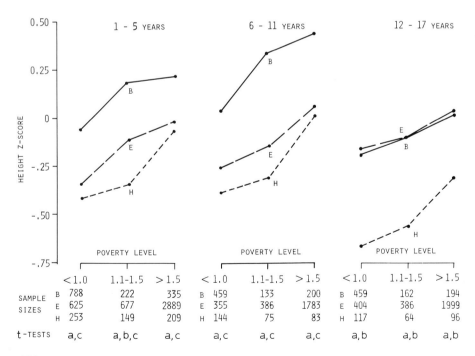

FIG. 5. Height z score by age, poverty, and ethnic group (B, Black; E, European; H, Hispanic). Lower-case letters refer to statistically significant t-tests ($p < 0.05$) as follows: a, Hispanic vs. Black; b, Hispanic vs. European; c, Black vs. European).

preschool Hispanics in the high-income group have average z scores nearly equal to 0, just as Europeans of non-Hispanic origin do.

Data for 6 to 11 years of age reveal the same basic picture as for 1 to 5 years. For 12 to 17 years, the differences are striking. Blacks become indistinguishable from Europeans, whereas Hispanics become smaller at all income levels.

The pattern in Hispanics is consistent with data from Guatemala (9,10). A careful study of two cohorts growing up in Guatemala, one with Guatemalan parents and grandparents and one with European or North American parents, revealed identical growth patterns in both cohorts prior to adolescence. Youths of Guatemalan origin had growth spurts of less intensity than their "foreign" playmates and fell to the 25th percentile at the end of the adolescent growth spurt, a level similar to that seen in U.S. Hispanics. For Hispanics, at least, genetic factors may be more important in adolescence than earlier as explanations for adult differences in stature.

Adolescents generally have healthier lives than younger children in poor societies. Access to food and food consumption are better, and rates of infection are very low. According to Eveleth and Tanner (14), adolescent growth rates are not markedly different in a variety of settings, and often differences are not larger than the 3 to 4-cm difference observed between wealthy children of Guatemalan and non-Guatemalan ancestry. An interesting study from India showed that increments from 5 to 17 years were similar in Indian children when compared to the NCHS pattern (43). The shorter stature of the Indian youths was largely the result of events prior to 5 years of age.

SUMMARY AND CONCLUSIONS

There are many interesting aspects to consider regarding adolescent growth, but our main concern is with preschool children. Figure 6 summarizes the following information:

1. The first four bars refer to the relationship between characteristics of the home and height z scores of children from rural Honduras (Fig. 2).
2. The last three bars refer to the relationship between the poverty index and height z scores in U.S. Hispanic children at ages 1 to 5 years (Fig. 5).

This figure summarizes the major points of this chapter. Where the level of socioeconomic development is low, we can expect stature to be heavily influenced by poverty, as in Honduras. At this level of development, the environment looms much larger as an explanation for population differences in stature than is the case for genetics.

As the level of socioeconomic development rises, the environment becomes less and less a factor limiting growth in stature. At this stage, it becomes easier to establish the extent to which genetics plays a role in explaining differences in stature among populations. For example, the information in Fig. 6 shows very clearly that preschool children of Hispanic origin should be expected to grow in stature

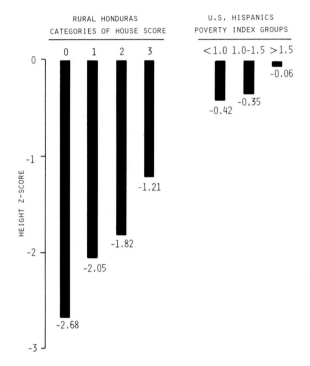

FIG. 6. Poverty and stature in two samples of preschool children: rural Honduras and U.S. Hispanics.

as in the NCHS reference curves. Earlier we mentioned that American blacks are expected to be slightly taller than the NCHS average but that this difference is too small to be concerned with.

In the case of Japanese and Chinese children, one would expect them to be smaller than the NCHS average, and many would attribute this difference to genetic factors. However, it may be that differences in infant-feeding practices between eastern and western cultures are part of the explanation for the differences in stature. It is also possible that the secular trend in western nations has all but stopped but that it will still continue in eastern nations and that eventually average heights will be somewhat increased.

These are interesting possibilities, but instead let us take the conservative position that all of the difference in stature between European, Chinese, and Japanese samples is a reflection of genetic origin. Then we would have a situation in which the largest difference in stature attributable to genetics is 3 to 4 cm, which would make average heights at age 5 to be near the 25th percentile of the NCHS norms. This difference is no longer trivial. However, it is many times smaller than what we can easily attribute to poverty in many populations.

We lack data about the stature of well-nourished children in many parts of the world. In many areas these data may underestimate growth potential, as several generations may be required for the effects of poverty to be removed (i.e., until the secular trend toward increased height ceases). As we collect more data, we will be able to document more clearly that genetic factors explain population differences in stature. We would be very surprised, however, if the effects we find turn out to be much larger than what we can maximally attribute to genetics by comparing European, Chinese, and Japanese children.

From what we know to date, we can clearly say that the growth potential of children from around the world is remarkably similar under conditions of adequate nutrition and health. Retardation in stature as a result of marked poverty is easy to demonstrate, and these effects are far greater than those we can possibly attribute to genetics. Stunting, we can say with confidence, is one of our best measures of social inequality. We know that its causes are deeply rooted in malnutrition and infection during the period of weaning. Thus, let us not go astray by hinging policy implications on the functional significance of stunting. Even if stunting proved to be largely harmless, let us keep in mind how children become stunted. Those who are prepared to argue that stunting has no policy implications must be prepared to defend social inequalities in income, diets, and the level of health.

ACKNOWLEDGMENTS

Supported in part by Grant MCJ-060518-01-0, Maternal and Child Health Research Grants Program, Bureau of Health Care Delivery and Assistance, Rockville, Maryland.

REFERENCES

1. Tanner JM. *A history of the study of human growth.* Cambridge: Cambridge University Press, 1981.
2. Hamill PVV, Drizd TA, Johnson CL, Reed RB, Roche AF, Moore WM. Physical growth: National Center for Health Statistics percentiles. *Am J Clin Nutr* 1979;32:607–29.
3. Damon A. Stature increase among Italian-Americans: environmental, genetic or both? *Am J Phys Anthropol* 1965;23:401–8.
4. Van Wieringen JC. Secular growth changes. In: Falkner F, Tanner JM, eds. *Human growth; vol 2: Postnatal growth.* New York: Plenum Press, 1978:445–73.
5. Martorell R, Kendall C, Foote DR. *Growth and poverty in Honduras.* Paper presented at the Fifty-Second Annual Meeting of the American Association of Physical Anthropologists. Indianapolis: April 1983 (unpublished).
6. Martorell R. Child growth retardation: a discussion of its causes and its relationship to health. In: Blaxter KL, Waterlow JC, eds. *Nutrition adaptation in man.* London, Paris: John Libbey, 1985:13–29.
7. Murillo Marques R, Berquo E, Yunes J, Marcondes E. *Crecimiento de é niños Brasileños: peso y altura en relación con la edad y el sexo y la influencia de factores socioeconomicos.* Washington, DC: Organización Panamericana de la Salud, 1975 (Publicación Cientifica no. 309).
8. Villarejos VM, Osborne JA, Payne FJ, Arguedas G. Heights and weights of children in urban and rural Costa Rica. *J Trop Pediatr Environ Child Health* 1971;17:31–43.
9. Johnston FE, Borden M, MacVean RB. Height, weight, and their growth velocities in Guatemalan private school children of high socioeconomic class. *Hum Biol* 1973;45:627–41.
10. Johnston FE, Wainer H, Thissen D, MacVean R. Hereditary and environmental determinates of growth in height in a longitudinal sample of children and youth of Guatemalan and European ancestry. *Am J Phys Anthropol* 1976;44:469–76.

11. Yarbrough C, Habicht J-P, Malina RM, Lechtig K, Klein RE. Length and weight in rural Guatemalan Ladino children: birth to seven years of age. *Am J Phys Anthropol* 1975;42:439–48.
12. Ashcroft MT, Lovell HG. Heights and weights of Jamaican children of various racial origins. *Trop Geogr Med* 1964;4:346–53.
13. Ashcroft MT, Heneage P, Lovell HG. Heights and weights of Jamaican schoolchildren of various ethnic groups. *Am J Phys Anthropol* 1966;24:35–44.
14. Eveleth PG, Tanner JM. *Worldwide variation in human growth*. Cambridge: Cambridge University Press, 1976.
15. Janes MD. Physical growth of Nigerian Yoruba children. *Trop Geogr Med* 1974;26:389–98.
16. Vijay Raghavan K, Singh D, Swaminathan MC. Heights and weights of well-nourished Indian school children. *Indian J Med Res* 1971;59:648–54.
17. Chang KSF, Lee MMC, Low WD, Kvan E. Height and weight of southern Chinese children. *Am J Phys Anthropol* 1963;21:497–509.
18. Prokopec M, Sachy J, Titlbachova S. Results of the third whole-state investigation of the youth in 1971 (Czech counties). *Cesk Pediatr* 1973;28:341–6.
19. Hagen W. Das Wachstrum in der Reifeperiode. *Internist (Berl)* 1967;8:282–91.
20. Tanner JM, Whitehouse RH, Takaishi M. Standards from birth to maturity for height, weight, height velocity and weight velocity; British children 1965. *Arch Dis Child* 1966;41:454–71.
21. Tuddenham RD, Snyder MM. *Physical growth of California boys and girls from birth to eighteen years*. Berkeley, Los Angeles: University of California Press, 1954.
22. Reed RB, Stuart HC. Patterns of growth in height and weight from birth to eighteen years of age. *Pediatrics* 1959;24:904–21.
23. Simmons K. The Brush Foundation Study of child growth and development. II. Physical growth and development. *Monogr Soc Res Child Dev* 1944;9:1–87.
24. McCammon RW. *Human growth and development*. Springfield, IL: Charles C Thomas, 1970.
25. Stuart HC, Meredith HV. The use of body measurements in the school health programs. I. General considerations and the selection of measurements. II. Methods to be followed in taking and interpreting measurements and norms to be used. *Am J Public Health* 1946;36:1365–86.
26. Garn SM. *Magnitude of secular trends in the Fels population*. Yellow Springs, OH: Fels Research Institute, 1967.
27. Knott VB. Stature, leg girth, and body weight of Puerto Rican private school children measured in 1962. *Growth* 1963;27:157–74.
28. King KW, Foucauld J, Fougere W, Severinghaus EL. Height and weight of Haitian children. *Am J Clin Nutr* 1963;13:106–9.
29. Barr GD, Allen CM, Shinefield HR. Height and weight of 7500 children of three skin colors. *Am J Dis Child* 1972;124:866–72.
30. Hamill PVV, Johnston FE, Grams W. *Height and weight of children: United States*. Washington, DC: US Government Printing Office, 1970 (Vital and Health Statistics; series 11; no. 104).
31. Hamill PVV, Johnston FE, Lemeshow S. *Body weight, stature and sitting height: white and negro youth 12–17 years: United States*. Washington, DC: US Government Printing Office, 1973; DHEW Publication no. (HRA) 74-1608 (Vital and Health Statistics; series 11; no. 126).
32. Krogman WM. Growth of the head, face, trunk, and limbs in Philadelphia white and Negro children of elementary and high school age. *Monogr Soc Res Child Dev* 1970;35:1–80.
33. Rauh JL, Schumsky DA, Witt MT. Heights, weights and obesity in urban schoolchildren. *Child Dev* 1967;38:515–30.
34. Verghese KP, Scott RB, Teixeira G, Ferguson AD. Studies in growth and development. XII. Physical growth of North American Negro children. *Pediatrics* 1969;44:243–7.
35. Kimura D, Tsai CM. Comparative studies of the physical growth in Formosans. I. Height and weight. *J. Anthropol Soc Nippon* 1976;75:11–18.
36. Greulich WW. Some secular changes in the growth of American-born and native Japanese children. *Am J Phys Anthropol* 1967;45:553–68.
37. Kondo S, Eto M. *Physical growth studies on Japanese-American children in comparison with native Japanese*. Proceedings of the Seminar of US–Japan Cooperative Research on Human Adaptabilities. Kyoto: Japan Society for the Promotion of Science and National Science Foundation, 1972.
38. Kovar MG, Serdula MK, Marks JS, Fraser DW. Review of the epidemiologic evidence for an association between infant feeding and infant health. *Pediatrics* 1984;74:615–38.
39. Tanner JM, Hayashi T, Preece MA, Cameron N. Increase in length of leg relative to trunk in Japanese children and adults from 1957 to 1977: comparison with British and Japanese Americans. *Ann Hum Biol* 1982;9:411–23.

40. Wheeler E, Tan SP. Trends in the growth of ethnic Chinese living in London. *Ann Hum Biol* 1983;10:441–6.
41. Kim YS. Growth status of Korean schoolchildren in Japan. *Ann Hum Biol* 1982;9:453–8.
42. Garn SM, Clark DC. Problems in the nutritional assessment of Black individuals. *Am J Public Health* 1976;66:262–7.
43. Satyanarayana K, Nadamuni Naidu A, Swaminathan MC, Narasinga Rao BS. Effects of nutritional deprivation in early childhood on later growth: a community study without intervention. *Am J Clin Nutr* 1980;34:1636–7.

DISCUSSION

Dr. Waterlow: I would like to start by referring to your Fig.1, on the height of children in Stockport in 1833. At that time the U.K. was a developing country. Nevertheless, we had good statistics even in those days, and it is interesting to recall that at that time, as reported in the very first volume of the *Lancet,* about 300 children per 1,000 born failed to reach the age of 5 years (1). What is striking to me is the enormous mortality in relation to what I would have thought was a rather small degree of stunting.

Dr. Martorell: Modern public health measures may be part of the answer. However, I think the level of stunting was quite high and in fact similar to what is observed today in many developing countries. It is interesting that the key indicator used by those concerned with child welfare in the U.K. at that time, when investigating the condition and quality of life of working children, was height. This is similar to what we do today.

Dr. Guesry: Could you not say that the difference in heights of British children 150 years ago and now represents a secular trend, as has been seen in Japan?

Dr. Martorell: That may be a way of describing it, but let me emphasize that secular trends are caused by environmental factors. The evidence from the United States and from a number of European countries is that since the 1960s secular trends in stature have ceased, and it seems that today's young people in many of the advanced countries are probably as tall as any future generation ever will be. Nevertheless, there is still a relationship between poverty and stature, as shown in Fig.5. The same relationship is found in England. The only societies that I know of in which there is no correlation between social class and growth are Scandinavian countries such as Sweden. Presumably, if one had a classless society all the children would grow optimally.

Dr. Guesry: In your Fig. 5 it seems that the first two groups, from 1 to 5 and from 6 to 11 years, belong to the same study and the third sample, from 12 to 17 years, belongs to another study. Is is possible that the differences observed were caused by some nutritional changes during the last 15 years in all ethnic groups in the United States?

Dr. Martorell: You may be quite right. However, this figure is based on data from HANES I and II, which were separated by a number of years, but there is no evidence of a secular trend in stature during that interval. If there had been a secular trend, one would have observed changes, particularly in the Hispanic group at ages 12 to 17 years, in which body sizes are consistently smaller.

Dr. Nabarro: Is the slope of the relationship between poverty and stature the same in all ethnic groups?

Dr. Martorell: Surprisingly, yes. The regressions predicting stature from poverty have similar coefficients.

Dr. Waterlow: What is the correlation coefficient? How much of the variance is explained?

Dr. Martorell: In the studies shown in Fig.5, the correlation coefficient is 0.1 to 0.15, not very high but significant because the samples were very large—thousands of children. In the Honduras sample, to give another example, the correlation between quality of housing and height was about 0.25.

Dr. Waterlow: Although in fact you have shown very clear relationships between these environmental factors and growth, the proportion of variance explained is very small.

Dr. Martorell: Yes, but I think that the percentage of variance explained can be misleading. A relationship can be very strong in biological terms even with a correlation as low as 0.25.

Dr. Mukherjee: We have conducted a longitudinal study of growth in the lower socioeconomic groups in Calcutta (2). We have found that even in the same socioeconomic groups, statistically highly significant correlations exist between growth and many environmental factors—nutrition, episodes of illness, sanitation, housing, size of the family, overcrowding, education, and maternal competence.

Dr. Martorell: That does not surprise me. In the final analysis, all these factors affect stature by limiting nutrient availability.

Dr. Waterlow: If I understood Dr. Mukherjee correctly, there were differences within his sample in spite of its being the same ethnic and socioeconomic group. You showed this very clearly within your Honduras sample.

Dr. Martorell: Yes, the sample of Honduran children belonged to the same ethnic group, and all were from the rural area. The differences in socioeconomic status that we identified are variations in what some call the microenvironment.

Dr. Aponso: It is not only poverty that determines the development of the child. My country, Sri Lanka, is one of the 12 poorest countries in the world. We all know that a high infant mortality rate (IMR) has been recognized not only as a yardstick of good health; it has been said to be an eloquent indicator of development. [Editor's note: Infant mortality rates are deaths during the first year of life per 1,000 live births.] Now in Sri Lanka, *per capita* income is only US$ 300, and our IMR is 34; in the United States, where the *per capita* income is US$ 4,000, the IMR is about 10. But in Saudi Arabia, with a *per capita* income only a little less than that of the United States, they still have an IMR of around 100; Pakistan, on the other hand, which has a *per capita* income only a little higher than that of Sri Lanka, still has an IMR of around 80 or 90. This is why people talking about development no longer talk only about *per capita* income or only about IMR; they talk about the physical quality of life based on IMR, life expectancy, and literacy. The social environment, customs, and village traditions could be modified by literacy. I think this is where poor countries can do something about this problem of malnutrition; the physical quality of life can be influenced by literacy. I submit to you that this is very important in addition to housing.

Dr. Martorell: I agree absolutely with you; it is not only a question of level of national income but of distribution of the income, of provision of health care, and so on. Certainly Sri Lanka and a number of other countries are really exceptions: they have used their resources wisely.

Dr. Waterlow: I have always found it astonishing that in the last 10 years Sri Lanka has shown such a large reduction in IMR and preschool children mortality without any increase in income, even with a decrease.

In support of what Dr. Aponso said about literacy, it is worth recalling that in Cravioto's study of a rural community in Mexico, the factors most clearly associated with good nutrition in the child were, as I recall, maternal literacy and listening to the radio.

Dr. Keller: In Sri Lanka a high correlation between IMR and female literacy has been found (3). It is the highest one can find. But there is a low correlation between IMR and stunting.

Dr. Waterlow: That is a very important point in relation to the efforts that are being made to develop a set of indicators of the quality of life.

Dr. Kraisid: I agree that poverty has to be defined at the microlevel as well as at the macrolevel. In the last 6 years we have had a national study on poverty and malnutrition in Thailand, in which we define poverty not only in economic terms, such as production per hectare of land, but also using a range of social indicators. These include prevalence of low birth weight and malnutrition: newborn babies in rural poor areas are 400 g lighter and 1.5 cm shorter than those born in Bangkok. At school age the difference in height is 10 to 15 cm. For 4 to 5 years now, the government has implemented "poverty eradication programs" in rural poor areas. The growth of children in terms of weight gain shows significant changes, and the prevalence of protein–energy malnutrition in children based on weight for age has also remarkably reduced from 51% to 30% (4). There were no data on height gain. Dr. Aree has done a study in one area in the northeast region where one of these poverty eradication programs was operating and showed that growth in weight and height showed little change until the program had been set up.

Dr. Waterlow: In this very intensive program, is there any relationship between indicators such as the nature of the house and more direct indicators of food intake and food availability?

Dr. Kraisid: Yes. When we looked at indicators such as soil quality, agricultural production, health statistics, social organization of people in clubs or groups, housing, or other indices of the quality of life, there was a good relationship between growth and housing conditions.

Dr. Keller: I want to warn against concentrating exclusively on one socioeconomic variable. The importance of housing as an indicator varies in different populations.

Dr. Martorell: This is good advice. However, in Honduras, the quality of the house is an excellent indicator of family resources and at the same time is easy to measure.

Dr. Milner: We have been discussing the interacting variables related to poverty. At the other end of the scale, in Western Europe today, the most common cause of stunting is probably psychosocial.

Dr. Rappaport: We have put emphasis so far on the effect of malnutrition on growth during the prepubertal period, but final height depends also on the pubertal growth spurt. Are you saying that during puberty nutrition is not important? There are some models that would not agree with that.

Dr. Martorell: Professor Waterlow referred to a very interesting Indian study (5) that showed that children who were short at 5 years were also short at 17 years. However, the amount of growth between 5 and 17 years was the same in short and tall children. This implies that adult stature in this area of India is determined by events before 5 years of age.

Dr. Waterlow: This is an important question. Is the growth that occurs at puberty affected differently from the growth occurring at earlier ages? This brings up the question of skeletal maturation.

Dr. Martorell: In Guatemala, mildly malnourished children are slightly retarded in biological age, so we would expect them to have some capacity for catch-up.

Dr. Waterlow: I was under the impression that maturation is less delayed than actual linear growth, so that it will be impossible to catch up completely once maturation is complete.

Dr. Davies: We have been discussing nutritional effects and secular trends in the growth of the skeleton, but there are also secular trends in head growth. British children have a head circumference about 1.5 cm greater than 25 years ago (6). Since an increase in head circumference of 1 cm is equivalent to an increase in intracranial content of approximately 20 to 30 ml, I wonder whether the brain size of children has also increased.

Dr. Martorell: You are right; there is a trend in head circumference, and maybe Dr. Colombo will comment on the possible significance for mental development.

Dr. Waterlow: Dr. Martorell has made a strong case for the overriding importance of environmental factors, summed up in the one word poverty, in determining linear growth, at least in young children. However, this does not entirely dispose of the genetic factor. As Monckeberg in Chile pointed out many years ago, some people may be poor because they are genetically less well endowed to cope with the problems of life. Hence, there would be a kind of indirect genetic selection for short stature.

REFERENCES

1. Edmonds TR. On the mortality of infants in England. *Lancet* 1835;1:690–4.
2. Mukherjee DK, Sethna NJ. The ecology of growth in underprivileged children. *Indian Pediatr* 1972;9:440–6.
3. Pabel M. Effects of health service and environmental factors on infant mortality: The case of Sri Lanka. *J Epidemiol Commun Health* 1980;34:76–82.
4. Tontisirin K. The nutrition situation and nutrition action programs in four ASEAN countries. *ASEAN Food J* 1985;1:162–8.
5. Satyanarayana K, Prasanna Krishna T, Narasinga Rao BS. Effect of early childhood undernutrition and child labour on growth and adult nutritional status of rural Indian boys around Hyderabad. *Hum Nutr Clin Nutr* 1986;40c:131–9.
6. Ounsted M, Moar VA, Scott A. Head circumference charts updated. *Arch Dis Child* 1985;60: 936–9.

Linear Growth Retardation in Less Developed Countries, edited by John C. Waterlow. Nestlé Nutrition Workshop Series, Vol. 14. Nestec Ltd., Vevey/Raven Press, Ltd., New York © 1988.

The Importance of Genetic Influences on Growth in Early Childhood with Particular Reference to Children of Asiatic Origin

D. P. Davies

Department of Paediatrics, The Chinese University of Hong Kong, Prince of Wales Hospital, Shatin, New Territories, Hong Kong

The growth of long bones and vertebrae, on which body stature largely depends, takes place through activities within the growth plate, a zone of dividing cartilage cells separating the primary from secondary ossification center that deposits substances containing mineral salts to form the bone matrix. As the rate of growth slows, the growth plate becomes narrower until eventually bone in the main shaft joins with bone in the epiphysis, eliminating the growth plate in the process. No further growth is then possible, the epiphysis being "closed." At the same time as bone growth takes place, constant remodeling and molding are also occurring in order to sustain the changes in shape demanded by the growing skeleton. For normal skeletal growth to take place, dividing cells must be provided with an optimum metabolic milieu supplying energy, amino acids, vitamins, minerals, and various endocrine secretions. Without balanced provision of these substances, growth will fail.

The growth curve of any child is the outward expression of the interaction between its genetic potential and environment. Its various stages—embryonic, fetal, neonatal adjustment, infancy, later childhood, and the adolescent climax—merge smoothly and imperceptibly with each other to provide, under normal conditions, a smooth continuum from conception to adulthood. In most instances this growth journey proceeds harmoniously, avoiding or at least mastering many potential obstacles on the way. On occasions, however, the journey is deviant, either setting off in the wrong direction (as might occur with genetic errors) or, more commonly, falling foul of environmental hazards, the most prevailing of which in the present world being a lack of food. These distortions lead to failure by the child to achieve its genetically endowed physical growth potential, becoming stunted. Faltering of linear growth rate is one of the most sensitive of all measures of socioeconomic adversity within any community.

The aim of this chapter is to provide some insight into how genetic makeup influences the linear growth program in both individuals and populations so as to see in perspective the problems of growth stunting, especially its epidemiology.

ONE OF MAN'S MOST HERITABLE TRAITS

In 1889, Francis Galton in his treatise *Natural Inheritance* (1) recognized the beautiful regularity in the stature of a population that shows "small dependence on differences of bringing up." Together with recognition of correlation of height with midparental size, he was among the first to document stature as one of man's most heritable traits and in so doing set the scene for the beginnings of a scientific appraisal of genetic influences in the control of growth. The importance of genetic influences, dictated by a plethora of genes of small effect residing on many chromosomes, is evident in many ways: variations of size between individuals within the same ethnic group; much higher coefficiency for height between monozygotic than dizygotic twins; the close relationship between the mean height of parents and mature stature of their offspring; and differences between the growth curves of boys and girls with the earlier puberty growth spurt in girls and in boys a higher peak growth velocity, to give but a few examples (2).

Where there is abnormal genetic makeup, stature is often affected. Some single-gene anomalies, as occur for example in achondroplasia, cause marked stunting and disproportionate growth. Girls with Turner syndrome (45,XO) grow at a slightly slower than average rate throughout childhood, fail to experience a puberty growth spurt, and end up as very short adults (3). Children with Down's syndrome (trisomy 21) grow slowly from fetal life through the early years after birth, resulting again in shorter than average adult stature (4). These examples, in both normal and abnormal children, leave no doubt as to the importance of genetic factors in controlling and directing the growth program, though how in individual children this genetic control, coded in the DNA template, is transcribed into actual growth processes is still incompletely understood. What we do know is that for the growth genotype to be allowed its optimum expression, growing cells must be provided with an adequate milieu supplying energy, amino acids, fatty acids, vitamins, minerals, and endocrine substances. (See R. D. G. Milner, *this volume,* and R. Rappaport, *this volume,* for a detailed consideration of the physiological determinants of growth.)

TIMING OF PHYSIOLOGICAL GENETIC INFLUENCES

In all living organisms there is an intrinsic "genetic momentum" that results in a minimal growth performance even under the most hostile environmental conditions.

In prenatal life, growth is heavily influenced by the mother through the intrauterine environment she provides for the fetus. At this focal point converge her own genetic makeup, nutrient intake, health (past and present), and lifestyle (in particular, cigarette consumption). So dominant are these intrauterine environmental influences that the fetal genome has been estimated to account for only about 20% of the variance in birth size (5). This powerful maternal control on fetal growth (totally dominating at this stage any paternal influences), recognized first by Walton and Hammond in their studies of Shetland pony/shire crosses in 1938 (6), has probably evolved in order to allow the safest possible conditions for parturition. For this to operate effectively, the fetal genotype must be subservient to local maternal environmental factors, especially those with the capacity to constrain growth. Thus, correlation between length at birth and midparental height is very small, only about 0.2 (2). This changes rapidly over the subsequent 18 months or so, when it reaches its adult value of 0.5. Correlation of length at birth with adult height is also small (about 0.3), but by the age of 3 it has risen to 0.8 (2). These improvements in height correlations with time are outward manifestations of genetic influences on growth rate, which somehow are brought into play once the child is freed at birth from prenatal maternal influences.

When considered against a background of conventional clinical centile standards, these genetically controlled "target-seeking and self-stabilizing" effects (7) are often seen as growth shifts with trajectories moving in either upward ("catch-up") or downward ("lag-down") directions. One study (8) from the late Professor David Smith and his colleagues in Seattle of well-nourished, healthy American children has shown that against a seven-point centile grid (97, 90, 75, 50, 25, 10, and 3), about two-thirds of children crossed more than one centile line over the first year. Those of extreme size at birth showed the greatest shift. Babies relatively long at birth (>90th centile) with a genetic makeup (judged by midparental stature) for smaller size tended to shift downwards after cruising for several months in the higher centile channels at their intrauterine growth rate. Where parental size was for greater stature, they tended to continue more in the centile channel in which they found themselves at birth. In most of the children, a "steady state" was achieved by about 18 months. In contrast, children small at birth (height <10th centile) born to tall parents showed "catch-up" growth that began almost immediately after birth, most accomplishing their growth shift by about 6 months. Small babies of smaller parents tended, on the other hand, to remain in the lower channels in which they were born. Possibly some of the most vivid of all examples illustrating the driving force of the offspring's genetic makeup in channeling early growth can be found where the prenatal environment has exercised a pathological influence on growth. The baby malnourished prenatally from maternal hypertensive disease will show very marked early "catch-up" growth. The baby grossly overgrown at birth as a result of poorly controlled maternal diabetes provides a mirror image of growth deceleration.

The first couple of years after birth must therefore be viewed as a time when the expression of genes controlling the growth program emerge out of the shadow of maternal intrauterine influences in order to direct the individual baby's growth trajectory into its genetically predetermined channel. It is this that underlies the remarkable heterogeneity in growth profiles in individual babies over this time. Thus, whenever growth shift occurs, it is worthwhile bearing in mind that genetic influences should be considered as a possible cause as well as those of environmental origin. Failure to do so may sometimes, in individual cases, give rise to mistaken diagnoses of growth failure or, even on occasions, of obesity. This statement will obviously apply less to children in poor countries, where environmental effects on growth will overshadow the more subtle genetic influences, than to children brought up in more privileged environments, but it is nonetheless an important principle to be aware of.

Why genes controlling the switch to "lag-down" should operate later than those influencing "catch-up" is not known. (Might it be that continued smallness is to the detriment of the small baby, whereas the big baby is not in so much haste to find its genetically determined channel?) What is important in day-to-day practice, however, is to recognize that "lag-down" or, as I consider it, "physiological growth failure" does occur and that its occurrence in an individual child should not automatically be considered stunting.

ARE THERE GENETIC ORIGINS TO DIFFERENCES THAT EXIST IN THE STATURE OF DIFFERENT RACIAL GROUPS?

It is against this background of genetic variation within individuals that I now turn to what seems a more contentious issue, namely, the extent to which genetic factors account for the diversity in physical size that exists between different races and ethnic groups.

Examining the physical attributes of the many groups of mankind can not fail to remind one of dramatic genetic influences. Color of skin, nature and distribution of body hair, body type, physical proportions, body composition, and rate of maturation are but a few examples of the ways in which various human subgroups have, over the eons of time, evolved and preserved through natural selection very varied physical characteristics to help accommodate and allow satisfactory adaptation to very diverse habitats. It therefore comes as some surprise to me to discover that where stature of young children is the physical characteristic under debate, this is considered by many authorities to be little affected by ethnic differences. The following statement from a paper by Habicht and his colleagues from Guatemala and published in the *Lancet* of 1974 introduces such an attitude: "From data collected among privileged groups of children in developing countries, we have concluded that child growth is mainly influenced by social economic status and not by race or ethnicity" (9). Yet no one can doubt the genetic origins of very obvious differences that exist between the adult heights of well-nourished and healthy different racial groups brought up in privileged environments that have allowed genetic potential achieve its full, uninhibited potential (10). Are protagonists of the equal or similar growth potential of various racial groups in early childhood implying that these differences emerge later in childhood?

Whether or not genetic factors are responsible for different patterns of growth between races is of interest not only in its own biological right. It is central to the continuing controversy of the appropriateness of reference growth standards to judge the adequacy of growth of individuals and populations and therefore ultimately to the definition of growth insufficiency (11). Those adhering to the view of equal growth potential during early childhood for children of all races inevitably favor the notion that growth standards developed from European populations in industrialized countries are appropriate for all child populations and can therefore be used as a tool to survey epidemiologically the problem of stunting.

SOME QUERIES

While admitting to the obvious, that appalling stunting of growth is caused by malnutrition and other environmental scourges (see elsewhere in this volume), can we put gene pools of different racial groups out into the cold in their differential influences on early growth? I believe not.

To argue my case I would first like to trace some of the recent history of this contentious issue. One of the key studies to which we are referred is that of Habicht and his colleagues in 1974 (9). They compared growth in height and weight over the first 5 years in samples of children (presumably) well nourished from developed countries (United States, Britain, Australia) with children in developing countries, urban and rural, assumed to be considerably undernourished (India, Colombia, Guatemala, Thailand). The overall differences between children's heights from developed countries were small, around 3%. In contrast, differences between these children and those living in poor urban and rural regions were much higher, approaching 12% and as high as 30% for weight. Differences related to race were therefore small compared with environmental effects. "We see no way to demonstrate with this kind of data that the small differences in growth found between different ethnic groups are due to genetic factors." The authors concluded that growth standards derived from well-to-do children in developed countries should serve as an optimum standard of reference for all children.

In 1981, Graitcer and Gentry analyzed heights and weights of 2,366 children aged 6 months to 5 years from privileged areas of Haiti, Egypt, and Togo (private day care centers, pediatricians offices, and families of government and military officials), populations representing principally peoples of African and Indo-Mediterranean origin (12). These were compared with the reference standards from the National Center for Health Statistics (NCHS) (healthy, noninstitutionalized American children) (13), the growth standard now widely used and recommended as a reference curve to judge the adequacy of growth in childhood (11). The authors found that the fifth, 50th, and 95th centiles were very close to those of the reference population and concluded, as had Habicht (9), that "when adverse environmental influences such as increased exposure to infection and decreased food intake are optimized, ethnic and geographical differences have little if any influence on growth." They likewise recommended the use of one reference for all countries to evaluate the impact of hostile environmental factors on the growth of preschool children. Professor John Waterlow, in a letter to the *Lancet* in 1980, wrote: "I am inclined to think that growth potential in the early years of life is not much affected by ethnic differences. If that is so, it seems justifiable to apply North American or European standards internationally" (14). A leading article in the *Lancet* in 1984 authoritatively seemed to put the lid on the argument with the statement that "the controversy of whether or not growth standards for children developed in Europe and North America are universally applicable appears now to be settled in favor of those who maintain that they are" (11). It reinforced the notion that the "growth of privileged groups of children in developing countries does not differ importantly from these standards." But this brings us to the kernel of the problem. What is important? How great must differences between ethnic groups be before they can be viewed as important? My contention is that any difference is important, however small, if it has an effect on professional opinion to influence and change dietary practices and other aspects of health care.

What is noteworthy, however, is that in the studies referred to, which have had considerable influence on recent thinking concerning genetic influences on early growth, little reference has been made to children whose origins are in the Far East—Chinese, Japanese, and Indo-Malays—who make up more than a quarter of mankind. These ethnic groups are currently classified as Asiatic (10), and it is this term that is used in this chapter. As adults brought up in fortunate socioeconomic circumstances, they are smaller than Europeans and Africans (10). But to what extent is this the consequence of variations in growth after birth during early childhood rather than later on? Before the case for a similar early genetic growth potential can be accepted for all races, with the crucial implications of such a statement for the definition of stunting, the early growth of these children must be analyzed in further detail and compared with that of other populations.

To this end I have analyzed eight sets of growth data published over the past 20 years from Japan (15,16), Hong Kong (17,18), Singapore (19), Korea (20), Thailand (P. Khanjanasthiti et al., *unpublished data*), and Taiwan (21). Children making up these studies were brought up in what were generally considered by the various authors to be favorable socioeconomic conditions. A growth curve has been constructed from mean heights at various ages over the first 5 years (1, 3, 6, 9, and 12 months, and 2, 3, 4, and 5 years) and compared with mean curves of linear growth from three sources chosen to provide a spectrum of growth profiles from other ethnic groups growing up in socioeconomically adequate environments: (a) NCHS curves (representing essentially a European pattern) (13); (b) Nigerian children from Ibadan (22); and (c) Northern Indian children from Delhi (representative of Indo-Mediterranean peoples) (23). The major source of comparison is with the NCHS data in view of the ubiquitous adoption of these curves as a reference (see elsewhere in this volume). I realize that there are several sources for error and inconsistencies in my approach to ethnic comparisons—differences in sizes of populations studied, different methods of measurement, diversities in environmental conditions, and variable time of assessment, to give but a few. Admitting to these, I do believe that the resulting mean growth curve is near to the truth for these Asiatic children.

Over the first year the average percentage differences in height measured at five different points (1, 3, 6, 9, and 12 months) between the biggest and smallest Asiatic populations is about 3%; from 1 to 5 years, about 4%. These differences are of similar magnitude to the differences between Habicht's privileged groups in European children of European origin (9). Figures 1 and 2 show the mean growth curves against a background of the range of heights of the Asiatic populations studied. Over the first few months or so, growth in length follows a pattern very similar in all study groups. Thereafter, there begins a very definite period of growth deceleration reflected as a downward shift, which continues for a few years. Figure 3 makes a more simplified comparison of the mean Asiatic curve with the NCHS data, showing a marked downward shift over the first few years after birth. Figure 4 gives a more detailed comparison of the Asiatic growth curve as a percentage of the NCHS median. The downward shift reaches to about 95%.

A more quantifiable and universally better applied measure of this downward shift can be obtained by analyzing changes in the standard deviation score (z score) of the NCHS reference (Fig. 5). Within the various populations studied, there was considerable variability in growth pattern, but all followed a similar downward trend. In both boys and girls there is, over the first 3 years, a shift of approximately 2 SD. Over the next 2 years, there is some upward shift, but not much.

The data in the studies referred to are widely used in their various countries as reference growth standards. It is not recorded that the children were anything other than healthy, although it is possible that within the group as a whole, some children's growth might have faltered for pathological reasons. It is difficult, therefore, in my opinion, to avoid concluding that the early growth pattern of Asiatic

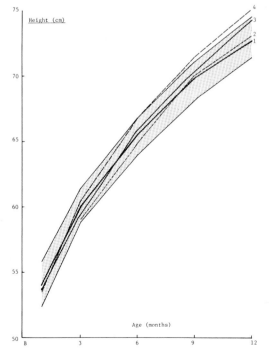

FIG. 1. Mean curves of growth in length from birth to 12 months in boys and girls of various racial groups. 1: Asiatic [Japan (15,16), Hong Kong (17,18), Singapore (19), Korea (20), Thailand (P. Khanjanasthiti et al., (*unpublished data*), and Taiwan (21)]. 2: Northern India (23). 3: NCHS (13). 4: Nigeria (22). The *hatched area* represents the range of means for Asiatic children (15–21; P. Khanjanasthiti et al., *unpublished data*).

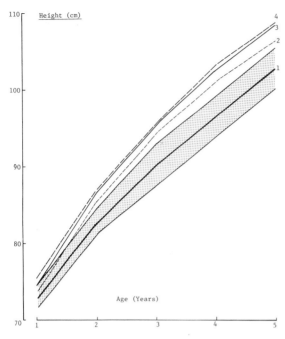

FIG. 2. Mean curves of growth in length from 1 to 5 years in boys and girls of various racial groups. Numbers 1–4, *hatched area,* and sources of data as in Fig. 1.

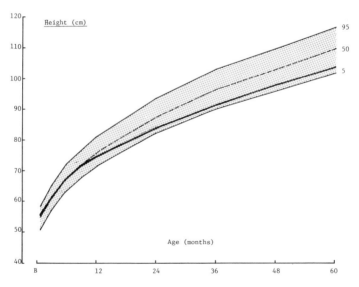

FIG. 3. Mean curve of growth in Asiatic children (*heavy curve*; refs. as in Fig. 1) compared with the NCHS centiles (11).

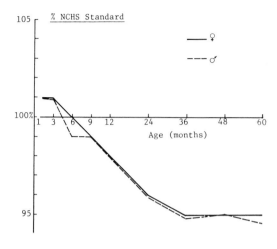

FIG. 4. Mean linear growth in Asiatic boys and girls (see Figs. 1 and 2) as percentage of the median of the NCHS standard.

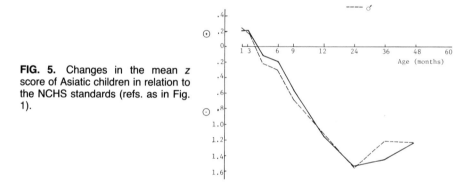

FIG. 5. Changes in the mean *z* score of Asiatic children in relation to the NCHS standards (refs. as in Fig. 1).

children is different from that of the NCHS reference. If the early period of growth faltering was caused by difficulties at weaning, catch-up would have been expected after this time with provision of a good, well-balanced diet. This does not take place.

A final comparison I wish to make is between the 3-monthly increments of the combined Asiatic data and those presented by Professor Waterlow (J. C. Waterlow, *this volume*) from several studies of poorly fed babies from developing countries (Fig. 6). There are some real similarities that might tempt one to speculate on nutritional reasons for the faltering of growth shown by the Asiatic children. I believe, however, that a sizable part of the faltering is of physiological origin. I propose that this downward shift after birth in Asiatic babies makes a sizable contribution to the eventual smaller adult size of Asiatic peoples.

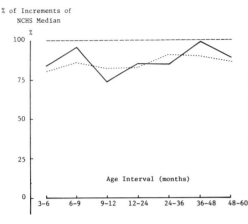

FIG. 6. Percentage of 3-monthly increments of the NCHS median (11). Comparisons between the combined Asiatic data (*solid curve;* refs. as in Fig. 1) and that from 10 studies from developing countries (*dashed curve;* J.C. Waterlow, *this volume*).

These views receive some indirect support from other published studies. In 1965 Ashcroft (24) in Jamaica studied the size of 5,000 children aged 11 to 17 years from similar upper and middle socioeconomic classes attending eight fee-paying secondary schools in Kingston. The statures of African, Afro-European, and European children were similar, indicating a similar potential for growth in height. That of the Chinese children was, however, consistently smaller. At 11 years the boys were 3 cm shorter. An earlier puberty growth spurt saw this narrow to about 2 cm at 13 years. The gap then widened until at 17 years the differences between the Chinese children and those of African and European origin amounted to about 7 cm. Ashcroft was firmly of the opinion that this difference was genetic in origin. Barr and his colleagues from San Francisco in 1972 (25) also showed in 7,500 children aged 5 to 14 years that, in general, children of "yellow skin" were markedly shorter and lighter than white and black children. Tanner, in his 1976 review of population differences in body size, shape, and growth rate, also concluded that genotypic differences did exist between Asiatic peoples and those of European and African origin (26).

CONCLUSIONS AND IMPLICATIONS

I wish now to summarize briefly my thesis of the relevance of genetic factors to linear growth in early childhood.

1. Differences in genetic makeup undoubtedly account for variations in size between individuals within any ethnic group who are brought up in comparable environmental conditions. This genotype has a particularly strong effect in the first few years after birth, when the child moves away from heavy maternal influences on prenatal growth. This will often result in considerable shifts in both upward as well as downward directions, which must be always borne in

mind in evaluating the profile of early growth in an individual child. These shifts are greater in children born at the extremes of size.

2. Variations in size between different racial groups, even allowing for hostile environmental factors, also frequently have a genetic basis. Pronouncements on the uniformity of genetic growth potential in infants and young children of the major racial groups are premature and do not apply when children of Asiatic origin are compared with those of European, African, and Indo-Mediterranean origin. The early growth characteristics of Asiatic children differ in their basic profile, showing a deceleration of growth rate over the first couple of years of postnatal life. Superimposed on standard growth curves, these show a downward shift and a continuation thereafter in lower-centile channels.

3. These characteristics of the Asiatic growth curve are likely to be more of genetic than environmental origin and make a major contribution to overall smaller adult stature. These children seem not to have a genetic potential "to approach the European/American norm" (14).

4. The magnitude of these differences of genetic origin do not under normal circumstances approach those that can be caused through malnutrition and other sources of environmental deprivation, where 10 to 20% differences from the NCHS median are being shown with shifts of up to -3 SD over the first few years. They should not, however, be disregarded.

5. They can, in the case of Asiatic children, be sufficient to query the validity of using the NCHS reference standard for these children to determine the prevalence of stunting. At the same time, failure to recognize a sizable physiological contribution to the period of early lag-down growth can lead to mistaken attitudes by professional people to such an extent that wrong feeding practices may be implemented in an attempt to reverse the trend. This is the case in Hong Kong, where the interpretation of faltering as being caused by nutritional deficiencies has questioned more traditional methods of feeding in early childhood.

6. If deviations from a widely accepted standard are such as to cause concern, then surely they are clinically important however small in comparison they might be. To recognize genetic differences is in no way to undermine the importance of environmental causes of growth faltering. It is to create a firmer scientific basis to allow us a more reliable epidemiologic survey of the problem of stunting. This will become increasingly important as faltering growth becomes acknowledged as an important objective measure of social and environmental disadvantage.

7. Further study is called for, including careful examination of growth patterns in Chinese and other children of Asiatic origin. Leaving aside the argument of an internationally accepted growth standard as an epidemiological tool for quantifying malnutrition in different countries, the use of such a standard in the routine day-to-day clinical use in individual children might lead to an inaccurate assessment of a clinical problem. Growth failure might be overdiagnosed, and its mirror image, obesity, underdiagnosed.

ACKNOWLEDGMENT

I thank Miss Angela Yan for her very patient perseverance in typing this manuscript.

REFERENCES

1. Galton F. *Natural inheritance*. London, New York: Macmillan, 1889.
2. Tanner JM. Physical growth and development. In: Forfar JO, Arneil GC, eds. *Textbook of paediatrics;* vol 1. 3rd ed. London: Churchill Livingstone, 1984: 278–329.
3. Lyon AJ, Preece MA, Grant DB. Growth curve for girls with Turner syndrome. *Arch Dis Child* 1985;60:932–5.
4. Cronk CE. Growth of children with Down's syndrome: birth to age 3 years. *Pediatrics* 1978;61:564–8.
5. Polani PE. Chromosomal and other genetic influences on birth weight variation. In: *Size at birth.* Ciba Foundation Symposium 27 (New Series). Amsterdam: Elsevier/Excerpta Medica, 1974:127–59.
6. Walton A, Hammond J. The maternal effects on growth and conformation in Shire horse–Shetland pony crosses. *Proc R Soc Biol* 1938;125:311–24.
7. Tanner JM. Regulation of growth in size of mammals. *Nature* 1963;199:845–7.
8. Smith DW, Truog W, Rogers JE, et al. Shifting linear growth during infancy and the genetics of growth in fetal life through infancy. *J Pediatr* 1976;89:225–34.
9. Habicht JP, Martorell R, Yarbrough C, et al. Height and weight standards for pre-school children. How relevant are ethnic differences in growth potential? *Lancet* 1974;1:611–5.
10. Eveleth PB, Tanner JM. *Worldwide variation in human growth*. Cambridge: Cambridge University Press, 1976.
11. Anonymous. A measure of agreement on growth standards [Editorial]. *Lancet* 1984;1:142–3.
12. Graitcer PH, Gentry EM. Measuring children: one reference for all. *Lancet* 1981;2:297–9.
13. Hamill PVV. *Growth curves for children, birth to 18 years, United States*. Hyattsville, MD: National Center for Health Statistics, 1977; Dhew Publication no. (PHS) 78-1650.
14. Waterlow JC. Child growth standards [letter]. *Lancet* 1980;1:717.
15. Department of Maternal and Child Health. *Physical status of Japanese children in 1970*. Tokyo: Institute of Public Health, Department of Maternal and Child Health, 1970.
16. Terada H, Hoshi H. Longitudinal study on the physical growth in Japanese. 4. Growth in lengths of extremities during the first three years of life. *Acta Anat Nippon* 1965;41:313–26.
17. Chang KSF, Lee MM, Low WD, Chai S, Chow M. Standards of height and weight of Southern Chinese children. *Far East Med J* 1965;1:101–9.
18. Medical and Health Department, Hong Kong, Family Health Service and Statistical Unit. *Survey on weight, height and head circumference of pre-school children in April 1978*. Hong Kong: Society of Community Medicine of Hong Kong Bulletin, 1980:45–57.
19. Wong HB, Tye CY, Quek KM. Anthropometric studies on Singapore children: 1. Heights, weights and skull circumference of preschool children. *J Singapore Paediatr Soc* 1972;14:68–89.
20. Korea Ministry of Health. Growth data of Korean children. *J. Korean Pediatr Assoc* 1967;10(suppl 4).
21. Shih SC, Wu TH, Chen KP. Growth charts of height, weight and chest and head circumference for children under 6 years of age in Taiwan. *J Form Med Assoc* 1966;65:313–25.
22. Janes MD. The effect of social class on the physical growth of Nigerian Yoruba children. *Bull Int Epidemiol Assoc* 1970;20:127–36.
23. Banik ND, Nayar S, Krishna R, Raj L. The effect of nutrition on growth of preschool children in different communities in Delhi. *Indian Paediatr* 1972;9:440–6.
24. Ashcroft MT, Heneage P, Lovell HG. Heights and weights of Jamaican school children of various ethnic groups. *Am J Physiol Anthropol* 1964;24:35–44.
25. Barr GD, Allen CM, Shinefield HR. Height and weight of 7,500 children of 3 skin colours. Pediatric Multiphasic Program: Report no. 3. *Am J Dis Child* 1972;124:866–72.
26. Tanner JM. Population differences in body size, shape and growth rate: a 1976 review. *Arch Dis Child* 1976;51:1–2.

DISCUSSION

Dr. Waterlow: I am totally convinced by your presentation, but at one point you used the words "optimal standards" for the NCHS standards. I think that is a misinterpretation. Let us call the NCHS standards a reference without questioning whether they are optimal or not. For various practical reasons, we need a reference. The question we are really asking is not related to children growing below the reference, except as a method of description, but to the differences in growth between different groups of children and the biological and practical meaning of those differences. Would you agree that we can get right away from the idea of an optimal standard?

Dr. Davies: Yes, I agree. The NCHS standard is a point of reference but not an optimal standard.

Dr. Martorell: The data suggest a lower growth potential for Asiatics. However, I was a little bit disturbed by the magnitude of the difference that your data suggest. You have data from as early as the 1960s. I think it is clear that in Japan as well as in China, there have been significant increases in stature over time. So I would be cautious in terms of the magnitude of the differences. At this stage, I would be willing to contemplate a recommendation that for Asiatic populations maybe the 25th centile ought to be the denominator rather than the 50th centile, but some of your samples showed medians closer to the fifth centile, and I think that is too low.

Dr. Davies: That was an "average" growth curve, as you say, with data collected between 1965 and 1978. The more recent data that I have from Hong Kong are based on 1978 information, which was collected in maternal and child health clinics. The overall downward shift in this sample over the first 2 years would put the median nearer to the 25th NCHS centile than the fifth centile. But it is the nature of the curve that I think is of interest, because in many ways it simulates quite closely the growth curve of children who are bigger at birth and who then drop down, as Smith et al. have shown (1).

Dr. Nabarro: Are you able to give us some rough idea of what your curves indicate in terms of velocity of linear growth? From looking at them quickly, there seems to be a consistent reduction in actual velocity compared with the expected velocity that one can derive from the NCHS figures. Is that correct?

Dr. Davies: I can't give you any absolute figures, but over the first couple of years, especially from 6 to 24 months, the velocity seems to be consistently lower, after which time there appears to be normal velocity.

Dr. Nabarro: Do you know roughly what the percentage of expected linear growth was?

Dr. Davies: No. What I have done is to compare the attained height at various ages; I haven't looked at velocities, only 3-month increments.

Dr. Nabarro: It may be necessary for us to think more about velocities. Several of us who have been working with economically disadvantaged Asian communities have observed variation in the velocity of linear growth, particularly in the first 2 years of life, dropping down sometimes to 50 to 60% of what is expected and then picking up again at the end of the second year. Dr. Davies' suggestion would imply that there is a reduction in the maximum potential for growth in some Asian populations, but at least the linear velocity remains relatively constant throughout the period. By contrast, those of us who find more variable velocities (compared with the NCHS reference) may well feel confident that we are dealing with something that is more environmental than genetic.

Dr. Martorell: That is a very good point; Japanese data, for example, show a constant distance from the NCHS 50th percentile.

Dr. Guesry: Could the slowdown of linear growth at the age of 3 to 4 years, which you observe in your cross-sectional data, not be caused by changes in the nutritional status of the population during the last 10 years? Wong Hock Boon in Singapore, for instance, mentioned that during the last 15 years there has been an increase in stature of about 5 cm in boys around 15 years of age (2).

Dr. Davies: Yes, I agree with that possibility. However, a study from Jamaica (3), made 20 years ago, looked at the heights of schoolchildren of Chinese, African, and European descent and was able to detect even then a difference of about 7 cm between Europeans on the one hand and Chinese on the other. I believe that the major differences in size between ethnic groups emerge in early childhood and not later on in life.

Dr. Aponso: Have you looked into genetic differences among races and ethnic groups not merely related to total length or height but to upper and lower segment? For example, are certain people taller or shorter because they have longer or shorter legs? Has this been looked into in different races?

Dr. Davies: All this is very well documented in Eveleth and Tanner's book (4). The smaller lower body segment of children of Asiatic origin is first observed at 18 months to 2 years; it is not evident in the first couple of years. I don't think that this differential growth of upper and lower body segments contributes to the initial decrease in linear growth.

Dr. Martorell: Professor Tanner and colleagues published a study on the secular trend in stature in Japan (5). The Japanese are now taller, and it is interesting that the increases in stature largely reflect increases in the length of the extremities, so that today the young people from Japan have body proportions similar to the British population. It has all been in leg growth.

Dr. Gopalan: In many of the Asian countries, there are such tremendous socioeconomic disparities that when we speak of populations considered to be living in specific socioeconomic conditions, it can be erroneous. The stratification in different classes—high and middle income, slum groups, and the truly affluent group—is extremely complex. In China, the differences between the North and the South are so wide that people are talking about using different standards. On the basis of certain population groups, to make a generalization about Asian children may perhaps be a bit premature. One has to see what sort of socioeconomic conditions we are talking about. Have the affluent groups really been in a position to express their full genetic potential?

Dr. Mukherjee: Growth is interrelated with social, environmental, and nutritional factors, especially in low socioeconomic groups (6). How could we differentiate the effects on growth of social and environmental factors and of genetic factors in low socioeconomic groups? How could we distinguish, among children from lower socioeconomic groups, those whose growth is poor because of social and environmental factors or because of genetic factors?

Dr. Davies: Your question is really very complex, and I am unable to answer it. What I'm trying to draw attention to in my chapter is that there is not a universal equal growth potential among all children, taking Asiatic children simply as an example.

Dr. Waterlow: In relation to Dr. Mukherjee's point, it has been suggested that more intelligent people tend to marry better. You could construct a model by which genetic factors have promoted a good environment. I don't know whether this would hold in India.

Somebody said that populations in Asiatic countries are bursting at the seams, and this I think is indeed true in such countries as Indonesia, Nepal, and India, whereas in Africa space and land seem not usually to be the limiting factors. Many African groups are nomads, living in the savannah. There was a question about body build: African legs are longer in adults than those of Europeans. So my question is: Would you regard the genetic smallness that you have described as a useful adaptation for survival in a highly over-crowded population with enormous pressure on food supply?

Dr. Davies: I wonder if it is an adaptation to shortage of food or perhaps to living in a warm climate? If you compare the growth patterns I described with patterns of growth in the Alaskan Eskimos, who are also of Asiatic stock, then there is a difference. There is not the same faltering. The American anthropologist Coon traced the origins of Asiatic peoples to the cold climates of northeast Asia; many of the physical characteristics of the Asiatic peoples are adapted to heat conservation. If these now migrate to climates where heat conservation is a disadvantage, biological changes might evolve. I wonder whether the pattern of physical growth that I've described is more an adaptation to an environmental climate change than an adaptation to overcrowding?

Dr. Martorell: I have always been amazed the other way around. Why, when there is an obvious advantage to being small, in requiring less food and so on, don't we see very clear genetic differences in growth potential? It seems that the human species does not em-phasize genetic mechanisms of adaptation but relies instead on phenotypic expression.

Dr. Tomkins: Have you any information on the way in which populations or subgroups within populations who are taller and shorter also vary over secular periods with respect to weight for height? Is there anything to back up Prof. Waterlow's point about the pastoralists who are very tall and thin and who are exposed to quite extreme changes in the temperature of the desert areas. How has body mass index or weight for height changed over a period of time in such populations? It would be rather interesting to see that in relationship to changes in height for age.

Dr. Davies: I don't have any data.

Dr. Keller: An analogous case is the Bushmen in the Kalahari Desert. The Bushmen are very thin and certainly do not have a build that would conserve heat even through the tem-perature differences between night and day are extreme in the Kalahari.

Dr. Nabarro: Dr. Martorell has expressed surprise that there appear to be no genetic differences in the ways in which populations respond to adverse environmental circum-stances. He has also suggested that there are circumstances in which it might be to people's advantage to grow less in length or height in order that they might eat less food. Professor Davies, your results indicate that the growth of some of the children with whom you have been working deviates from the NCHS reference figures. Do you believe it possible that different groups of children, subjected to similar adverse environmental circumstances, may show different characteristics? Might children in one group respond by reducing their rate of linear growth and maintain their ratio of lean tissue mass to height, whereas children in the other group maintain the expected linear growth rate but reduce their lean tissue mass-to-height ratio?

Dr. Davies: I don't know how many generations would be needed before these changes take place. It is certainly likely that if you have a group of people who are biologically distinctive in their growth characteristics, they may well respond differently, but I don't know in which direction.

Dr. Martorell: What about the old idea that children with a faster growth potential have therefore greater needs and are thus more at risk for severe malnutrition under conditions of relative lack of food?

Dr. Waterlow: That is what I suggested to Prof. Davies. It might be a positive advantage when food supplies are limited. On the other hand, should we not agree that everybody has the "right" to fulfill his genetic potential, which presumably includes growth in the same way as, under the United Nations Declaration of Human Rights, he has a "right" to health? I think there is evidence, certainly crude evidence, that for adults, it is smart to be small. It was shown in the prisoner of war camps during the last war that the small soldiers survived much better than those who were big. I've always tried to promote the slogan, "it is smart to be small," but that's for adults; you need less clothing, food, and space.

Dr. Keller: I have recently analyzed data that were collected from laborers during the second World War in Germany: body mass indices decreased progressively in parallel with the deterioration of the rationing, and this affected the tall people much more than the short people.

Dr. Davies: If the growth curve that we observe in Asiatics is truly a biological characteristic, how right are we in applying the NCHS standards? Dr. Keller, I wonder if part of the darker areas on the world map of stunting that you showed (Fig. 1 of W. Keller, *this volume*) can perhaps be accounted for by what I have just described?

Dr. Keller: The trouble is that what you call Asiatics make up a very small part of that, because I showed only data on that part of the world from the Philippines and Indonesia, which wouldn't really fit, and Singapore, which didn't show up because it is so small. Thus, only Thailand, Burma, and part of Nepal are left.

REFERENCES

1. Smith DW, Truog W, Rogers JE, et al. Shifting growth during infancy and the genetics of growth in fetal life through infancy. *J Pediatr* 1976;89:225–34.
2. Wong HB, Tye CY, Quek KM. Athropometric studies on Singapore children. *J Singapore Paediatr Soc* 1972;14:68–89.
3. Ashcroft MT, Lovell HA. Heights and weights of Jamaican children of various racial origins. *Trop Geogr Med* 1964;4:345–53.
4. Eveleth PB, Tanner JM. *Worldwide variation in human growth.* New York: Cambridge University Press, 1976.
5. Tanner JM, Hayashi T, Preece MA, Cameron N. Increase in leg length relative to trunk in Japanese children and adults from 1957 to 1977: comparison with British and with Japanese Americans. *Ann Hum Biol* 1982;9:411–23.
6. Mukherjee DK, Sethna NJ. The ecology of growth in underprivileged children. *Indian Pediatr* 1972;9:440–6.

Linear Growth Retardation in Less Developed Countries, edited by John C. Waterlow. Nestlé Nutrition Workshop Series, Vol. 14. Nestec Ltd., Vevey/Raven Press, Ltd., New York © 1988.

Determinants of Growth *in Utero*

R. D. G. Milner

Department of Paediatrics, University of Sheffield, the Children's Hospital, and the Jessop Hospital for Women, Sheffield S10 2TH, England

In a logical approach to the subject of determinants of growth *in utero,* genetic influences should be considered separately, since they are fixed at the time of conception and immutable. Then the fetus, the placenta, and the mother should be taken in that order, because it is helpful to review first how the fetus exerts control over its own development, assuming a normal and stable intrauterine environment. The placenta is central to the theme not only because it is the eye of the needle through which nutrient must pass from mother to fetus but also because placental hormone production influences fetal growth directly and also indirectly by altering maternal metabolic patterns. Maternal influences on fetal growth are in one sense peripheral but in another the most important, since they may be amenable to direct intervention by clinicians wishing to optimize intrauterine growth to minimize perinatal mortality and morbidity.

GENETICS

Normal fetal growth and development are the result of a precisely organized sequence of gene activation and suppression under the control of a biological clock. This is poorly understood (1). Chromosomal abnormalities that give rise to recognizable syndromes such as Turner's syndrome (45,XO) or Down's syndrome (trisomy 21) characteristically produce small babies. This is thought to be the result of a reduced rate of cell division (2), and in the case of Turner's syndrome intrauterine blighting has lifelong consequences since birth weight is the most powerful single predictor of adult height (3).

Multiple gene loci contribute to the birth weight of the normal fetus. Models have been developed that partition the contribution of genetic and environmental factors in determining birth weight (Table 1) (4). Variation in birth weight can be roughly partitioned: one-third to genetic factors, one-third to recognizable environmental factors, and one-third unknown. Of the 38% that is genetic, the maternal genotype (20%) is more important than the fetal genotype (15%), and the paternal contribution is solely via the fetal genotype.

TABLE 1. *Partitioning of birth weight variation*[a]

Genetic		
Maternal genotype	20%	
Fetal genotype	16%	
Fetal sex	2%	
		38%
Environmental		
General maternal environment	18%	
Immediate maternal environment	6%	
Maternal age and parity	8%	
Unknown	30%	
		62%

[a]Derived from Polani (4).

THE FETUS

The human fetus undergoes the equivalent of some 42 succesive mitotic divisions in pregnancy in progressing from a fertilized ovum to a term infant, with only five more divisions being necessary to achieve adult size (5). Maximal growth velocity in length occurs at approximately 20 weeks of gestation, and in weight at 34 weeks. This reflects developmental changes in growth by cell number and size: in the first trimester growth is by increase in cell number, in the second there is a stable rate of cellular division accompanied by an increase in cell size, and in the third trimester growth in cell number slows, and that in cell size accelerates (6).

Adipocyte lipid becomes an important contributor to body weight in the last trimester. It is worth remembering that the first 1.5 kg of the 3.0 kg that a term infant weighs takes two-thirds of pregnancy to develop. In the first 1.5 kg there is about 50 g fat, whereas the second 1.5 kg acquired in the last 12 weeks of gestation includes 500 g fat (7). Lipid accumulation by the fetus in the third trimester, which is largely controlled by glucose-sensitive insulin secretion, is the most important single contributor to a term infant being overweight or underweight (8).

If fetal growth is compromised in the first trimester, the end result is usually abortion; in the second trimester, growth retardation results in shortness and underweight that are largely irreversible, whereas growth failure originating in the third trimester produces a long skinny baby who can catch up postnatally if nutrition is optimal.

Adequate cellular delivery of nutrient is an overriding condition for normal intrauterine growth. Nutrient oversupply is not known to influence growth before 28 weeks but may modulate weight gain in the third trimester by stimulating pancreatic B cell ontogeny and insulin secretion (9). Our understanding of the contribution of insulin, other hormones, and peptide growth factors to the control of fetal growth has advanced dramatically in recent years with an important shift from a traditional concept of endocrine growth control to one in which endocrine hormones interact with peptide growth factors that function in a paracrine or autocrine manner.

The placenta is impermeable to peptide hormones, and the peptides involved in fetal growth control originate in the fetus or the fetal side of the placenta. The balance of evidence indicates that growth hormone (GH) plays little part in human fetal growth (10). Thyroid hormones are important in both neuronal development and osseous maturation but are not essential for tissue development overall (11). Candidates for a central part in the overall control of intrauterine cellular growth are insulin, placental lactogen, and the logically acting tissue growth factors. All growth factors induce a positive pleiotypic response in the target tissue, which includes glucose and amino acid uptake and DNA, RNA, and protein synthesis, and all are mitogens. Some, such as the somatomedins (insulin-like growth factors), epidermal growth factor, and nerve growth factor, induce differentiation of the target tissue, whereas others such as the transforming growth factors and fibroblast growth factor do not. A combination of growth factors is required to stimulate a cell to replicate (Fig. 1) (12).

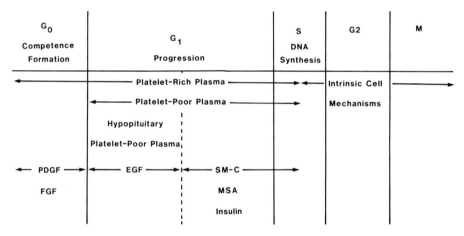

FIG. 1. Sequence of events and their endocrine control leading to cell replication in BALB/c–3T3 fibroblasts. Cells growth-arrested in G_0 are made to enter G_1, where they progress to DNA synthesis in S phase. This is followed by preparation for G_2 and the process of mitosis (M). The sequential addition of competence and progression factors are required for the full cycle of events, and both are contained in platelet-rich human plasma. Platelet-poor plasma has only progression activity but will result in DNA synthesis if added following transient exposure of the cells to the competence factors platelet-derived growth factor (PDGF) or fibroblast growth factor (FGF). Platelet-poor plasma from GH-deficient subjects, which lacks somatomedins, allows progression over the initial part of G_1 only, but full G_1 progression is restored if such plasma is followed by exposure to somatomedin C (SM-C), multiplication-stimulating activity (MSA), or supraphysiological concentrations of insulin. The need for SM-deficient platelet-poor plasma in early G_1 is obviated by exposure of the cells to epidermal growth factor (EGF). These cells can therefore be induced to traverse the cycle of proliferation in serum-free medium by sequential exposure to PDGF or FGF, EGF, and a SM or insulin. (Adapted from Van Wyk et al., ref. 12).

In man more is known about the somatomedins than about other growth factors. There are two predominant classes of somatomedin: insulin-like growth factor I (IGF I), otherwise known as somatomedin C (SM-C), and IGF II. The analogous peptide to IGF II in the rat is called multiplication-stimulating activity (MSA). The IGFs are so called because they have structural and functional similarities with insulin and proinsulin. This has led to the concept that they are all members of a family of insulin-like molecules, more distant relatives in which are relaxin and nerve growth factor (13). This relationship helps explain the limited biological cross reactivity, insulin being a weak growth factor for fibroblasts and the IGFs enhancing glucose oxidation in isolated adipocytes (14). Insulin may therefore have a dual role in fetal growth, on the one hand behaving like the somatomedins and stimulating mitosis and on the other acting as a classical hormone controlling carbohydrate and lipid metabolism in the third trimester with important implications for term body weight.

The concentration of IGF I in human cord blood is one-half or less of that present in the normal adult (15) despite the rapid rate of fetal growth, but cord IGF I levels do correlate with both fetal age and body weight, whereas those of IGF II do not. The IGF II levels in cord blood are the same as or slightly lower than those in the adult. But it is naive to seek a biological link between cord IGF levels in fetal growth for a number of reasons. The total IGF concentration in the blood does not reflect the IGF free to react with receptor, since most IGF is bound to a carrier protein. In the adult and in neonates of 30 weeks or more gestation, this has a molecular weight of approximately 150,000, whereas in infants under 27 weeks of gestation it is approximately 40 kilodaltons in size (16). The ontogeny of binding protein form and affinity may control the amount of IGF available to the tissues.

The action of IGF and other growth factors depends as much on the ontogeny of receptors as on the messenger peptide. The apparent paradox of rapid fetal growth in the face of low circulating levels of IGF could be resolved if fetal tissues were more sensitive than postnatal tissues to the action of IGF. Most human fetal tissues possess receptors for both IGF I and IGF II, though the liver is said to have IGF II receptors only (17). Circulating monocytes from cord blood have a greater IGF I binding capacity than those in the adult circulation (18).

A major difference between pre- and postnatal life is that in the adult IGFs are synthesized mainly in the liver and are transported via the circulation to act in an endocrine fashion on cartilage growth plates, whereas in the fetus most if not all tissues synthesize IGFs, which are released to act locally in a paracrine or autocrine fashion (19). Some IGF I has been recovered from all tissues tested from human fetuses 9 to 19 weeks of gestation (Table 2) (20). Lung and intestine had the highest concentration, and liver the lowest. Complementary evidence of human fetal tissue IGF has been obtained by immunohistochemistry (21). The circulation therefore probably represents a sump receiving IGF overflow from all the tissues, and there seems to be little of biological import to be gained from analyzing blood IGF concentrations.

TABLE 2. *Mean (± SEM) insulin-like growth factor 1 in human fetal tissues*[a]

Lung	166 ± 35
Intestine	160 ± 20
Kidney	132 ± 18
Skin	127 ± 10
Pancreas	101 ± 12
Muscle	99 ± 7
Thymus	98 ± 25
Brain	82 ± 11
Heart	79 ± 10
Adrenal	76 ± 10
Liver	67 ± 16

[a]All results are expressed in milliunits per gram. Between five and 26 determinations were made on tissues from fetuses of 9 to 19 weeks of gestational age. Mean plasma concentration: 270 ± 20 mU/ml. From D'Ercole et al. (20).

The control of fetal growth factor synthesis and release is clearly fundamental to an understanding of fetal growth control overall. What follows is of necessity speculative, since the evidence from which generalizations are made is based on *in vitro* experiments on cellular growth and replication. A circular but plausible argument has been advanced that links delivery of nutrient to the fetal cell, fetal insulin secretion, and the synthesis of IGFs (8). If either of the first two variables is increased or decreased, a predictable change occurs in the others. The trio of nutrient, insulin, and IGF should now be enlarged to a quartet by the addition of human placental lactogen (HPL), a peptide secreted by placental trophoblasts that has amino acid sequence homology with both GH and prolactin. Ovine HPL is released into both fetal and maternal circulations. From 80 to 100 days, the level is higher in the fetus, but by term at 145 days, the maternal level has risen and the fetal level fallen to give a maternofetal ratio approximately 10 (22). A conventional view is that HPL influences fetal growth indirectly by acting as an insulin antagonist in the mother, stimulating the mobilization of metabolites, and increasing nutrient delivery to the fetus (23). There is indirect evidence that HPL also stimulates maternal IGF synthesis and release. Normal women have elevated IGF I levels in late pregnancy, and these fall following parturition (24). A GH-deficient woman was shown to have normal circulating levels of IGF I and II at 35 weeks of gestation, which fell rapidly postpartum in parallel with the disappearance of circulating HPL (25). Recent work suggests that HPL may also have a direct action on IGF synthesis and release in the fetal compartment.

Adams et al. (26) were the first to show that fetal rat fibroblasts release MSA in response to ovine PL but not to GH. Postnatally, rat fibroblasts were responsive to both hormones. We have shown that HPL is capable of stimulating amino acid uptake and thymidine incorporation by human fetal fibroblasts and myoblasts (27) and that this can be inhibited but not abolished by IGF I antibody. We have also shown that HPL, but not GH, stimulates human fetal fibroblasts and myoblasts to release IGF I into the culture medium in a dose-dependent manner (28). In contrast, both HPL and GH simulate DNA synthesis and IGF I release by isolated human fetal hepatocytes (29). A possible direct link between HPL and insulin has been suggested by the observation that insulin stimulates HPL release from isolated cultured trophoblasts in a dose-dependent manner (30).

These findings can be woven into a working hypothesis that fetal cellular growth is dependent first on delivery of nutrient (e.g., glucose, amino acids, and fatty acids). The uptake of nutrient by the fetal cell is stimulated by insulin. Fetal insulin secretion is stimulated by amino acids up to 28 weeks of gestation and by amino acids and glucose thereafter (9). Cellular anabolism progresses to replication under the influence of growth factors. Growth factor synthesis and release are stimulated not only by intracellular events such as the delivery of fuel, which is augmented by insulin, but also by HPL, which may be acting on many fetal tissues in a manner analogous to GH acting on the hepatocyte postnally. Finally, there is a long loop in which insulin reinforces the anabolic process by stimulating HPL secretion.

THE PLACENTA

The influence of the placenta on fetal growth is twofold. First, there is a mechanistic role involving the transfer of nutrients and oxygen to the fetus and the removal of waste products. In this must be considered not only placental macro- and microanatomy but fetal and maternal blood flows, which are themselves controlled elsewhere. Then there are the metabolic and endocrine aspects of placental function, which include most importantly HPL production and steroid hormone metabolism.

The placenta grows faster than the fetus and reaches maximum weight at about 33 weeks of gestation, though surface area and vascularity continue to develop thereafter (31). Although there is a positive relationship between placental and fetal weights, this is unlikely to be linear as term approaches. In theory, if a fetoplacental weight ratio is assumed at which fetal growth is optimal, an increase of placental weight does not augment growth, which in these circumstances is under endogenous fetal control, but a reduction in placental weight can become rate limiting. In undergrowth there is interaction between fetus and placenta, as the majority of placental weight is fetal in origin, and there is some evidence that fetal abnormality can inhibit placental growth. In anencephaly placental weight is reduced (32).

Morphological abnormalities such as a bilobate or reniform placenta or a placenta with an accessory lobe do not appear to influence fetal development, but abnormalities of the umbilical cord do. Reduced birth weight is commonly associated with velamentous insertion of the cord or battledore placenta and also with a single umbilical artery, which is, however, often a clinical marker of other abnormal fetal morphology. Microscopic changes in the placenta are often associated with fetal growth retardation. There may be intervillous thromboses, placental infarction, and degeneration of the syncytiotrophoblast in preeclamptic toxemia (33). Placental pathology of this kind may arise from maternal disease such as hypertension or habits such as smoking and drug abuse.

The principal determinants of fetal placental perfusion are cardiac output and the distribution of blood in the fetal circulation. The fetal placenta has a low vascular resistance and receives about half the cardiac output. The umbilical arterial wall is muscular and is not thought to be innervated outside the abdomen but is sensitive to circulating vasoactive peptides. Important umbilical artery vasoconstrictors include angiotensin, vasopressin, bradykinins, serotonin, adrenergic agonists, and the prostaglandins. Angiotensin II may exert a tonic vasoconstrictor action, since saralasin, an angiotension II antagonist, has been shown to decrease ovine umbilicoplacental vascular resistance (34) when injected intravenously into the fetus. A corollary is that increased renin–angiotensin secretion in maternal hypertension might cause reduced umbilical flow and thereby fetal growth retardation (35).

Umbilical blood flow is highly dependent on fetal heart rate since there is little variation in stroke volume. Flow increases with body size but not proportionately, since in late gestation a greater fraction perfuses fetal organs. Hypoxemia causes a redistribution of blood flow between fetal organs but little alteration in umbilical vascular resistance. In early gestation hypoxemia causes fetal tachycardia and increased umbilical blood flow, whereas later on there is bradycardia coupled with increased arterial pressure, which helps to preserve umbilical flow (36). Morphine and other central nervous system depressants cause fetal bradycardia. The resulting fall in umbilical blood flow may partly explain the intrauterine growth retardation seen in the offspring of drug abusers.

Placental gaseous exchange is by passive diffusion. The major physiological determinants of oxygen delivery to the fetus are maternal and fetal blood flow and the relative affinities of fetal and maternal hemoglobin for oxygen. If placental surface area is reduced or the diffusion distance increased by thickening of the placental membrane, reduction in the overall oxygen diffusion capacity may restrict fetal growth. This can occur as a result of placental infarction or intervillous fibrin deposition.

A variety of transport mechanisms exists for nutrient delivery across the placenta. Glucose crosses the placenta by facilitated diffusion, and the major determinant of fetal glucose supply is maternal blood glucose concentration with lesser contributions from maternal blood flow and placental size. Maternal glucose was thought to be quantitatively the most important contributor to fetal energy supply. Recent evidence, reviewed by Battaglia and Hay (37), indicates that not only is the placenta an important consumer of maternal glucose but also that lactate produced from placental glucose metabolism passes largely into the fetal circulation. Maternal lipid also contributes to the fetal energy supply (38). The relative amounts of glycerol, free fatty acids, and ketone bodies crossing to the fetus at different stages of human pregnancy are unknown, but it seems likely that some of the lipid stores of the newborn infant are derived directly from the mother, since they reflect the fatty acid pattern of the maternal diet (39).

Placental amino acid transport is active, carrier mediated, and largely uphill (40). The pattern of amino acids in the maternal circulation varies with gestation and with pregnancy-related illness such as preeclamptic toxemia. The relationship between the maternal aminogram and fetal development deserves further study in view of the observations that the total plasma free amino acids during the third trimester are positively correlated with birth weight (41) and that the maternal amino acid profile is related to fetal malnutrition as early as 25 weeks of gestation (42). Maternal hyperaminoacidemia, specifically hyperphenylalaninemia, may also damage fetal development (43).

The complicated way in which HPL influences fetal growth has been dealt with in the section on the fetus. The other important contribution of the placenta involves the secretion and metabolism of steroid hormones. In pregnancy, maternal cardiac output increases. This is in part because of an increase of maternal blood volume, which in turn is the result of an increase in plasma volume and erythrocyte mass. It has been argued that maternal placental perfusion is proportional to the increase in blood volume (44), and therefore factors controlling the latter play an important if indirect part in the control of fetal growth. Pregnenolone synthesized in the placenta is converted to dehydroepiandrosterone sulfate by the fetal adrenal, and this in turn is metabolized to estradiol-17α and estrone by the placenta. These steroids pass into the maternal circulation, where they stimulate the renin–angiotensin system, causing retention of fluid and expansion of the maternal vascular compartment. Maternal erythropoiesis in pregnancy is stimulated by HPL (45).

THE MOTHER

Maternal influences on fetal growth can be subdivided for practical convenience into those that are unalterable, such as maternal age, parity, and genotype, and those that reflect maternal life pattern. The latter include socioeconomic factors and disease and are very important since they are potentially manipulable in order to optimize fetal growth. Of all the influences on variation in birth weight (Table 1), the unalterable maternal contribution accounts for more than 28% (maternal genotype 20%, maternal age and parity 8%, plus an unknown proportion of maternal environment). The alterable maternal contribution could account for up to 54% (general maternal environment 18%, immediate maternal environment 6%, plus an unknown 30%) but is probably less than this.

The best-known examples of immutable maternal influences on fetal growth are uterine shape and size. In the crossing of Shire horses and Shetland ponies, the birth weight of the foals reflected maternal uterine size, those born to Shetland dams being much smaller than those born to Shire dams (46). The possible contribution of dwarf genotype in this kind of experiment was excluded in later experiments in which fertilized eggs were transplanted from dwarf pigs into normal-size sows or vice versa. Genotypically normal piglets growing in dwarf sows were about half the expected size at birth, whereas dwarf piglets implanted in normal sows were twice as big as expected (47). A similar if less dramatic illustration of this phenomenon can be seen in man when birth weight is compared between different ethnic groups or examined as a function of maternal height. In man adult uterine size may be influenced by factors affecting postnatal growth; a plausible hypothesis is that infantile malnutrition compromises uterine growth, leading to suboptimal intrauterine development of the next generation and the vertical transmission of small stature (48).

Uterine size is important to fetal growth because the uterus is the site where the placenta interfaces the fetus and mother. Anything that adversely influences implantation and placental growth will reduce fetal development. This is part of the explanation for the progressive reduction in birth weight with increasing birth number in man. Anatomical abnormalities such as a bicornuate uterus are commonly associated with impaired prenatal growth, as is abnormal placental implantation; lower-segment implantation is associated with a reduction in birth weight of about 200 g (49).

The maternal influences on fetal growth that are amenable to intervention all act on the delivery of nutrient and oxygen to the fetus. The mechanism may be by alteration of the concentration in the maternal circulation or of placental perfusion and transfer. The adverse effect of low maternal socioeconomic status can be considered first, since there is a clear-cut relationship with low birth weight (50). But detailed analysis shows that the disadvantage can be explained in terms of specific factors such as nutrition, smoking, and disease associated with low socioeconomic status and that, in Western society at least, lower social class per se has no significant effect in its own right (51). Social class or socioeconomic grouping is a useful form of categorization for program planning to improve prenatal growth but is of limited value in scientific analysis.

Fetal caloric requirements in man are 95 kcal/kg per day, of which 40 are committed to growth and 55 are oxidized (52). This is accounted for by the small gross overall cost of pregnancy to the mother, 100 kcal/day, who nevertheless experiences profound metabolic and body tissue changes in preparation for parturition (53). Despite this relatively high optimal plane of maternal nutrition, underfeeding has a relatively small effect on fetal growth (54). Starvation, as experienced in Holland in 1944–1945, led to a fall in birth weight only when maternal intake was less than 1,500 calories/day in the third trimester (55). Of more contemporary relevance is the observation that food supplementation during pregnancy led to an increase in birth weight in a poor Guatemalan community (56).

It is a moot point whether maternal alcohol ingestion should be considered as nutrition or as a drug. A sustained high alcohol intake is now accepted as the specific cause of a clinical syndrome of fetal underdevelopment in which there are craniofacial, limb, and cardiac anomalies and psychomotor retardation (57). Less deviant patterns of drinking in pregnancy have also been alleged to reduce birth weight independently of any effect on maternal caloric intake (58). Ethanol and its metabolite acetaldehyde may inhibit growth by a direct toxic action on fetal cellular mitosis or indirectly by inhibiting placental hormone synthesis (59) or causing fetal hypoperfusion and acidosis (60). Other drugs that the mother may take of her own volition include those characteristic of drug abuse, such as opiates, and those readily available for symptom relief, such as aspirin. Maternal drug abuse retards fetal growth. There is a 50% incidence of low birth weight in the offspring of women taking heroin, though whether this a direct effect or secondary to maternal malnutrition and other related factors is not clear (61).

There is an extensive literature on drugs used therapeutically during pregnancy (62), since in every instance the prescriber must consider possible side effects on the fetus. Many drugs are known to inhibit fetal growth and development and are avoided; these include all kinds of cytotoxic and immunosuppressive agents. Examples of drugs more likely to be used are salicylates and glucocorticoids. The daily ingestion of aspirin during pregnancy is associated with an increased stillbirth rate and reduction in birth weight (63). The effect may be mediated by inhibition of prostaglandin synthesis, resulting in uterine vasoconstriction (64). Glucocorticoids when used in pregnancy are usually required in pharmacological doses. In animals this is teratogenic; in man there is no clear-cut evidence of teratogenicity, but there is a reduction in birth weight (65). Whether the fetal growth retardation results from the steroid or from the maternal disease for which it was prescribed is unresolved.

Drugs that alter nutrient delivery to the fetus deliberately or fortuitously are particularly relevant to this review. These can be illustrated by the β-sympathomimetics and β-blockers, both of which cross the placenta freely. The β-mimetics are commonly used to suppress premature uterine contractions and may be administered for periods ranging from hours to weeks. Brettes et al. (66) reported improved fetal growth of small-for-dates infants whose mothers were treated with ritodrine and claimed that this was because of increased uterine blood flow and improved fetal nutrition, an interpretation that has subsequently been queried (67). Ritodrine is said to induce maternal carbohydrate intolerance, but when glucose tolerance of mother and baby was tested in control and ritodrine-treated pregnancies, no significant difference was found (68). An alternative explanation is that lipid metabolism may be altered. Isoxuprine, another β-mimetic, caused a large rise in plasma free fatty acids and insulin when given to newborn rabbit pups (69). It is possible that the fetal growth-promoting effect claimed for β-mimetics may result from stimulation of lipolysis and increased transplacental passage of lipid constituents, a mechanism already proposed for infants of diabetic mothers (70). Propranolol is the most commonly employed β-blocker and may be used in pregnancy for the treatment of hypertension, cardiac arrhythmias, or thyroid disease. Chronic fetal exposure to propranolol results in reduced body and placental weight (71). A suggested explanation is reduced uterine blood flow because of a fall in maternal cardiac output and increased uterine muscle tone coupled with reduced blood flows in the fetus (72). To this must be added a metabolic action; propranolol blocks cold-induced thermogenesis and may inhibit mobilization of nutrient from mother to fetus.

Although nicotine is a drug, smoking is sufficiently prevalent and preventable to merit consideration separate from toxic drug actions in the fetus. Fetal growth retardation is directly proportional to the number of cigarettes smoked by the mother; 20 a day brings the birth weight down by 200 g. This is not related to associated malnutrition (73). Placental weight may be increased, and there is a characteristic placental pathology—obliterative endarteritis, villous cytotrophoblastic hyperplasia, and necrosis of the decidua basalis—all of which are compatible with hypoperfusion (74). These adverse effects are caused by both nicotine and carbon monoxide. High concentrations of nicotine in the circulation can increase uterine vascular resistance and decrease blood flow, leading to fetal hypoxia and hypercapnia (75). Nicotine has also been shown to depress human placental amino acid transfer *in vitro* (76). Inhaled carbon monoxide leads to tissue hypoxia by the formation of carboxyhemoglobin in both mother and fetus. Carbon monoxide also binds to cytochrome and therapy may impair active placental transport of nutrients.

Maternal disease influences fetal development by altering placental perfusion or by producing placental transfer of abnormal molecules. Impaired delivery of oxygen to the placenta occurs in maternal cyanotic heart disease or chronic debilitating lung disease. Maternal pregnancy-associated hypertension is often associated with poor intrauterine growth. This may be related to thromboses in the placental microvasculature or to associated renal involvement (77). A corollary is that factors increasing uterine blood flow, such as bed rest, stimulate fetal growth (78). Maternal undernutrition severe enough to affect fetal development is certainly an illness, but one that has been more appropriately considered in the context of socioeconomic factors. Maternal metabolic disorders characterized by excess circulating concentrations of one or more metabolites might be expected to affect fetal growth, the most often cited example being phenylketonuria (43). There are a group of conditions that have in common immunoglobulin overproduction. The placenta is permeable to IgG, and fetal tissue damage results from the transplacental passage of immunoglobulin in systemic lupus erythematosus (79). The baby born thyrotoxic as a result of the passage of long-acting thyroid stimulator (LATS) is often small and may have experienced thyrotoxicosis *in utero* (80).

Maternal infections have a spectrum of harmful effects on the fetus. Malaria inhibits fetal growth principally by impairing placental blood flow (81). Any serious maternal illness, especially an infectious one, in the first trimester usually results in abortion. Serious systemic bacterial infection, particularly gram-negative septicemia, at any stage of pregnancy may kill the fetus, whereas viral or protozoal infections such as rubella, cytomegalovirus, or toxoplasmosis all cause fetal tissue damage and growth retardation along with specific pathology characteristic of the infecting agent (82).

The only environmental factor with an unequivocal effect on human fetal development is altitude. Infants born at 15,000 ft have a mean birth weight 16% lower than do infants born at 500 ft (83). Fetal growth retardation in these circumstances results from decreased oxygen delivery.

ACKNOWLEDGMENTS

Any review is of necessity derivative, and this one has drawn particularly on the comprehensive account of the regulation of fetal growth by Gluckman and Liggins (84). I am grateful to Dr. D.J. Hill for helpful discussion.

REFERENCES

1. Holliday R, Pugh JE. DNA modification mechanisms and gene activity during development. *Science* 1975;187;226–32.
2. Robson EB. The genetics of birthweight. In: Falkner, F, Tanner JM, eds. *Human growth: principles and prenatal growth, vol 1*. New York: Plenum Press, 1978:285–97.
3. Park E, Bailey JD, Cowell CA. Growth and maturation of patients with Turner's syndrome. *Pediatr Res* 1983;17:1–7.
4. Polani PE. Chromosomal and other genetic influences on birth weight variation. In: Elliott K, Knight J, eds. *Size at birth*. Ciba Foundation symposium 27 (new series). Amsterdam: Elsevier, 1974:127–64.
5. Liggins G.C. The drive to fetal growth. In: Beard RW, Nathanielsz PW, eds. *Fetal physiology and medicine*. 1st ed. London: WB Saunders, 1976:254–70.
6. Widdowson EM, Crabb DE, Milner RDG. Cellular development of some human organs before birth. *Arch Dis Child* 1972;47:652–6.
7. Widdowson EM. Changes in body composition during growth. In: Davis JA, Dobbing J, eds. *Scientific foundations of paediatrics*. 2nd ed. London: W Heinemann, 1981:330–42.
8. Milner RDG. Fetal growth control: the role of insulin and related peptides. In: Aynsley-Green A, ed. *Paediatric endocrinology in clinical practice*. Lancaster: MTP Press, 1984:125–48.
9. Milner RDG. The role of insulin and glucagon in fetal growth and metabolism. In: Visser HKA, ed. *Nutrition and metabolism of the fetus and infant*. The Hague: Martinus Nijhoff, 1979:3–18.
10. Hill DJ, Milner RDG. The role of peptide growth factors and hormones in the control of fetal growth. In: Chiswick ML, ed. *Recent advances in perinatal medicine 2*. London: Churchill Livingstone, 1985:79–102.
11. Maenpaa J. Congenital hypothyroidism. Aetiological and clinical aspects. *Arch Dis Child* 1972;47:914–23.
12. Van Wyk JJ, Underwood LE, D'Ercole AJ, et al. Role of somatomedin in cellular proliferation. In: Ritzen M, Aperia A, Hall K, Larsson A, Zetterberg A, Zetterstrom R, eds. *Biology of normal human growth*. New York: Raven Pres, 1981:223–39.
13. Blundel TL, Humbel RE. Hormone families: pancreatic hormones and homologous growth factors. *Nature* 1980;287:781–7.
14. Phillips LS, Vassilopoulou-Selli R. Somatomedin, Parts 1 and 2. *N Engl J Med* 1980;302:371–80,438–46.
15. Gluckman PD, Barrett-Johnson JJ, Butler JH, Edgar B, Gunn TR. Studies of insulin-like growth factor I and II by specific radioligand assays in umbilical cord blood. *Clin Endocrinol* 1983;19:405–13.
16. D'Ercole AJ, Wilson DF, Underwood LE. Changes in the circulating form of somatomedin-C during fetal life. *J Clin Endocrinol Metab* 1980;51:674–6.
17. Sara VR, Hall K, Misaki M, Fryklund L, Christensen L, Wetteberg L. Ontogenesis of somatomedin and insulin receptors in the human fetus. *J Clin Invest* 1983;71:1084–94.
18. Rosenfeld R, Thorsson A, Hintz RL. Increased somatomedin receptor sites in newborn circulating mononuclear cells. *J Clin Endocrinol Metab* 1979;48:456–61.
19. Brown AL, Graham DE, Nissley SP, Hill DJ, Strain AJ, Rechler MM. Developmental regulation of insulin-like growth factor II mRNA in different rat tissues. *J Biol Chem* 1986;261:13144–50.
20. D'Ercole AJ, Hill DJ, Strain AJ, Underwood LE. Tissue and plasma somatomedin C/insulin-like growth factor I (SM-C/IGF I) concentrations in the human fetus during the first half of gestation. *Pediatr Res* 1986;20:253–5.
21. Han VKN, Hill DJ, D'Ercole AJ, et al. Immunolocalization of somatomedins/insulin-like growth factors in human fetal tissues [Abstract]. *J Endocrinol* 1986;108(suppl):A2–17.

22. Gluckman PD, Kaplan SL, Rudolph AM, Grumbach MM. Hormone ontogeny in the ovine fetus. II Ovine chorionic somatomammotropin in mid- and late gestation in the fetal and maternal circulations. *Endocrinology* 1979;104:1828–33.

23. Grumbach MM, Kaplan SL, Sciarra JJ, Burr I. Chorionic growth hormone–prolactin (CGP): secretion, deposition, biological activity in man, and postulated function as the 'growth hormone' of the second half of pregnancy. *Ann NY Acad Sci* 1968;148:501–31.

24. Furlanetto RW, Underwood LE, Van Wyk JJ, Handwerger S. Serum immunoreactive somatomedin-C is elevated in late pregnancy. *J Clin Endocrinol Metab* 1978;47:695–8.

25. Merimee TJ, Zapf J, Froesch ER. Insulin-like growth factor in pregnancy: studies in a growth hormone-deficient dwarf. *J Clin Endocrinol Metab* 1982;54:1101–3.

26. Adams SO, Nissley SP, Handwerger S, Rechler MM. Development patterns of insulin-like growth factor I and II synthesis and regulation in rat fibroblasts. *Nature* 1983;302:150–3.

27. Hill DJ, Crace CJ, Strain AJ, Milner RDG. Regulation of amino acid uptake and DNA synthesis in isolated human fetal fibroblasts and myoblasts: effect of human placental lactogen, somatomedin C, multiplication stimulating activity and insulin. *J Clin Endocrinol Metab* 1986;62:753–60.

28. Hill DJ, Crace CJ, Milner RDG. Incorporation of (^{3}H)thymidine by isolated human fetal myoblasts and fibroblasts in response to human placental lactogen (HPL): possible mediation of HPL action by release of immunoreactive Sm-C. *J Cell Physiol* 1985;125:337–44.

29. Strain AJ, Hill DJ, Swenne I, Milner RDG. Stimulation of DNA synthesis in isolated human fetal hepatocytes by insulin-like growth factor I, placental lactogen and growth hormone [Abstract]. *J Endocrinol* 1986;108(suppl)A142.

30. Hochberg Z, Perlman R, Brandes JM, Benderli A. Insulin regulates placental lactogen and estradiol secretion by cultured human term trophoblast. *J Clin Endocrinol Metab* 1983;57:1311–3.

31. Alexander G. Factors regulating the growth of the placenta: with comments on the relationship between placental weight and fetal weight. In: Naftolin F, ed. *Abnormal fetal growth: biological bases and consequences*. Berlin: Abakon Verlagsgesellschaft, 1978:149–64.

32. Honnebier WJ, Swaab DF. The influence of anencephaly upon intrauterine growth of fetus and placenta and upon gestation length. *J Obstet Gynaecol Br Commonw* 1973;80:577–88.

33. Rolschau J. Infarctions and intervillous thrombosis in placenta, and their association with intrauterine growth retardation. *Acta Obstet Gynecol Scand [Suppl]* 1978;72:22–7.

34. Tulenko TN, Millard RW. Evidence for a physiological role for fetal angiotensin II in the regulation of the umbilicoplacental vasculature. *Ann Rech Vet* 1977;8:484–5.

35. Tulenko TN. Regional sensitivity to vasoactive polypeptides in the human umbilicoplacental vasculature. *Am J Obstet Gynecol* 1979;135:629–36.

36. Boddy K. Fetal blood flow to and from the placenta. In: Chamberlain GVP, Wilkinson AW, eds. *Placental transfer*. Tunbridge Wells: Pitman Medical, 1979:45–59.

37. Battaglia FC, Hay WW Jr. Energy and substrate requirements for fetal and placental growth and metabolism. In: Beard RW, Nathanielsz PW, eds. *Fetal physiology and medicine*. 2nd ed. New York: Marcel Dekker, 1984:601–28.

38. Milner RDG. Fetal fat and glucose metabolism. In: Beard RW, Nathanielsz PW, eds. *Fetal physiology and medicine*. 2nd ed. New York: Marcel Dekker, 1984:153–76.

39. Widdowson EM, Dauncey MJ, Gardner DMT, Jonxis JHP, Petikan-Filipkova M. Body fat of British and Dutch infants. *Br Med J* 1975;1:653–5.

40. Mestyan J, Soltesz G. Maternal, fetal, and neonatal amino acid and protein metabolism. In: Beard RW, Nathanielsz PW, eds. *Fetal physiology and medicine*. 2nd ed. New York: Marcel Dekker, 1984:177–209.

41. Kamran S, Churchill JA, Kurrie D. Relationship of the maternal amino acids and protein to fetal growth and mental development. *Am J Obstet Gynecol* 1975;123:398–407.

42. McClain PE, Metcoff J, Crosbie WM, Costiloe JP. Relationship of maternal amino acid profiles at 25 weeks of gestation to fetal growth. *Am J Clin Nutr* 1978;31:401–7.

43. Lenke RR, Levy HL. Maternal phenylketonuria and hyperphenylalaninemia: an international survey of the outcome of untreated and treated pregnancies. *N Engl J Med* 1980;303:1202–8.

44. Lango LD. Intrauterine growth retardation: a "mosaic" hypothesis of pathophysiology. *Semin Perinatol* 1984;8:62–72.

45. Johnson JD. Regulation of fetal growth. *Pediatr Res* 1985;19:738–41.

46. Walton A, Hammond J. The maternal effects on growth and conformation in Shire horse–Shetland pony crosses. *Proc R Soc Lond [Biol]* 1938;125B:311–35.

47. Smidt D, Steinbach J, Scheven B. Die Beeinflussung der pro- und post-natalen Entwicklung durch

Grosse und Körpergewicht der Mutter, largesteller an Ergebnissen reziproker Eitransplantationen zwischen Zwergschweinen und Grossen Hausschweinen. *Monatsschr Kinderheilkd* 1967;115:533–45.

48. Ounsted M, Scott A, Ounsted C. Transmission through the female line of a mechanism constraining human fetal growth. *Ann Hum Biol* 1986;13:143–51.
49. Higginbottom J, Slater J, Porter G. The low-lying placenta and dysmaturity. *Lancet* 1975;1:859.
50. Illsley R, Mitchell RG. *Low birth weight: a medical, psychological and social study.* Chichester: John Wiley & Sons, 1984.
51. Ounsted M, Ounsted C. On fetal growth rate. *Clin Dev Med* 1973;46:9–11.
52. Sparks JW, Girard JR, Battaglia FC. An estimate of the caloric requirements of the human fetus. *Biol Neonate* 1980;38:113–9.
53. Emerson K Jr, Saxena BN, Poindexter BL. Caloric cost of normal pregnancy. *Obstet Gynecol* 1972;40:786–94.
54. Metcoff J. Association of fetal growth with maternal nutrition. In: Falkner F, Tanner JM, eds. *Human growth: principles and prenatal growth, vol 1.* New York: Plenum Press, 1978:415–60.
55. Smith CA. The effects of maternal undernutrition upon the newborn infant in Holland (1944–45). *J Pediatr* 1947;30:229–43.
56. Lechtig A, Habicht JP, Delgado H, Klein RE, Yarbrough C, Martorell R. Effect of food supplementation during pregnancy on birth weight. *Pediatrics* 1975;56:508–20.
57. Jones KL, Smith DW, Ulleland CN, Streissgath AP. Patterns of malformation in offspring of chronic alcoholic mothers. *Lancet* 1973;1:1267–71.
58. Hansen JW, Streissgath AP, Smith DW. The effects of moderate alcohol consumption during pregnancy on fetal growth and morphogenesis. *J Pediatr* 1978;92:457–60.
59. Wunderlich SM, Baliga BS, Munro HM. Rat placental protein synthesis and peptide hormone secretion in relation to malnutrition from protein deficiency or alcohol administration. *J Nutr* 1979;109:1534–41.
60. Mann LI, Bhaktharathsalan A, Liu M, Makowski P. Placental transport of alcohol and its effect on maternal and fetal acid–base balance. *Am J Obstet Gynecol* 1975;122:837–44.
61. Kandall SR, Albin S, Lowinson J, Berle B, Eidelman AI, Gartner LM. Differential effects of maternal heroin and methadone use on birthweight. *Pediatrics* 1976;58:681–5.
62. Peterson RG. Pharmacology. In: Boyd R, Battaglia FC, eds. *Perinatal medicine.* London: Butterworths, 1983:131–44.
63. Turner G, Collins E. Fetal effects of regular salicylate ingestion in pregnancy. *Lancet* 1975;2:338–9.
64. Rankin JHG, McLoughlin MK. The regulation of the placental blood flows. *J Dev Physiol* 1979;1:3–30.
65. Reinisch JM, Simon NG, Karow WG, Gandelman R. Prenatal exposure to prednisone in humans and animals retards intrauterine growth. *Science* 1978;202:436–8.
66. Brettes JP, Renaud R, Gandar R. A double blind investigation into the effects of ritodrine on uterine blood flow during the third trimester of pregnancy. *Am J Obstet Gynecol* 1976;124:164–8.
67. Lunell NO, Sarby B. Utero-placental blood flow. Methods of determination, clinical application and the effect of beta mimetic agonists. In: Sutherland HW, Stowers JW, eds. *Carbohydrate metabolism in pregnancy and the newborn 1978.* Berlin: Springer-Verlag, 1979:86–101.
68. Blouin D, Murray MAF, Beard RW. The effect of oral ritodrine on maternal and fetal carbohydrate metabolism. *Br J Obstet Gynaecol* 1976;83:711–5.
69. Cser A, Girard JR, Goode M, Leach FN, Assan R, Milner RDG. Effects of racemic, dextro-, laevopropranolol and isoxuprine on the metabolic and endocrine response to cold in the newborn rabbit. *Eur J Clin Invest* 1977;7:491–6.
70. Szabo AJ, Szabo O. Placental free fatty acid transfer and fetal adipose tissue development. An explanation of fetal adiposity in infants of diabetic mothers. *Lancet* 1974;2:498–9.
71. Pruyn SC, Phelan JP, Buchanan GC. Long-term propranolol therapy in pregnancy: maternal and fetal outcome. *Am J Obstet Gynecol* 1979;135:485–9.
72. Oakes GK, Walker AM, Ehrenkranz RA, Chez R. Effect of propranolol infusion on the umbilical and uterine circulations of pregnant sheep. *Am J Obstet Gynecol* 1976;126:1038–42.
73. Persson P, Grennert L, Gernser G, Kullander S. A study of smoking and pregnancy with special reference to fetal growth. *Acta Obstet Gynecol Scand [Suppl]* 1978;78:33–9.
74. Naeye RL. Effects of maternal cigarette smoking on the fetus and placenta. *Br J Obstet Gynaecol* 1978;88:732–7.

75. Suzuki K, Honguchi T, Comas-Urratia AC, Mueller-Henbach E, Morishima HO, Adamsons K. Pharmacological effects of nicotine upon the fetus and mother in the rhesus monkey. *Am J Obstet Gynecol* 1971;111:1092–101.

76. Barnwell SL, Sastry BVR. Inhibition of the uptake of amino acids in human placental villus by nicotine, cocaine and morphine [Abstract]. *Fed Proc* 1980;39:861.

77. Novy MJ. Regulation of placental blood flow and oxygen transfer in relation to fetal growth. In: Naftolin F, ed. *Abnormal fetal growth: biological bases and consequences.* Berlin: Abakan Verlagsgesellschaft 1978:229–56.

78. Morris N, Osborn SB, Wright HP. Effective uterine blood flow during exercise in normal and preeclamptic pregnancies. *Lancet* 1985;2:481–4.

79. Tozman ECS, Urowitz MB, Gladman DD. Systemic lupus erythematosus and pregnancy. *J Rheumatol* 1980;7:624–32.

80. Mahoney CP, Payne GE, Stamm SJ, Bakke JL. Neonatal Grave's disease. *Am J Dis Child* 1964;107:516–22.

81. Galbraith RM, Fox M, Hsi B, Galbraith GMP, Bray RS, Faulk WP. The human materno-fetal relationship in malaria. II. Histological, ultrastructural and immunopathological studies of the placenta. *Trans R Soc Trop Med Hyg* 1980;74:67–72.

82. Remington JS, Klein JO, eds. *Infectious diseases of the fetus and newborn infant.* Philadelphia: WB Saunders, 1976.

83. Kruger H, Arias Stella J. The placenta and the newborn infant at high altitudes. *Am J Obstet Gynecol* 1970;106:586–91.

84. Gluckman PD, Liggins GC. Regulation of fetal growth. In: Beard RW, Nathanielsz PW, eds. *Fetal physiology and medicine.* 2nd ed. New York: Marcel Dekker, 1984:511–58.

DISCUSSION

Dr. Tomkins: Could I ask you to expand on why it is that socioeconomic status affects birth weight? As I understand it, there are many factors. The one that I would be particularly interested to hear about is the interaction with activity, which did not appear in your analysis. The reason I ask is that when we look at birth weight in relation to poor socioeconomic status, the women who are the poorest are often working the hardest, e.g., in agriculture or cleaning factories in Scotland, even though they are not malnourished by body mass index or fat stores. I wonder if you have any information, experimental or otherwise, on the effect of activity on placental blood flow, on hormone release, or anything like that?

Dr. Milner: That is a very good point that I have omitted to emphasize and is a corollary of what is accepted in current clinical practice. If maternal placental perfusion is jeopardized for whatever reason, whether because of maternal essential hypertension or preeclamptic toxemia, the surest way of improving it is maternal rest. That is totally compatible with what you are saying; i.e., the more active a pregnant woman has to be, certainly through the second and third trimesters, the more this could have an adverse effect on fetal nutrition as a result of a reduction in maternal placental perfusion.

Dr. Tomkins: David Saunders in Zimbabwe *(personal communication)* describes what they call ''maternity villages'' where mothers come at least for the last month of pregnancy and where everything is done for them. I don't know how widespread this is in developing countries, but it is certainly not my experience in West Africa, where women have to keep going until delivery.

Dr. Rappaport: My understanding is that maternal rest at the end of pregnancy, at least in European countries, results in a decreased incidence of prematurity but not of intrauterine growth retardation (IUGR) and that the number of small-for-date children has decreased much less than the number of premature babies. In developing countries there are probably many other factors that could affect the fetal growth. Has anybody tried to differentiate prematurity and IUGR, and their causes, in developing countries?

Dr. Milner: I believe that one of the problems commonly experienced is difficulty in being confident about gestational age.

Dr. Keller: In WHO we recently reviewed the literature on low birth weight. It seems that very little is actually known about the possible effect of maternal physical work on birth weight and on the development of the fetus. That hypothesis is very interesting because it would be a more plausible explanation for the very high rate of small-for-date babies, mostly in developing countries, than the hypothesis of a deficient calorie supply to the mother, which is the usual one.

Dr. Milner: That goes along with a mild but chronic intrauterine growth retardation; once you have got that as a piece of pathophysiology, then you are going to have a different kind of conceptus, and the implications for postnatal catch-up are adverse, whereas if the problem begins from, say, 28 weeks onwards, you may end with a baby that still weighs only 2.2 kg but with very good implications for postnatal catch-up, assuming that the extrauterine environment is favorable.

Dr. Waterlow: You used the phrase, "maternal placental perfusion." I have never been able to understand the idea that the fetus, during the third trimester of pregnancy, could not get enough nutrients from the mother. I tried to calculate from what we know of fetal oxygen consumption and fetal protein turnover rates what proportion of the nutrients that are circulating through the placental blood are actually taken up by the fetus. If I remember correctly, for amino acids, glucose, and even oxygen, it might come to something of the order of 10% of the supply. I find it very difficult to understand how a mother, for example, one who might have a slightly low blood amino acid concentration, would still not have a plentiful supply if only 10% had to be taken up? Do you have any comments on the arithmetic of the situation?

Dr. Milner: In the maternal–fetal transfer across the placenta of the three classes of nutrients, protein, fat, and carbohydrate, each differs from the other. Glucose crosses by facilitated diffusion. Amino acids cross by active transfer, where the fetal concentrations are always higher than the maternal and the fetomaternal differential increases towards term. Fatty acid transfer is now accepted to be more important in total fetal caloric accretion than was previously thought to be the case, specifically in respect to different classes of essential fatty acids. If the molecules can actually get to the maternofetal interface at the hemochorial junction, the fetus can pick up the molecule from the maternal side. The block to adequate delivery of nutrients to the fetus, in so far as the concept is acceptable, is in perfusion failure on the maternal side of the placenta.

Dr. Gopalan: What do you think of maternal anemia? Anemia is one of the most common conditions in developing countries. In particular, I would like your comment on the claims that folic acid supplementation to the mother brings about an increase in birth weight. If supplements have to be given, what would be the supplement? What would be the optimal time for the introduction of these supplements?

Dr. Milner: Your question makes it perfectly clear to everybody why I took refuge in simple concepts. When we turn back to real life, we know from the onset that your question, which is a very straightforward and legitimate one to ask, is nonetheless very difficult to answer because maternal anemia does not exist in isolation. So, to what extent anemia is responsible, and to what extent coexistence of adverse influences is responsible, I do not know.

Dr. Gopalan: Do you believe that iron supplementation could be an answer to the problem of low birth weight?

Dr. Milner: I am very pleased you introduced the word "believe." I do not know of evidence in support of that specific statement. There is increased maternal erythropoiesis to keep up with the increase in the maternal circulating blood volume. So although the hemoglobin concentration falls, the total circulating red cell mass increases. With respect to folate and other vitamin supplements, the question is also very complicated.

Dr. Valyasevi: We have some data on iron deficiency anemia and on the effects of iron supplements in about 300 pregnant mothers with moderate iron deficiency anemia (hemogloblin concentration around 8 g/dl). We could not demonstrate any difference in birth weight between the unsupplemented and the supplemented group with a hemoglobin level of about 12 g/dl.

Dr. Milner: When one thinks of the oxygen-binding capacity of fetal hemoglobin versus maternal hemoglobin, I would be surprised if maternal anemia, be it iron deficiency or a macrocytic anemia, is an important variable in determining fetal cellular development.

Dr. Kraisid: You said that fetal growth can be divided into three trimesters characterized by an increase in cell numbers and size. You used muscle tissue as an example. Can the same be applied to other organs such as bone and brain?

Dr Milner: Information is available on liver, heart, lung, and skeletal muscle. It is not available on brain, but Dobbing and Sands (1) have information on the brain in which neuronal and neuroglial tissue follow different patterns of cellular growth. I do not know of analogous information pertaining to prenatal skeletal growth in man.

Dr. Kraisid: In your opinion, what would be the critical period for supplementation in terms of all nutrient supplementation? Should we supplement poor pregnant women during the first, second, or third trimester?

Dr. Milner: If I had a very limited amount of food to give as supplementation, I would be more concerned that it went in trimesters 1 and 2 and less concerned about trimester 3.

Dr. Guesry: I think it is very difficult to give a clear answer to this very important question. For example, if you want to reduce the incidence of neural tube defects, it seems that the vitamin supplements need to be given even before conception.

Dr. Davies: You said that intrauterine size possibly holds a key position. A recent study from Sweden (2) has shown that the "terminal flattening" (slowing down of fetal growth in the last few weeks of gestation) is now much less than previously. I wonder whether you can fit this in with your hypothesis of small uterine size having a constraining effect on growth: that the reason for the high incidence of small-for-date babies in women who themselves have been malnourished may simply be that the uterus is too small to allow optimum growth expression. The opposite would apply to the Scandinavian women who have enjoyed excellent nutrition throughout their lives.

Dr. Milner: There is a circularity in this argument, and it is almost seductive in its plausibility; on the other hand, it does not have to be wrong. The statement that you make does not surprise me. The point that I find interesting is that it would take a number of generations to get a secular trend, which could appear partly prenatally as well as postnatally.

Dr. Nabarro: In countries where there is a pronounced seasonal variation in infections and in the availability of nutrients, and where there probably are 3 or 4 months that are considered to be totally adverse by the local population, the timing of conception and birth would appear to be of extreme importance in determining the potential for linear growth. There is a need to examine cohorts of children born in different seasons to study their linear growth rates and to relate these to the season of birth.

Dr. Guesry: Do we have any information on this from the Dutch famine in 1944–1945? It seems that starvation during the last trimester had the most severe effect.

Dr. Milner: I accept that starvation experienced in the last trimester would have a dramatic effect on body weight, and that 500 g of fat would just not appear, but those babies would not be permanently disadvantaged, whereas the ones who experience the same starvation during the first trimester and who are not aborted—and of course fertility goes down—are the ones who might have lifelong disadvantages.

Dr. Colombo: Could you comment on the effect of alcohol? I think it is a bigger problem than usually thought, at least in Chile. Could the amount of alcohol necessary to affect fetal growth be less than what is usually said?

Dr. Milner: Social drinking as opposed to alcoholism is quite sufficient to have an adverse effect on cellular development *in utero,* and this, as is also the case with smoking, is not related to a reduction in total caloric intake, which is being compensated for by ethanol intake.

Dr. Martorell: Another possible environmental factor is smoke, cooking smoke. One of the first things the very poor, who live in single-room huts, do when they have money is build a separate kitchen. The effect of cooking smoke on intrauterine growth has never really been studied seriously.

Dr. Milner: That is an excellent example of what I had to end up thinking about. In our vast area of ignorance, there are possibly all sorts of other factors that could have an adverse effect on growth throughout pregnancy. I was thinking of some of the herbal medicines that are taken because they are reputed to be beneficial for pregnancy, but some of them plainly are not.

REFERENCES

1. Dobbing J, Sands J. Quantitative growth and development of human brain. *Arch Dis Child* 1973;48:757–67.
2. Rooth G, Meirik O, Karlberg P. Estimation of the "normal" growth of Swedish infants at term. *Acta Paediatr Scand* [Suppl] 1985;319:76–9.

Linear Growth Retardation in Less Developed Countries, edited by John C. Waterlow. Nestlé Nutrition Workshop Series, Vol. 14. Nestec Ltd., Vevey/Raven Press, Ltd., New York © 1988.

Endocrine Control of Growth

Raphaël Rappaport

Research Unit on Developmental Biology and Growth, INSERM U. 30, Hôpital des Enfants-Malades, Paris 15, France

It is generally accepted that adequate nutrition is a prerequisite for normal postnatal growth. Hormones such as growth hormone (GH), insulin, thyroxine, and sex steroids play a pivotal role in controlling musculoskeletal growth, as proven in a number of well-described clinical conditions (Fig. 1). However, it has been observed that the *in vitro* stimulatory effect of hormones on cell metabolism or cell multiplication is often less impressive than their *in vivo* effect, suggesting that their action at the cellular level could involve other factors. This led to the discovery of many cell growth factors. The most extensive studies concerned the somatomedins (Sm) or insulin-like growth factors (IGF) isolated from human plasma and believed to mediate the growth-promoting action of GH. The measurement of their concentration in tissue, biological fluid, and principally in blood provided numerous data concerning growth and nutrition in various clinical conditions.

In a developmental perspective, growth regulation, particularly the regulation of skeletal growth, presents considerable differences according to age from the perinatal period to adolescence. Hormonal changes play an important role in the adaptation to nutritional alterations by limiting the growth rate. Their role in catch-up growth is still under investigation.

GROWTH HORMONE AND SOMATOMEDINS

A major difference between pre- and postnatal life is the switch, at the time of or just before birth, to the GH dependence of statural growth. At the same time it can be hypothesized that there is a shift from an autocrine or paracrine to a more endocrine type of control of growth. In fact, after birth the events that control skeletal growth and more specificallly cartilage activity are largely dependent on GH, although there is presently some debate on the significance of experiments that showed a direct effect of GH on this tissue.

Control of Growth Hormone Secretion

Growth hormone secretion is regulated by both stimulatory and inhibitory factors of hypothalamic origin. Growth hormone-releasing factor (GRF) is well iden-

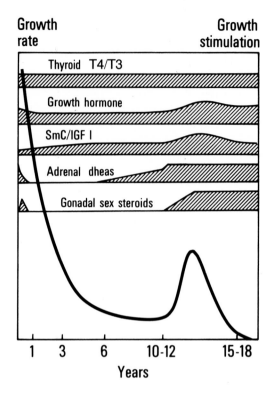

FIG. 1. Schematic representation of growth rate and levels of the main circulating hormones from birth until adolescence. dheas, dehydroepiandrosterone sulfate.

tified among the first group, and somatostatin (SRIF) belongs to the latter. The availability of human GRF for clinical studies and eventually for therapeutic use has stimulated much interest in this area. Presently much has been done to evaluate the somatotrophic cell responsiveness to GRF. The relationship that exists between hypothalamic regulation of GH secretion and changes in growth rate in relation to age and sex has also attracted much attention.

Much of our knowledge of the physiological roles of endogenous somatostatin and GRF in the control of GH secretion has been provided by experimental studies on the rat (1,2). The elegant studies of Tannenbaum and Ling in freely moving rats demonstrated that the episodic pulses of GH secretion in male rats were partly dependent on episodic release of GRF and, more importantly, related to the intermittent withdrawal of a tonic inhibition of GH secretion by hypothalamic somatostatin (3). Similar findings in humans are consistent with this hypothesis, as intermittent pulsatile GH secretion was observed during human GRF (hGRF) infusion (4). Further evidence that endogenous somatostatin in the rat plays a role in controlling GH secretion is provided by the administration of somatostatin antiserum, which reverses the inhibition of GH secretion induced by starvation and streptozotocin diabetes (5,6). In fact, tonic somatostatin inhibition has been postulated in man during starvation. This could in part explain the elevated concentrations of circulating GH that are frequently found in malnutrition. The concentration of circulating IGF I could also be involved in this feedback. This peptide stimulates somatostatin release from rat hypothalami *in vitro* (7) and exerts a potent direct inhibitory effect on GRF-stimulated GH release in cultured pituitary cells (8). Low circulating values of IGF_1 are observed in contrast to the high concentrations of GH in Laron-type dwarfism as well as in children with kwashiorkor (9). There is also strong evidence that GH itself is capable of regulating its own secretion through a short-loop feedback mechanism (10,11).

Furthermore, it has been shown, at least in rats, that the normal GH response to GRF is not a simple phenomenon (12): glucocorticoids enhance the GH response to GRF, probably by modulating the pituitary sensitivity; similarly, testosterone increases the GH response, but estrogens do not; and chronic hypothyroidism inhibits the GH response to GRF *in vivo*. Therefore, the whole endocrine status of the animal must be considered when evaluating the GH response to GRF. To what extent this can be applied to the child remains to be seen.

Growth Hormone Secretion in Relation to Age and Puberty

Plasma GH levels are higher in fetuses and newborns than in later life. Growth hormone does not play a central role in the control of growth in the fetus. In only a few isolated cases of complete genetic deficiency of GH and/or IGF I may a moderate growth retardation occur *in utero*. Fetal GH deficiency can therefore be largely compensated by other growth-stimulating mechanisms. However, in cases with complete GH deficiency, cessation of growth is observed during the early weeks following birth (Fig. 2). This indicates that GH takes over the control of

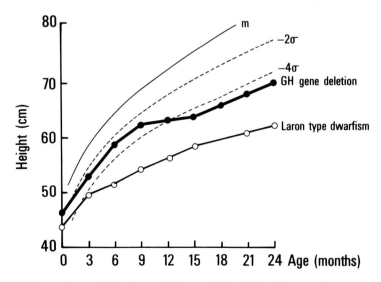

FIG. 2. Early growth retardation in two children with the clinical features of complete GH deficiency caused either by GH gene deletion or by absence of somatomedin generation (Laron-type dwarfism).

growth in extrauterine life. The so-called "basal GH values," more precisely the episodic pattern of plasma GH concentrations, is changing at the time of puberty under the influence of gonadal steroids. Recently it was shown that puberty, at least in boys, is accompanied by an increase in GH pulse height and frequency, although considerable individual variations were observed (13). The stimulatory effect of estrogens, although less convincing in physiological conditions, is also likely to occur, as mean plasma GH levels are higher in women than in adult men (14). It can therefore be firmly concluded that GH secretion is stimulated by sex steroids and plays a major role in the pubertal growth spurt.

During the first semester of life, infants present with a pubertal-like spurt of testosterone secretion and, although to a lesser extent, of estradiol. These steroids might play a role in the maintenance of higher GH levels in neonates. The effect of these on skeletal growth, if it occurs in infants, is probably blunted in the presence of an already maximal, although decelerating, growth rate. Precise longitudinal studies have shown that boys grow faster than girls during the first part of the first year, coincidentally with elevated plasma testosterone levels. However, acceleration of bone age does not occur at that time (14).

Clinical Assessment of Growth Hormone Secretion: Difficulties and Limits

Because of large age-dependent inter- and intraindividual variations in the 24-hr profile of plasma GH concentrations, there is no simple way to assess GH secretion routinely in physiological conditions. There are strict methodological and practical requirements for this evaluation during physical exercise or during sleep. Preliminary data have shown a positive relationship between height and the integrated 24-hr GH concentration in healthy children (15). For practical reasons, GH secretion is commonly estimated by the response to pharmacological stimulation including the injection of synthetic human GRF.

In children with retarded growth, when pituitary dwarfism has been ruled out, there remains, according to the degree of GH response to stimulation, a spectrum of clinical conditions ranging from normal pituitary function to overt hypopituitarism. To what extent the degree of responsiveness can be correlated with the individual growth rate remains unclear. Furthermore, the usefulness of this evaluation in deciding to use human growth hormone (hGH) or GRF therapy in nonhypopituitary children is questionable, as it does not make it possible to predict the growth response. Other factors such as the nutritional status and the age of the child might influence the response to hGH, as observed in hypopituitary children.

In the normal child with short stature, there is some evidence that a prepubertal transient decrease of GH secretion may contribute to growth retardation and cause pubertal delay (16). Whether such children would benefit from hGH administration remains to be demonstrated by long-term studies.

Growth Hormone Deficiency

The availability of hGRF to test the pituitary response was expected to facilitate greatly the differential diagnosis between GH deficiency of pituitary and hypothalamic origin. This has turned out to be an oversimplification. A tentative classification, maintaining that approach, of conditions with GH deficiency has been proposed. It takes into account other aspects of GH/somatomedin regulation:

1. Neuroendocrine control: the hypothalamic and pituitary regulation of GH secretion.
2. Cellular response to GH: the effect of GH on somatomedin-producing tissues, principally the liver. This effect depends on the binding of GH to its receptors, postreceptor events, and IGF production. It is largely influenced by nutrition.
3. The equilibrium between the circulating somatomedins and peptides acting as inhibitors of the somatomedin activity. This equilibrium is closely related to the nutritional status.
4. The cellular response to somatomedins and hormones in skeletal tissues such as cartilage and bone.

It is beyond the scope of this chapter to comment on the efficacy of hGH therapy in hypopituitary children (17). However, from the many studies evaluating the effects of hGH, it is remarkable that complete catch-up growth is seldom achieved, as would be expected from a fully substitutive therapy (as, for example, in hypothyroidism). Several factors could explain this situation: (a) our inability to mimic fully the true episodic GH secretion, which, at least in the animal, has been shown to be necessary for normal growth; (b) the occurrence of permanent cartilage lesions caused by GH deficiency; however, this has not been demonstrated in animals; (c) one could also speculate on the metabolic and nutritional condition of the children—it is known that hGH administration cannot accelerate the growth rate in extreme cases when calorie intake is insufficient; (d) growth response to hGH could be age related, as it decreases in older children when epiphyseal cartilage is close to fusion. However, quite unexpectedly, we did not observe a better catch-up growth in treated children with a bone age below 3 years than above (18). This inability to recover fully from severe growth retardation (greater than 2 SD) could simply reflect inadequate hGH therapy. Again, these poor results contrast with the full catch-up growth obtained in growth-retarded children with celiac disease when put on a gluten-free diet. They probably recover within a few weeks and have a normal cartilage responsiveness to the circulating somatomedin activity (Fig. 3).

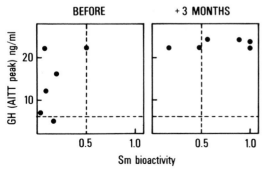

FIG. 3. Changes in GH secretion assessed by the response to the arginine-insulin tolerance test (AITT) and plasma somatomedin bioactivity in children with celiac disease before and after 3 months of gluten-free diet. The most consistent finding is the normal value of somatomedin activity in treated children.

Somatomedins and Growth

The somatomedins, also called insulin-like growth factors (IGF), are polypeptide growth factors named for their functional and structural similarity to insulin. They mediate the growth-promoting action of GH; they have an insulin-independent insulinomimetic effect on adipocytes and stimulate chondrocyte sulfation and cell multiplication in a variety of other cultured cell types. One of these, IGF I or SmC, stimulates skeletal growth when administered to hypopituitary rats (19). It is produced by the liver but has also been isolated from other tissues (20). Circulating levels and tissue content of this peptide in hypophysectomized rats definitely depend on GH (20). This again brings up the concept of paracrine and autocrine control of somatomedins reaching target cells to regulate growth and puts theoretical limits on the clinical significance of circulating SmC levels.

Measurements of IGF I by radioimmunoassay enable easy discrimination between acromegaly and hypopituitarism in adults (21). In children it is necessary to take into account factors such as age and puberty to define normal values. The IGF I concentrations are low at birth and correlate positively with birth weights. They remain in the low range during the first 2 years of life. This is surprising in view of the very high growth rates observed during this period. An increased target tissue ''sensitivity'' has therefore been suggested from studies on cartilage responsiveness in animals and on SmC receptors on circulating monocytes in newborns. It is also possible that during the early postnatal period the fetal paracrine control still has preeminence over endocrine control mechanisms. Plasma IGF I values increase progressively to adult values with a sharp but transient peak at the time of puberty in both sexes (22). As already mentioned for the pattern of pulsatile secretion of GH, there is also a significant correlation between IGF I levels and the stature of the child. This could partly account for the large cross-sectional age-related variations observed in normal children.

The clinical usefulness of IGF I measurements is quite limited. In children between 5 or 6 years of age, they do not give any information on the level of GH secretion. Only normal values are of diagnostic significance in older children, as plasma IGF I can be low in many pathological situations, particularly in undernutrition. In fact, IGF I evaluation has not become a routine technique. However, circulating IGF I values bear some significance by comparison with the level of GH secretion as usually assessed. High GH values contrasting with low IGF I levels are definitely suggestive of nutritional problems such as protein–calorie deficiency. Furthermore, it is not clear whether the IGF I levels should be interpreted with respect to chronological age or to developmental age expressed by bone age or stage of puberty. It may be preferable to use developmental age. Longitudinal studies need to be conducted to analyze the relationship between statural growth and circulating IGF I/SmC levels.

Finally, it is also worth mentioning that some hypopituitary children present with normal growth in the absence of GH secretion but with normal IGF I levels. Growth in these children may have been caused by obesity with hyperinsulinism and/or hyperprolactinemia (24). Other examples of discordance between growth rates and GH/SmC concentrations have been reported (25).

OTHER HORMONES INTERVENING IN SKELETAL GROWTH

The other hormones definitely differ, from a clinical point of view, in their effects on linear growth and bone maturation. Insulin seems to play a role closely similar to other cellular growth factors. Thyroxine is necessary for growth at all ages and has a major effect on bone maturation. The role of hydrocortisone at physiological levels is unclear. Sex steroids dramatically change the course of growth during puberty and accelerate the epiphyseal maturation.

Thyroxine

Thyroid hormones do not play a significant role in the linear skeletal growth of the fetus. As a matter of fact, newborns with thyroid aplasia are of normal size at birth. However, congenital hypothyroidism after birth results immediately in retarded growth (26). The major characteristic and consequence of fetal and postnatal hypothyroidism is the severe retardation of osseous development. Thyroxine (T_4) and/or triiodothyronine (T_3) have a permissive role on and influence the secretion of GH by the pituitary gland as well as the cellular response to somatomedin. Growth hormone does not stimulate growth in hypothyroid children in spite of an increase in SmC levels (27). The most important site of action of thyroid hormones therefore seems to be at the level of the cartilaginous growth plate (28).

Insulin

Insulin deficiency, as observed in inadequately treated diabetes mellitus and in malnutrition, is associated with growth failure (29). Increased insulin levels may contribute to accelerated growth in obese children. Most authors are of the opinion that the primary role of insulin is to regulate fuel homeostasis, enabling other factors to fully control linear growth.

Glucocorticoids

The role of hydrocortisone on growth in normal children is unknown. It has been shown, in pathological situations during treatment with glucocorticoids, that growth is impaired by a minimal excess of corticoid activity. This is largely because of a direct action of corticoids on the target tissue. Incomplete catch-up growth in some of these children is thus probably caused by permanent cartilage damage.

Sex Steroids

The stimulation of growth by gonadal sex steroids depends on the dosage and duration of administration. When given at pharmacological doses, they always cause a disproportionate stimulation of epiphyseal maturation. Their ultimate effect, before puberty, is loss of growth potential and diminished final height. Interestingly, when given at low doses, anabolic steroids, which are considered weak androgens, stimulate growth without modifying GH secretion or circulating SmC levels (30).

In the perinatal period boys grow faster than girls, but their skeletal maturation is slower (14). In view of the higher plasma levels of testosterone in boys, this could indicate that skeletal maturation in the perinatal period does not respond to testosterone (Table 1). This would fit the observation that newborns with congenital adrenal hyperplasia do not exhibit advanced bone age at birth.

Adrenal androgens, which are weak androgens, may be responsible for the mild growth spurt demonstrated at the age of 7 years, which is essentially an acceleration of the growth of the long bones (31).

Analysis of pubertal growth provides a model for the study of the interaction among GH, Sm, and gonadal steroids. Growth hormone plays an undoubtedly major role during puberty by causing the pubertal rise of IGF I. Androgens increase the amplitude of secretory pulses of GH (13). It is likely that estrogens similarly promote GH secretion in girls. There is also some evidence for a direct skeletal action of sex steroids: estrogens, given at very low doses, stimulate the growth of long bones in agonadal girls without modifying circulating IGF I levels (32); in Laron-type dwarfs, characterized by a genetic deficiency of IGF production, a pubertal growth spurt has been reported. More recently, *in vitro* studies in our laboratory have shown that estradiol and testosterone can stimulate chondrocyte

TABLE 1. *Sex differences in growth of infants: boys compared to girls* [a]

	Length	Weight	Skinfolds (subscap.)
Distance			
Birth	+ +	+	
3 months	+ + +	+ + +	−
12 months	+ + +	+ + +	−
Velocity			
0.5 month	−		
2 month	+ + +	+ + +	+
7.5 month	0	+	0
10.5 month	0	0	0

[a]Data adapted from the Zurich longitudinal growth study (14).
+ or − means significantly higher or lower values for boys than for girls.
$0.001 < p < 0.05$.

metabolism in cultured cells taken from pubertal animals. Thus, the pubertal growth spurt might be caused by a complex sequence of events eventually modulated by the level of circulating steroids. In addition, a direct action of GH on epiphyseal cartilage has also been demonstrated in hypophysectomized rats (33). Growth hormone could play a role by stimulating local production of growth factors.

ENDOCRINE ADAPTATION TO NUTRITIONAL ALTERATION

Many studies and monographs have addressed this topic. Our comments are largely derived from the recent review article by Philipps and Unterman (34).

Growth Hormone and Somatomedin-C

Normal growth does not occur in malnutrition despite the presence of normal or increased circulating GH levels (Table 2). This apparent paradox is even more pronounced in protein deficiency. In addition, administration of GH does not benefit children with malnutrition. Acute starvation, chronic enteropathies such as celiac disease (Fig. 3), anorexia nervosa (Fig. 4), and of course protein deficiency and marasmus provide human models for the study of this situation. Anthropometric measurements such as skinfold thickness, arm circumference, body weight, and height changes as well as the measurement of plasma proteins, red blood cell counts, and bone mineralization have been used as indices of the nutritional deficiency. However, we still need a simple and reliable index that could be sensitive enough to detect minimal changes in the nutritional status. Plasma SmC/IGF I is a candidate for this role, especially in children with unexplained short stature whose nutritional status might be suboptimal. Severe malnutrition is associated with very low level of somatomedin by bioassay or SmC by radioimmunoassay and eventually with the presence of circulating sulfation inhibitory peptides. The changes in

TABLE 2. *Clinical conditions characterized by low SmC/IGF I and normal or elevated GH secretion*

Genetic absence of IGF_I/IGF_{II} (Laron dwarfism)
GH dependent dwarfism with normal immunoreactive GH
Idiopathic short stature
Starvation/suboptimal nutrition
    Acute starvation
    Low-calorie/low-protein diet
    Celiac disease
    Psychological dwarfism
    Anorexia nervosa
    Chronic nutritional deficiency

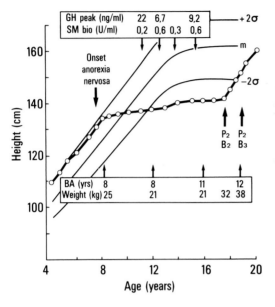

FIG. 4. Slowing down of growth in a girl with anorexia nervosa. Late weight gain was associated with pubertal onset and growth resumption. For several years, the patient exhibited low levels of somatomedin; furthermore, she did not respond to a hGH therapeutic trial (data not shown) performed at the age of 14 years. BA, bone age.

plasma SmC–IGF I levels during fasting correlate positively with changes in nitrogen balance (Fig. 5); they are unresponsive to hGH administration and increase dramatically during refeeding (35). It is likely that similar changes occur in chronic illnesses and kidney diseases, which are usually accompanied by comparable nutritional alterations. More remains to be done to evaluate the information provided by changes of SmC levels in different states of malnutrition of variable intensity (Fig. 6).

FIG. 5. Changes in plasma SmC/IGF₁ and cumulative nitrogen balance in response to nutritional therapy in six patients with Crohn's disease, relapsing pancreatitis, or postgastrectomy syndrome. (From Clemmons et al., ref. 35.)

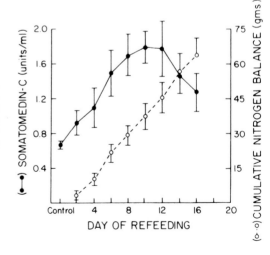

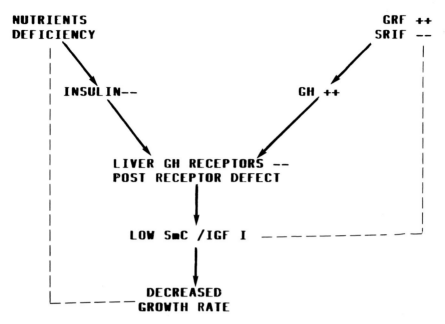

FIG. 6. Sequence of events likely to occur during malnutrition and starvation. Changes at the level of hepatic receptors for GH and the inability to secrete adequate amounts of IGF/SmC play a central role. GH, growth hormone; GRF, growth hormone-releasing factor; SRIF, somatostatin; SmC, somatomedin; IGF I, plasma somatomedin.

Insulin

Hypoinsulinemia plays a role in the adjustment of the metabolic machinery to the growth failure induced by undernutrition. Insulin appears to be linked to the IGF system and to growth in many ways: it regulates cellular nutrition and may stimulate the release of growth factors by increasing the sensitivity to GH (36). Actually, changes in hepatic binding of the growth hormone under conditions of altered nutrition raise the possibility that this could be one of the mechanisms responsible for the changes in IGF I/SmC (37,38).

Cortisol

Catabolism may increase somewhat in marasmus because of the high cortisol levels observed in these patients. This might contribute to the increased loss of muscle protein in children given low-protein diets.

Thyroid

Reduced peripheral conversion of T_4 to T_3 is characteristic of starvation and chronic malnutrition. The organism, as it were, attempts to conserve energy by reducing metabolic expenditure. This is associated with an increased production of reverse T_3.

A paradoxical blunting of the release of thyroid-stimulating hormone in response to thyroid-releasing hormone is also observed. There is thus little evidence to support the diagnosis of hypothyroidism in malnutrition. However, the effects on growth of the low levels of T_3 have not been adequately documented yet. In view of the critical role of T_3 in the control of growth, these changes are probably important for survival.

CONCLUSION

The most important endocrinological findings in malnutrition relate to the GH–somatomedin system. Changes observed appear to be acute markers of change in nitrogen balance and energy intake. It appears likely that the binding capacity of GH binding sites, mainly in the liver, is one of the main regulating factors. This area of clinical investigation and experimental research shows promise as a means for evaluating the impact of nutrition on growth of children.

REFERENCES

1. Wehrenberg WB, Ling N, Böhlen P, Esh F, Brazeau P, Guillemin R. Physiological roles of somatocrinin and somatostatin in the regulation of growth hormone secretion. *Biochem Biophys Res Commun* 1982;109:562–7.
2. Wehrenberg WB, Bloch B, Philips BJ. Antibodies to growth hormone-releasing factor inhibit somatic growth. *Endocrinology* 1984;115:1218–20.
3. Tannenbaum GS, Ling N. The interrelationship of growth hormone (GH)-releasing factor and somatostatin in generation of the ultradian rhythm of growth hormone secretion. *Endocrinology* 1984;115:1952–7.
4. Vance ML, Kaiser DL, Evans WS, et al. Pulsatile growth hormone secretion in normal man during a continuous 24-hour infusion of human growth hormone releasing factor (1–40). Evidence for intermittent somatostatin secretion. *J Clin Invest* 1985;75:1584–90.
5. Tannenbaum GS, Epelbaum J, Colle E, Brazeau P, Martin JB. Antiserum to somatostatin reverses starvation-induced inhibition of growth hormone but not insulin secretion. *Endocrinology* 1978;102:1909–14.
6. Tannenbaum GS. Growth hormone secretory dynamics in streptozotocin diabetes: evidence of a role of endogenous circulating somatostatin. *Endocrinology* 1981;108:76–82.
7. Berelowitz M, Szabo M, Frohman LA, Firestone S, Chu L, Hintz RL. Somatomedin-C mediates growth hormone negative feedback by effects on both the hypothalamus and the pituitary. *Science* 1981;212:1279–81.
8. Brazeau P, Guillemin R, Ling N, Van Wyk J, Humbel R. Inhibition par les somatomédines de la sécrétion de l'hormone de croissance stimulée par le facteur hypothalamique somatocrinine (GRF) ou le peptide de synthèse hpGRF. *C R Acad Sci* [III] 1982;295:651–4.
9. Daughaday WH. Growth hormone and the somatomedins. In: Daughaday WH, ed. Endocrine control of growth. New York: Elsevier, 1983:1–24.
10. Abrams RL, Grumbach MM, Kaplan SL. The effect of administration of human growth hormone on the plasma growth hormone, cortisol, glucose, and free fatty acid response to insulin: evidence for growth hormone autoregulation in man. *J Clin Invest* 1971;50:940–50.
11. Mendelson WB, Jacobs LS, Gillin JC. Negative feedback suppression of sleep-related growth hormone secretion. *J Clin Endocrinol Metab* 1983;56:486–8.

12. Vale W, Vaughan J, Yammoto G, Spiess J, Rivier J. Effects of synthetic human pancreatic (tumor) GH releasing factor and somatostatin, triiodothyronine and dexamethasone on GH secretion in vitro. *Endocrinology* 1983;112:1553–5.
13. Miller JD, Tannenbaum GS, Colle E, Guyda HJ. Daytime pulsatile growth hormone secretion during childhood and adolescence. *J Clin Endocrinol Metab* 1982;55:989–94.
14. Prader A. Biomedical and endocrinological aspects of normal growth and development. In: Boems J, Hanspie R, Sand A. Susanne C, Hebbelinick M, eds. *Human growth and development*. New York: Plenum Press, 1984:1–22.
15. Albertson-Wikland K, Rosberg S, Westphal O. 24 hour-secretory pattern of growth hormone in tall and short children [Abstract]. *Pediatr Res* 1984;18:102.
16. Gourmelen M, Pham-Huu-Trung MT, Girard F. Transient partial hGH deficiency in prepubertal children with delay of growth. *Pediatr Res* 1979;13:221–4.
17. Milner RDG, Russell-Fraser T, Brook CGD, et al. Experience with human growth hormone in Great Britain: the report of the MRC working party. *Clin Endocrinol* (Oxf) 1979;11:15–38.
18. Mugnier E, Ployard F, Roy MP, Fermanian J, Rappaport R. Résultat du traitement par l'hormone de croissance humaine chez les insuffisants hypophysaires âgés de moins de 7 ans. Etude de 26 observations. *Arch Fr Pediatr* 1985;42:671–6.
19. Schoenle E, Zapf J, Humbel RE, Froesch ER. Insulin-like growth factor I stimulates growth in hypophysectomized rats. *Nature* 1982;296:252–3.
20. d'Ercole AJ, Stiles AD, Underwood LE. Tissue concentration of somatomedin-C: further evidence for multiple sites of synthesis and paracrine or autocrine mechanisms of action. *Proc Natl Acad Sci USA* 1984;81:935–9.
21. Furlanetto RW, Underwood LE, Van Wyk JJ, d'Ercole AJ. Estimation of somatomedin-C levels in normals and patients with pituitary disease by radioimmunoassay. *J Clin Invest* 1977;60:648–57.
22. Bala RM, Lopatka J, Leung A, McCoy E, McArthur RG. Serum immunoreactive somatomedin levels in normal adults, pregnant women at term, children at various ages, and children with constitutionally delayed growth. *J Clin Endocrinol Metab* 1981;52:508–12.
23. Gourmelen M, Le Bouc Y, Girard F, Binoux M. Serum levels of insulin-like growth factor (IGF) and IGF binding protein in constitutionally tall children and adolescents. *J Clin Endocrinol Metab* 1984;59:1197–203.
24. Bucher H, Zapf J, Torresani T, Prader A, Froesch ER, Illig R. Insulin-like growth factors I and II, prolactin, and insulin in 19 growth hormone-deficient children with excessive, normal or decreased longitudinal growth after operation for craniopharyngioma. *N Engl J Med* 1983;309:1142–6.
25. Reiter EO, Lovinger RD. The use of a commercially available somatomedin-C radioimmunoassay in patients with disorders of growth. *J Pediatr* 1981;99:720–4.
26. Letarte J, Dussault JH, Guyda H, Fouron C, Glorieux J. Clinical and laboratory investigations of early detected hypothyroid infants. In: Collu R, Ducharme JR, Guyda H, eds. *Pediatric endocrinology*. New York: Raven Press, 1981:433–64.
27. Chernausek SD, Underwood LE, Utiger RD, Van Wyk JJ. Growth hormone secretion and plasma somatomedin-C in hypothyroidism. *Clin Endocrinol* 1983;19:337–44.
28. Froesch ER, Zapf J, Audhya TK, Ben-Porath E, Segen BJ, Gibson KO. Non suppressible insulin-like activity and thyroid hormones: major pituitary-dependent sulfation factors in chick embryo cartilage. *Proc Natl Acad Sci USA* 1976;73:2904–8.
29. Lunn PG, Whitehead RG, Cole TJ, Austin S. The relationship between hormonal balance and growth in malnourished children and rats. *Br J Nutr* 1979;41:73–84.
30. Link K, Blizzard RM, Evans WS, Kaiser DL, Parker MW, Rogol AD. The effect of androgen on the pulsatile release and the twenty four hour mean concentration of growth hormone in peripubertal males. *J Clin Endocrinol Metab* 1986;62:159–64.
31. Molinari L, Largo RH, Prader A. Analysis of the growth spurt at age seven (mid-growth spurt). *Helv Paediat Acta* 1980;35:325–34.
32. Ross JL, Cassorla FG, Skerda MC, Valk IM, Loriaux DL, Cutler GB. A preliminary study of the effect of estrogen dose on growth in Turner's syndrome. *N Engl J Med* 1983;309:1104–6.
33. Isaksson OGP, Jansson JO, Gause IAM. Growth hormone stimulates longitudinal bone growth directly. *Science* 1982;216:1237–9.
34. Phillips LS, Unterman TG. Somatomedin activity in disorders of nutrition and metabolism. *Clin Endocrinol Metab* 1984;13:145–89.
35. Clemmons DR, Underwood LE, Dickerson RN, et al. Use of plasma somatomedin-C/insulin

growth factor I measurements to monitor the response to nutritional repletion in malnourished patients. *Am J Clin Nutr* 1985;41:191–8.
36. Baxter RC, Bryson JM, Turtle JR. Somatogenic receptors of rate liver: regulation by insulin. *Endocrinology* 1980;107:1176–81.
37. Postel-Vinay MC, Cohen-Tanugi E, Charrier J. Growth hormone receptors in rat liver membranes: effects of fasting and refeeding and correlation with plasma somatomedin activity. *Mol Cell Endocrinol* 1982;28:657–69.
38. Maes M, Underwood LE, Gerard G, Ketelslegers JM. Relationship between plasma somatomedin-C and liver somatogenic binding sites in neonatal rats during malnutrition and after short and long term refeeding. *Endocrinology* 1984;115:786–92.

DISCUSSION

Dr. Martorell: When you refer to undernutrition in developing countries, do you mean severe malnutrition? What evidence do we have that there are endocrine disturbances, in milder forms of undernutrition and that these endocrine disturbances, if they exist, are involved in stunting?

Dr. Rappaport: Of course, many of the studies to which I referred are either acute studies on fasting or related to the problem of short stature, in which we still question whether nutritional factors play a role or not. How much are these models relevant to stunting in developing countries? It is difficult to answer that question, but I would imagine that stunting is associated with disturbances of the whole system that regulates skeletal growth, i.e., cartilage activity and bone formation. One of the long-lasting examples that we know of is anorexia nervosa. Anorexia nervosa sometimes occurs in young children, from 5 years onwards. We know that the hormones control growth from the very first weeks or months of life and that the same mechanisms (might) control growth before and after the age of 5. Thus, the same mechanisms could be responsible for growth retardation between the ages of 0 and 5 as well as after 5 years of age. Some children with anorexia nervosa present with total cessation of growth, sometimes as early as 8 years of age and eventually until the age of 19, and only at that time does growth resume if they gain weight and if puberty begins. I would thus assume that this model is appropriate.

Dr. Golden: We have recently been looking at somatomedin-C in Jamaican malnourished children. It follows closely the pattern you have described for patients with celiac disease: it is very low in malnourished children on admission, together with a very high growth hormone level, which comes down although the somatomedin doesn't start to rise for about 30 to 35 days in longitudinal measurements; then it goes up to really quite high levels. We couldn't demonstrate any difference between the somatomedin-C in edematous and non-edematous children. Dr. Smith recently brought specimens from Nigeria to Jamaica and analyzed them at the same time to try to get comparative data on somatomedin-C levels between the Nigerian marasmic kwashiorkor children and the Jamaican ones. She found exactly the same pattern in longitudinal samples taken from Nigeria and Jamaica.

Dr. Milner: It is nearly 20 years since we demonstrated, in the same unit, high GH and low plasma insulin levels and inappropriately low insulin responses to glucose and amino acid challenges (1,2). The loop of the circle has been closed as a result of recent work with rats (3). The maintenance of the GH receptor on the hepatocyte is insulin dependent, and this closes the conceptual circle, because if there is insulin deficiency and failure of maintenance of GH receptors on the hepatocyte, there is a block to GH making somatomedin.

Dr. Rappaport: Until recently all our interest lay in the changes in GH levels that we see in malnourished children: some have very low values, comparable to those found in hypopituitarism, and some have very high values. Our interest has now shifted to the circulating growth factor, somatomedin ($Sm-C/IGF_1$), yet we don't know exactly what its levels mean. We have to be very careful because we do not know exactly what the active and nonactive parts are in the circulating somatomedin that we measure. Somatomedin is bound to proteins, and we don't know how much of it is really active; furthermore, at present we really don't know exactly how the skeleton is able to pick up the somatomedin from the circulating blood in order to grow. There are data showing that local growth factors, including Sm-C, which are produced in many tissues and eventually in the cartilage, are of great importance in the regulation of its growth. So it might turn out that what we see in the blood does not have much relevance and that most of the events occur at a cellular level, in which case it is almost impossible to get an insight. Circulating cells and fibroblasts can be looked at, but we cannot perform biopsies of skeletal tissue in these patients. However, rat models do exist.

Dr. Gopalan: In a comparison of the pattern of adolescent growth in the malnourished and well-nourished, Tanner has made the point that menarche is delayed while the duration of the adolescent growth spurt is prolonged in the undernourished, with the result that they are allowed to grow, for example, until 19 years of age instead of 16 or 17 years, as in well-to-do populations. I would like to know the hormonal mechanism through which this is mediated.

Dr. Rappaport: I don't know of a clear study on hormonal changes comparing these conditions. It has been shown that when the growth spurt occurs later in case of undernutrition or in case of spontaneous delay of puberty—again I don't know to what extent these two conditions are similar—the growth spurt is somewhat less important, and the final height is the same as in normal adolescents. However, this is not relevant to all models. When pubertal growth is very much delayed, the total growth during puberty may not be as important as expected, and these patients might end up with a final height below normal. That is what we see in a small number of patients with anorexia nervosa: the total gain in height during the pubertal growth spurt is less when puberty occurs very late.

Dr. Nabarro: Several workers have noted that there are seasonal differences in the rates of weight gain and length increment in children. In our situation, weight gain appears to be greatest in the months around harvest, and length gain is greatest about 3 months later. We suspect that children with a small postharvest weight gain rate also have a low rate of length increment. Perhaps children are resistant to GH during the preharvest month and need to gain weight subsequently to overcome this resistance and develop adequate somatomedin levels for increased skeletal growth. This would explain the observed interval of about 2 to 3 months between the period of greatest weight gain and the period of greatest height increment.

Dr. Rappaport: I cannot go that far. Your example is unique because we don't have many opportunities to relate these events, weight and height gain, over the years at a population level. One might hypothesize that in your model we could find the sequence of changes in GH and somatomedin that has been described in acute conditions. The point is whether studies of circulating somatomedin would provide more information. Some believe that it is a very sensitive index and that it could be used to monitor very precisely the adequacy of the nutritional supply. However, we are still at the very beginning of using this parameter, and I would not be overenthusiastic about it.

Dr. Martorell: In Bangladesh, it seems to me that what children did first when the food situation improved was to put on weight because they had a low weight for height, and after they had achieved that, then they grew in length. Is that the same as you found?

Dr. Nabarro: Identical. It is about 2 months earlier where we are working than in Bangladesh, but that is because the harvest takes places 2 months earlier.

Dr. Rappaport: May I make a comment on the question of low weight for height. I am still puzzled by the condition in which weight for height is normal and yet the children are undernourished. Here again I come back to the models that I know, although I am not sure that they are relevant in other situations—celiac disease for example. Celiac disease presents itself in two ways. Either it is an acute disease that is clinically diagnosed during the first months of life; these children have diarrhea and are underweight, in which case there is no problem. Or, quite a number of children present with just normal weight for height and look like hypopituitary children. Celiac disease in these children is diagnosed at 5, 6, or 7 years of age, and in fact they are investigated because they are very short. That is puzzling to me for two reasons. First, I don't know how they achieve this equilibrium between weight and height, and sometimes they are even slightly fat; second, several studies have been done—a Belgian group (4) found consistently low values of GH secretion in these children, as in hypopituitarism. In our experience, 80% of the children we have been able to study had normal or high levels of GH (5). Thus, GH secretion is probably extremely variable according to age or to other factors that I don't know about. We can only speculate that all these children have probably an impaired "production" of cellular growth factors. Malnourished children frequently present with normal weight for height. What does a normal weight for height mean, compared to low weight for height, in terms of risk or metabolic balance? It seems to me that hormonal changes are just superimposed, but I don't think they explain what is happening.

Dr. Tomkins: You mentioned two studies on GH in celiac disease, yours and someone else's, which showed different results. Could the difference not be attributed to differences in food intake in the week preceding the measurement? Quite a number of studies in celiac disease have shown a profound decrease in food intake (30%), certainly in teenagers and adults, comparable to the poor nutrient intake in chronic diarrhea, which is indeed associated with longitudinal growth faltering. What do you think is the effect of differences in food intake as opposed to nutritional status, weight for height, or height for age? Could these explain the differences?

Dr. Rappaport: That is a good point. I have absolutely no data on the food intake at the time of the study in either case. All I can say is that none of these children had any diarrhea at the time of the study. Thus, the mechanisms explaining the limitation of the nutrient supply, which I suppose exists in these children, is still unclear.

Dr. Hernandez: Do you have any data about the 24-hr secretion of GH in these celiac patients or about the response to the GRF stimulus?

Dr. Rappaport: I have no data on the 24-hr secretion of GH in these patients. Regarding your second question, a Chilean study showed that the response to GRF in undernourished children was normal, but I don't know exactly the details of the population that was studied.

Dr. Waterlow: I found fascinating the attempt in the discussion to see how we could bring Professor Rappaport's models, which are basically clinical, close to those of the Third World. This has given us a tremendous stimulus to look for an appropriate model in the light of the data Dr. Rappaport describes. What about the effect on growth of mild iodine deficiency, which is very common throughout large parts of Asia, Africa, and South America? Of course, severely iodine-deficient infants present with stunted growth. What, however, is the effect of mild iodine deficiency and reduced thyroid hormone production on the growth factors you have been discussing?

Dr. Rappaport: Extreme situations are much better documented than milder deficiencies. Extreme hypothyroidism induces GH deficiency and eventually also somatomedin deficiency, which is probably secondary to GH deficiency. When a hypothyroid child is treated with thyroid hormone, he thereafter has a normal GH secretion. However, it is not clear whether catch-up growth, which is very rapid in the treated hypothyroid child, occurs prior to normalization of GH secretion and somatomedin levels. There are very few data, especially longitudinal data, on this aspect.

Dr. Davies: Would you care to speculate why birth seems to switch the control of growth from one largely autocrine and paracrine to one more endocrine? In those infants who are born very prematurely, does this switch take place at the same time? Is this simply part of a maturational march, or is there another reason for the switch?

Dr. Rappaport: Even when a child is born prematurely, TSH and thyroid function mature in the first 24 hr, as they would in a child who is born at term. There is a switch. Most people working in developmental biology are looking for a change in the genetic expression at the time of birth, just before, or just after, explaining why some signals appear all of a sudden at birth. For instance, there are two growth factors: somatomedin-C, or IGF I and IGF II. The IGF II is more important for fetal growth; it has been demonstrated in the rat that IGF II decreases after birth, when it probably becomes less important than IGF I, which is totally GH dependent. Thus, the GH dependence of growth that occurs at birth goes along with a rapid increase of IGF I. Although these data cannot be transferred to the human yet, they give some information about possible changes in the genetic expression for the synthesis of these growth factors that could explain how the body at the time of birth comes under the control of GH, which prior to birth is of no importance. Dr. Milner, would you like to comment further on this?

Dr. Milner: I think the switch is related to parturition, in particular, to the switch to enteric nutrition as opposed to intravenous nutrition via the umbilical cord, and to the removal of placental lactogen. Everything else you said I agree with.

Dr. Kraisid: Has any relationship between the level of physical activity or exercise and growth factors been documented? Since changes in growth velocity are observed during various seasons when children could increase or decrease their physical activity, is there any evidence that hormonal changes also occur during periods of increased activity?

Dr. Rappaport: I am not very familiar with the relationship between hormones and physical activity. Here again, we always look at very extreme models. Athletes are one of the extreme models of intensive physical activity. These people are probably in a very special situation: they present with something like a nutrient deficiency because they behave very much like anorexia nervosa patients and on top of it have a strenuous physical activity. As a result, they frequently grow less than normal, puberty is delayed, and they sometimes end up shorter. However, I have no data on regular physical activity in undernourished populations; it might be a totally different situation.

REFERENCES

1. Milner RDG. Metabolic and hormonal responses to glucose and glucagon in patients with infantile malnutrition. *Pediatr Res* 1971;5:33–9.
2. Milner RDG. Metabolic and hormonal responses to oral amino acids in infantile malnutrition. *Arch Dis Child* 1971;46:301–5.

3. Binoux M, Lassère C, Hardouin M. Somatomedin production by rat liver in organ culture. III. Studies on the release of insulin-like growth factor and its carrier protein measured by radioligand assays. Effects of growth hormone, insulin and cortisol. *Acta Endocrinol* 1982;29:422–30.
4. Vanderschueren-Lodeweyckx M, Wolter R, Molla A, Eggermont E, Eeckels R. Plasma growth hormone in coeliac disease. *Helv Paediatr Acta* 1973;28:349–57.
5. Bresson JL, Prévot C, Rappaport R, Czernichow P, Rey J. Activité somatomédine circulante et sécrétion d'hormone de croissance. II. Modifications au cours de la maladie coeliaque à révélation tardive et effets du traitement. *Arch Fr Pediatr* 1979;36(suppl 9):XIII–XVIII.

Linear Growth Retardation in Less Developed Countries, edited by John C. Waterlow. Nestlé Nutrition Workshop Series, Vol. 14. Nestec Ltd., Vevey/Raven Press, Ltd., New York © 1988.

Nutritional Growth Retardation: Experimental Studies with Special Reference to Calcium

D. R. Fraser

Dunn Nutritional Laboratory, University of Cambridge and Medical Research Council, Cambridge CB4 1XJ, England

A universal observation in vertebrate biology is that a low plane of nutrition in early life slows the rate of growth and, if it persists may result in small stature at maturity. The retardation in length of long bones can be attributed directly to diminished growth of epiphyseal cartilage, which becomes narrow with a decreased rate of chondrocyte proliferation (1–3). The synthesis of bone matrix collagen in particular appears to be depressed (4,5), although the incorporation of bone mineral is apparently unaffected (2–4) and resorption of bone mineral is similarly unimpaired (3,4). If the undernourished animals are subsequently rehabilitated, bone growth returns to normal, although in pigs, growth ceases at the same chronological age as in those animals that were adequately fed (6), so that the adults are stunted. Although bone structure is restored on rehabilitation, teeth may remain small, with permanent abnormalities in their fine structure (7). It has also been found that bones of pigs growing after protein deficiency may become bent and twisted, whereas such deformities are infrequent in recovery from deficiency of calories alone (8).

Young rats with maximum growth rate have been compared with those having a marginal degree of undernutrition by the simple technique of raising litters with large or small numbers of rat pups (9). Here the slower growth was associated with skeletons that were not only smaller but had poor structural development.

These changes in hard tissues are part of the general response of the whole body to gross nutritional deficiency and are inevitable consequences of cell malfunction when cells are starved of the molecules required for tissue growth. How much more likely are growth failure and abnormal development of bone with selective deficiency of the specific mineral elements required for bone structure itself? Experimental studies bearing on this question are reviewed in this chapter.

CALCIUM HOMEOSTASIS

One of the unifying characteristics among vertebrates is the presence in all of sensitive control mechanisms for maintaining a constant extracellular ionized calcium (Ca^{2+}) concentration (10). Although the mechanisms differ between aquatic and land vertebrates, in every species examined Ca^{2+} concentration in serum is kept close to 1.25 mM. Any tendency for this level to rise causes excretory pathways to remove the excess. On the other hand, with a tendency for Ca^{2+} concentration to decline, an adaptive capacity develops for enhanced absorption of calcium from the environment (diet), and sometimes internal calcium stores are mobilized as well. The sensitivity of nerve, muscle, and endocrine cells in particular to changes in extracellular Ca^{2+} concentration requires that that concentration be kept constant.

When there is a deficiency of calcium during growth, competition exists between the calcium that is required for incorporation into bone and that required to maintain the extracellular ion pool. The importance of the latter for the function of all cells gives it precedence over bone mineralization. Hence, with a prolonged inadequate supply of calcium, either bone would be undermineralized or its growth would have to cease.

However, just as constancy of extracellular Ca^{2+} concentration is important for cells in general, so also is it important for the bone-forming role of chondrocytes and osteoblasts. Deficiency of dietary calcium would not only starve bone of its substrate for growth but could lead to defective function of bone cells.

Thus, in principle, calcium deficiency could provoke two alternative responses:

1. Growth continues at a rate commensurate with the supply of other nutrients (energy and protein), but the bone is undermineralized with a defective structure.
2. Growth is retarded to a rate at which the limited calcium supply allows normally structured and mineralized (but smaller) bone to be formed.

EXPERIMENTAL INVESTIGATION OF THE CONSEQUENCES OF CALCIUM DEFICIENCY ON BONE GROWTH

Despite a large body of research accumulated over many years on the effect of variable calcium supply on bone growth in laboratory and other animals, very little of this has related the actual supply of calcium to the rate of growth. Most studies have created severe deficiency, suddenly imposed, and usually observed for a relatively short time of a few days or a few weeks. The long-term consequences of continuous deprivation of calcium during the total period of growth have seldom been investigated. Many of the published experiments have been concerned with the effect of calcium deficiency on the metabolism and function of vitamin D. Many were aimed at devising an experimental, diet-induced osteoporosis model to compare with the widespread osteoporosis of postmenopausal women (e.g., 11).

Any significance of a lack of calcium has been overshadowed by the observation that phosphorus deficiency has a much more striking effect on growth and development than does calcium deficiency. The importance of calcium supply is often assessed in relation to the dietary calcium : phosphorus ratio. For most species, variation in the calcium : phosphorus ratio away from an optimum value leads to impaired growth and development of bones. However, because the influence of phosphorus on variable bone growth is more apparent than that of calcium, any specific effect of calcium may have been neglected. For growing children, phosphorus deficiency has not been identified as a practical problem, yet calcium intake well below recommended values is commonly found in malnourished communities.

Farm animal studies of undernutrition are often concerned with the efficiency of production rather than long-term consequences for adult life. Hence, the effect of calcium and phosphorus supply on food intake and the efficiency of food conversion are of prime importance (12). An undergrown farm animal is a poor economic unit, so interest lies in the optimization of diet and growth rate, and there is little incentive to follow the long-term consequences of malnourished curiosities, which predictably have low economic prospects.

Studies in Man

Poor growth in children is a characteristic of chronic illness, particularly in renal failure and inflammatory bowel disease. The etiology of stunting in renal disease is complex and multifactorial (13), and undernutrition is seldom the major cause of the problem. On the other hand, growth retardation in celiac disease can be more directly linked to intestinal malabsorption in the face of an apparently adequate diet. As Samuel Gee wrote in 1888 (14): "while the disease is active, children cease to grow; even when it tends slowly to recovery, they are left frail and stunted." Nevertheless, although calcium absorption can be markedly diminished with the abnormal intestinal mucosa, the bone of the affected children appears to be normally mineralized for their height and weight (15). Furthermore, analysis of all the many factors influencing growth in chronic malabsorption suggests that insufficiency of energy is of greater significance than protein, vitamin, or mineral deficiencies (16). Therefore, where there is an inadequate supply of several nutrients, it does appear that lack of calcium is not the limiting factor for growth.

One further complication in attempting to assess the role of nutrients on bone growth and mineralization is that nutritional and endocrine factors are not the only ones involved. Repetitive exercise and physical activity also enhance the density of bone (17). The influence of mineral nutrient supply on the long-term growth of bone in humans is not readily apparent from investigations so far.

Studies in Animals

Scattered in the earlier literature are reports of experiments in which dietary calcium was restricted for growing rats (18), puppies (19), and kittens (20). In each instance, the efficiency of retaining dietary calcium was much greater on a low-calcium diet, but bone abnormalities were surprisingly unspectacular. However, severe calcium deficiency, with a dietary content of only 0.03 to 0.05% dry weight, did induce gross skeletal retardation in rats (18) and kittens (20,21), and marked osteopenia was observed (21).

The effect of calcium deprivation is clearly different between adult and growing animals. Adult rats fed a low-calcium, high-phosphorus meat diet survived with little or no sign of abnormality. On such a diet, weanling rats stopped growing after a few weeks and then died (22). The skeletons of these young rats with calcium deficiency had become severely demineralized and often showed fractures.

If, however, the diet were supplemented with 0.2% calcium for 14 days, the rats grew at almost the normal rate, and their bones were of similar size and shape to those given a continuous and adequate supply of calcium. Yet the bone mineral content of these calcium-deprived rats was only about 50% that of the controls (22). Only when the bone ash had decreased to 30% or less of the control values did the rate of growth decline. In the rat, therefore, it appears that growth takes precedence over the mineralization of bone and that bone continues to grow even though the incorporation of mineral is low.

Such a study relating calcium supply and bone mineralization to growth has apparently not yet been done in man. Nevertheless, the dimensions, composition, and density of bones from communities with a low calcium intake are reported to be similar to those where calcium supply is deemed to be adequate (23). Furthermore, such diets were not associated with the development of osteoporosis.

ADAPTATION TO LOW-CALCIUM DIET

The necessity for vitamin D when there is enhanced calcium absorption has been known for more than 50 years, but the discovery in the past 15 years of the functional metabolism of vitamin D has partly revealed the mechanism by which this adaptation takes place. Nicolaysen postulated that there existed an endogenous factor that stimulated calcium absorption when calcium supply was inadequate (24). It is now clear that Nicolaysen's factor is mainly, if not entirely, the metabolite 1,25-dihydroxyvitamin D [$1,25(OH)_2D$]. When there is an increased requirement for calcium, the synthesis of $1,25(OH)_2D$ in the kidney is increased (25). This metabolite passes into the circulation and is taken up by many cell types in which it associates with specific, high-affinity binding proteins ("receptors"). This protein complex with $1,25(OH)_2D$ is then thought to mediate the vitamin D effect by inducing new protein synthesis in the manner of the standard steroid hormones.

The action of $1,25(OH)_2D$ in the cells of the intestinal mucosa is to increase the capacity for active transport of calcium. Hence, the central concept in the mechanism of adaptation is an endocrine loop. During growth, pregnancy, and lactation, when there is an increased demand for calcium, $1,25(OH)_2D$ synthesis is also increased, and the intestinal absorption capacity for calcium rises. As the demand for calcium declines, the synthesis of $1,25(OH)_2D$ also declines.

If growth suddenly ceases because of insufficient supply of protein or energy, the absorptive capacity for calcium declines abruptly (26,27). This would be predicted by the theory of an endocrine loop, and it is assumed (but has not been demonstrated) that in undernutrition the synthesis of $1,25(OH)_2D$ is suppressed although the synthesis of other metabolites, 25-hydroxyvitamin D [25(OH)D] and 24,25-dihydroxyvitamin D [$24,25(OH)_2D$] are apparently unaffected (28).

There is, however, a problem with this interpretation of the adaptation being mediated entirely by $1,25(OH)_2D$ according to the prevailing need for calcium. It has been shown that in growing children the synthesis of $1,25(OH)_2D$ is not just regulated according to the demands of calcium homeostasis. The concentration of $1,25(OH)_2D$ in the plasma of children has been found to be directly related to the concentration of its precursor, 25(OH)D (29). Hence, not only does variation in calcium status control the synthesis of $1,25(OH)_2D$, it is also determined by the vagaries of vitamin D status [25(OH)D level in plasma]. The absolute level of $1,25(OH)_2D$ cannot then be linked directly to the degree of response in the target cells.

From this it follows that homeostatic regulation of calcium absorption may depend on some other factor acting in concert with $1,25(OH)_2D$ in the intestine. Such a factor (or factors) might modify the number of receptors for $1,25(OH)_2D$ (30) or might modulate the activity of proteins induced by $1,25(OH)_2D$ in the mucosal cells. However, because in other circumstances the production of $1,25(OH)_2D$ has been clearly shown to be related to growth (31,32), it must nevertheless be the major influence in the adaptation to a low-calcium diet.

Of course, in vitamin D deficiency the ability to absorb calcium is greatly impaired, and the rate of bone growth is markedly reduced (33). However, as vitamin D functions in such a wide variety of cells, the effect of its absence must compromise growth in a multiplicity of ways other than merely interfering with the utilization of dietary calcium for the growth of bone.

AVAILABILITY OF DIETARY CALCIUM

The proportion of dietary calcium that is actually retained is seldom more than 50% and usually, in adults, is no more than 30% (34). There are two explanations for any variation in the limited amount of calcium that is absorbed. As described above, the adaptive increase in absorptive capacity can improve the availability of calcium. The other modifying factor is variable interaction of calcium with other dietary components in the lumen of the gut.

In general, such interaction tends to decrease the availability of calcium. However, in the special case of milk and milk products, calcium absorption is promoted by the presence of other constituents. Lactose specifically enhances the uptake of Ca^{2+} across the brush border of mucosal cells (35,36). The mechanism by which this occurs is unknown, but there is some evidence to suggest that lactose diminishes the sodium content of the mucosa with a resulting hyperpolarization of the brush border membrane, favoring the entry of calcium. Casein also promotes calcium absorption, mediated by phosphopeptides produced during proteolytic digestion (37,38). These phosphopeptides form soluble complexes with Ca^{2+} and increase its availability for absorption in the ileum.

Apart from dairy products, dietary calcium comes mainly from fruit, vegetables, and cereal grains. Three components of plant foods are known to form complexes with calcium that decrease its availability. These are complexes with phytate (39), oxalate (40), and unavailable carbohydrate (dietary fiber) (41,42). In comparison with milk, plant foods have a lower content of calcium, much of which is unavailable for absorption by the small intestine.

Although an increased absorptive capacity of the small intestine can, in principle, provide more calcium for bone growth and development, if this calcium is complexed in an unavailable form, then the increased absorptive capacity will be ineffective in raising the calcium supply.

Adaptation to a low-calcium diet is usually considered to be a capability of the small intestine only, yet the colon also has some capacity for absorbing calcium. Calcium deficiency in experimental rats and in humans with the short bowel syndrome leads to an increased absorption of calcium by the colon (43,44). As with the small intestine, this adaptation in the colon is mediated by $1,25(OH)_2D$ (45). Because bacteria in the colon are able to break down any fiber and phytate that has resisted enzymatic digestion in the small intestine, the complexed calcium carried into the colon could then be available for absorption. If children on a persistently low calcium intake have an adaptive increase in calcium absorption by the colon, then the availability of calcium from cereal, vegetable, and fruit diets may be much higher than has hitherto been considered likely. Such a possibility has yet to be investigated.

INFLUENCE OF CALCIUM DEFICIENCY ON VITAMIN D STATUS

With the discovery of 25(OH)D, it has been possible to determine the adequacy of vitamin D supply. The concentration of 25(OH)D in plasma reflects the amount of vitamin D obtained from the environment (46). By comparing seasonal variation in the plasma levels of 25(OH)D to variation in both the oral intake of vitamin D and the exposure of skin to ultraviolet light, it is evident that in western Europe vitamin D status is determined mainly by solar irradiation. Dietary vitamin D at less than 5 μg per day has little significance in adults except when vitamin D reserves are very low (46).

It is therefore a paradox that those areas of the world where vitamin-D-deficiency rickets is more common, such as India (47), Egypt (48), Saudi Arabia (49), and Greece (50), are regions where the sun shines in abundance. Such observations raise the possibility of some other factor in these sunny countries that might reduce the efficiency of utilization of the vitamin D formed in skin.

Research in our laboratory has recently demonstrated in rats that deficiency of calcium enhances the hepatic destruction of vitamin D and, depending on the supply, leads sooner or later to vitamin D deficiency. With secondary hyperpara-thyroidism, the production of $1,25(OH)_2D$ is increased, and this metabolite acts in the liver, stimulating the metabolic inactivation of vitamin D.

Vitamin D deficiency is most often found in those countries where both the intake and the availability of dietary calcium are low. Of course, vitamin D deficiency causes a more acute response on bone development than does a prolonged low intake of calcium, and the effect of simple vitamin D deficiency is readily apparent. What might not be so obvious is any deleterious influence on growth of combined low status of vitamin D and calcium. In communities where calcium intake is low, the possibility of such a combined deficiency should be considered.

GENERAL CONCLUSIONS

From the experimental research summarized in this chapter, a number of problems can be identified concerning the influence of a low calcium intake on the growth of children.

The recommended dietary allowance for calcium ranges between 500 and 1,200 mg/day. If milk is not included in the diet, it is difficult to see how such levels could be achieved without food fortification. Because many populations receive considerably less than the recommended intake of calcium, it is necessary to determine whether these apparently low supplies have deleterious consequences. More information is needed on whether adaptation by children to calcium intakes significantly below those recommended is able to compensate for the shortfall. Although balance data on well-fed individuals on a Western diet do indicate the amount of dietary calcium that is retained, such information may not be applicable to malnourished children. Certainly, when young children are recovering from malnutrition, the amount of dietary calcium that is retained may be as high as 87% (51).

Studies in the rat indicate that, provided the diet is not severely deficient in calcium, growth takes precedence over bone formation. There is no information about whether children with a low supply of calcium also have normal stature but bone undermineralization.

If children are receiving inadequate amounts of energy or protein, does a superimposed dietary deficiency of calcium further promote their failure to thrive?

The relationship between calcium supply and long-term growth has not been studied in experimental animals. To decide whether calcium deficiency is a cause of stunting requires that this possibility be specifically investigated in children.

REFERENCES

1. Pratt CWM, McCance RA. Severe undernutrition in growing and adult animals. 12. The structure of the long bones in pigs. *Br J Nutr* 1964;18:393–408.
2. LeRoith D, Pimstone BL. Bone metabolism and composition in the protein-deprived rat. *Clin Sci* 1973;44:305–19.

3. Kuramitsu N, Matsui T, Yano H, Kawashima R. The influence of protein and/or energy deficiency on the growth of long bone in rats. *J Nutr Sci Vitaminol (Tokyo)* 1985;31:189–96.
4. Dickerson JWT, McCance RA. Severe undernutrition in growing and adult animals. 8. The dimensions and chemistry of the long bones. *Br J Nutr* 1961;15:567–76.
5. Nakamoto T, Miller SA. The effect of protein–energy malnutrition on the development of bones in newborn rats. *J Nutr* 1979;109:1469–76.
6. Lister D, McCance RA. Severe undernutrition in growing and adult animals. 17. The ultimate result of rehabilitation: pigs. *Br J Nutr* 1967;21:787–99.
7. McCance RA, Owens PDA, Tonge CH. Severe undernutrition in growing and adult animals. 18. The effects of rehabilitation on the teeth and jaws of pigs. *Br J Nutr* 1968;22:357–68.
8. Adams P. The effect of experimental malnutrition on the development of long bones. *Bibl Nutr Dieta* 1969;13:69–73.
9. Dickerson JWT, Widdowson EM. Some effects of accelerating growth. II. Skeletal development. *Proc Roy Soc Lond [Biol]* 1960;152:207–13.
10. Urist MR. The regulation of calcium and other ions in the serums of hagfish and lampreys. *Ann NY Acad Sci* 1963;109:294–311.
11. Shah BG, Krishnarao GVG, Draper HH. The relationship of Ca and P nutrition during adult life and osteoporosis in aged mice. *J Nutr* 1967;92:30–42.
12. Field AC, Suttle NF, Nisbet DI. Effect of diets low in calcium and phosphorus on the development of growing lambs. *J. Agr Sci* 1975;85:435–42.
13. Hodson EM, Shaw PF, Evans RA, et al. Growth retardation and renal osteodystrophy in children with chronic renal failure. *J Pediatr* 1983;103:735–40.
14. Gee S. On the coeliac affection. *St Bartholomew's Hosp Rep* 1888;24:17–20.
15. Exner GU, Sacher M, Shmerling DH, Prader A. Growth retardation and bone mineral status in children with coeliac disease recognized after the age of 3 years. *Helv Paediatr Acta* 1978;33:497–507.
16. Kirschner BS, Voinchet O, Rosenberg IH. Growth retardation in inflammatory bowel disease. *Gastroenterology* 1978;75:504–11.
17. Emiola L, O'Shea JP. Effects of physical activity and nutrition on bone density measured by radiographic techniques. *Nutr Rep Int* 1978;17:669–81.
18. Sherman HC, MacLeod FL. The calcium content of the body in relation to age, growth and food. *J Biol Chem* 1925;64:429–34.
19. Gershoff SM, Legg MA, Hegsted DM. Adaptation to different calcium intakes in dogs. *J Nutr* 1958;64:303–12.
20. Roberts AH, Scott PP. Nutrition of the cat. 5. The influence of calcium and iodine supplements to a meat diet on the retention of nitrogen, calcium and phosphorus. *Br J Nutr* 1961;15:73–82.
21. Scott PP, Greaves JP, Scott MG. Nutrition of the cat. 4. Calcium and iodine deficiency on a meat diet. *Br J Nutr* 1961;15:35–51.
22. Moore T, Impey SG, Martin PEN, Symonds KR. Meat diets. II. Effect of the age of rats on their ability to withstand the low calcium intake induced by a diet of minced beef. *J Nutr* 1963;80:162–70.
23. Walker ARP. The human requirement of calcium: should low intakes be supplemented? *Am J Clin Nutr* 1972;25:518–30.
24. Nicolaysen R. The absorption of calcium as a function of the body saturation with calcium. *Acta Physiol Scand* 1943;5:201–12.
25. Fraser DR. Regulation of the metabolism of vitamin D. *Physiol Rev* 1980;60:551–613.
26. Adams PH, Hill LF, Wain D, Taylor C. The effects of undernutrition and its relief on intestinal calcium transport in the rat. *Calcif Tissue Res* 1974;16:293–304.
27. Younoszai MK, Ghishan FK. In vivo intestinal calcium transport in infant rats: Normal and growth retarded. *J Nutr* 1979;109:573–9.
28. Philbrick D-J, Hollis BW, Draper HH. Effects of a protein deficiency on plasma levels of 25-hydroxyvitamin D and 24,25-dihydroxyvitamin D in the rat. *Am J Clin Nutr* 1980;33:2174–6.
29. Stern PH, Taylor AB, Bell NH, Epstein S. Demonstration that circulating 1-alpha,25-dihydroxyvitamin-D is loosely regulated in normal children. *J Clin Invest* 1981;68:1374–7.
30. Bar A, Rosenberg J, Hurwitz S. Induced changes in the affinity of 1,25-dihydroxyvitamin-D_3 receptors in chick intestine. *FEBS Lett* 1983;163:261–4.
31. Bushinsky DA, Favus MJ, Coe FL. Elevated $1,25(OH)_2D_3$, intestinal absorption, and renal mineral conservation in male rats. *Am J Physiol* 1984;246:F140–F145.

32. Bar A, Hurwitz S. Relationships between cholecalciferol metabolism and growth in chicks as modified by age, breed and diet. *J Nutr* 1981;111:399–404.
33. Halloran BP, DeLuca HF. Effect of vitamin D deficiency on skeletal development during early growth in the rat. *Arch Biochem Biophys* 1981;209:7–14.
34. Nordin BEC, Horsman A, Marshall DH, Simpson M, Waterhouse GM. Calcium requirement and calcium therapy. *Clin Orthop* 1979;140:216–46.
35. Pansu D, Bellaton C, Bronner F. Effect of lactose on duodenal calcium-binding protein and calcium absorption. *J Nutr* 1979;109:508–12.
36. Favus MJ, Angeid-Backman E. Effects of lactose on calcium absorption and secretion by rat ileum. *Am J Physiol* 1984;246:G281–5.
37. Lee YS, Noguchi T, Naito H. Phosphopeptides and soluble calcium in the small intestine of rats given a casein diet. *Br J Nutr* 1980;43:457–67.
38. Mykkänen HM, Wasserman RH. Enhanced absorption of calcium by casein phosphopeptides in rachitic and normal chicks. *J Nutr* 1980;110:2141–8.
39. Wise A. Dietary factors determining the biological activities of phytate. *Nutr Abstr Rev A* 1983;53:791–806.
40. Johnston FA, McMillan TJ, Falconer GD. Calcium retained by young women before and after adding spinach to the diet. *J Am Diet Assoc* 1952;28:933–8.
41. James WPT, Branch WJ, Southgate DAT. Calcium binding by dietary fibre. *Lancet* 1978;1:638–9.
42. Cummings JH, Hill MJ, Jivraj T, Houston H, Branch WJ, Jenkins DJA. The effect of meat protein and dietary fiber on colonic function and metabolism. 1. Changes in bowel habit, bile acid excretion, and calcium absorption. *Am J Clin Nutr* 1979;32:2086–93.
43. Favus MJ. Factors that influence absorption and secretion of calcium in the small intestine and colon. *Am J Physiol* 1985;248:G147–57.
44. Hylander E, Ladefoged K, Jarnum S. The importance of the colon in calcium absorption following small-intestinal resection. *Scand J Gastroenterol* 1980;15:55–60.
45. Grinstead WC, Pak CYC, Krejs GJ. Effect of 1,25-dihydroxyvitamin D_3 on calcium absorption in the colon of healthy humans. *Am J Physiol* 1984;247:G189–92.
46. Fraser DR. The physiological economy of vitamin D. *Lancet* 1983;1:969–72.
47. Pramanik AK, Gupta S, Agarwal PS. Rickets in protein calorie malnutrition. *Indian Pediatr* 1971;8:195–9.
48. Golal OM, El Nabawy MI, Hassan A. Incidence of rickets in two children populations in Egypt. *Ain Shams Med J* 1970;21:133–40.
49. Elidrissy ATH, Sedrani SH. Infantile vitamin D deficiency rickets in Riyadh. *Calcif Tissue Int* 1980;33:47–52.
50. Lapatsanis P, Deliyanni V, Doxiadis S. Vitamin D deficiency rickets in Greece. *J Pediatr* 1968;73:195–202.
51. de Portela ML, Zeni S, Piazza N, Rio ME. Calcium balance in infants recovering from undernutrition. *Nutr Rep Int* 1982;26:1045–51.

DISCUSSION

Dr. Rappaport: You didn't mention a problem that might be of interest to discuss: How do we evaluate clinically the calcium status of malnourished children? What is supposed to be a reliable index of the calcium status in various conditions of severe or less severe undernutrition? You did not mention urinary calcium.

Dr. Fraser: That is a very good point. The evaluation of calcium status is a particularly tricky thing; it has usually been done by inference, that if the calcium supply is low, then calcium status must be low, and it is well known that calcium supply is low in a large number of populations. Probably the most effective way of measuring calcium status is by measuring the mineralization of bone; the only really efficient way of doing this is by taking the bone and ashing it, which of course is not a practical prospect in population studies. There is, however, the technique of single-photon absorptiometry of bone, which I think might be of great significance. This is a process by which one can measure the attenuation of a photon beam going through bone and, by computation, calculate from this attenuation the amount of mineral that is actually in the bone. This can be done very easily with little interference with the subject. We have been doing this type of work, looking at the mineralization of the radius in children in Gambia and in Great Britain, but the data have not been analyzed yet. Looking at the raw figures, it seems that there is very little difference between the mineralization of the bones in children in Gambia, on a very low calcium intake, and that of the bones of children in Cambridge. The conclusion from this would have to be either that children were growing more slowly in Gambia, which does not appear to be the case (provided that other nutrients have been supplied in reasonable amounts), or they are absorbing calcium in their diet much more efficiently than one would have predicted from what we know of calcium balance of children in affluent societies.

Dr. Waterlow: Is it not the case that Pettifor, in South Africa, has described vitamin D deficiency consequent to low calcium intake?

Dr. Fraser: Yes, this is true. The studies that he did (1) were with young children who, to his surprise, had clear signs of rickets in the face of adequate 25-hydroxyvitamin D levels. It is probably true that if the supply of substrate for bone formation is greatly diminished, then the clinical effect or the radiological appearance of the bone is very similar to that produced by frank vitamin D deficiency. Except in children during times of rapid growth, frank calcium deficiency probably doesn't produce exactly the same effects on bone as vitamin D deficiency.

Dr. Waterlow: You discussed plasma phosphorus levels in animals on a low-calcium diet, and I couldn't quite grasp what was happening to the phosphates. Could you elaborate on that?

Dr. Fraser: The plasma phosphate in those animals was elevated. This is somewhat surprising because in the face of hyperparathyroidism, which would enhance the excretion of phosphorus by the kidney, one could imagine that the plasma phosphorus, if anything, would be low. But these animals were on an extremely low calcium diet, and they were still growing; in fact, their growth rate was only marginally less than that of the controls. Their bone mineralization was greatly reduced, and I think the plasma phosphorus had been elevated merely because the bone mineral had been so rapidly resorbed that the rate of delivery of phosphorus to the plasma was greater than the rate of excretion of phosphorus by the kidney.

Dr. Valyasevi: Could you comment on the situation that exists in rural northeast Thailand, where there is endemic bladder stone disease. The oral phosphate intake in that area is extremely low, as well as the urinary excretion, about 1/10 of what is measured in children from Bangkok. Calcium intake is low too, 200 to 250 mg/day in preschool children, but phosphate intake is even less than that. We did a survey of about 200 preschool children living in the village. Of these, we found four or five cases of radiological rickets; serum alkaline phosphatase was high in general. To prevent bladder stone disease, we gave a supplement of phosphate, about 60 mg of phosphorus per kilogram per day, roughly 600 mg per day. If we give this supplement on a long-term basis, will it have any kind of undesirable effect on bone mineralization? In such cases, with an extremely low intake, how do adaptation mechanisms operate?

Dr. Fraser: The situation in man may be different from that in experimental animals. In rats, when you increase the amount of phosphorus in the diet, it has a negative effect on the absorption and availability of calcium, but in man this doesn't seem to be quite so important; the phosphorus content of the diet probably has to go up considerably more in man to cause an impairment of calcium absorption. On the other hand, if the calcium supply is very low, this will probably enhance the availability of phosphorus when the phosphorus supply is also limited. So it may well be that in children who have got both a low calcium supply and not a very high phosphorus intake, their phosphorus availability could be enhanced because of the low calcium in the diet. If the rickets, which you say is present in this community, is really because of a low vitamin D status and not any other cause, that could be related to the low calcium supply. The easiest way of treating this would be merely to enhance the availability of calcium without supplying extra vitamin D. Because these children are presumably also vitamin D deficient, the way to correct this is of course to insure that they get exposed to sunlight.

A particular puzzle has been to explain why vitamin D deficiency seems to occur in regions where there is plenty of sunlight. We know that most vitamin D comes from the effect of sunlight on vitamin D formation in skin. The two things can be taken together: sufficient sunlight and sufficient calcium. If you are on a low-calcium diet, you have a greater requirement for vitamin D, and if you are not exposed to adequate sunlight, either for cultural or any other reason, then this will put you at more risk of vitamin D deficiency. Thus, you can reduce the requirement for vitamin D by increasing the calcium supply, but nevertheless vitamin D still has to be provided, so the two things should go together.

Dr. Waterlow: I have learned three things in the last few days. First, that stunting is very common in northeast Thailand; secondly, that phosphate deficiency is very common in northeast Thailand; and thirdly, and I quote from you, phosphate deficiency is probably more important in affecting the growth of bone than calcium deficiency. Is it reasonable to put these things together and to suggest that phosphate deficiency might be a cause of stunting?

Dr. Fraser: In theory, phosphate deficiency is a cause of stunting. If it were possible for you to do the unethical experiments of putting children on a phosphorus-deficient diet, I would be very surprised if it did not produce growth failure because it does so in every domestic and experimental animal. Phosphorus deficiency in cattle and sheep, for instance, is a cause of profound growth failure. What I don't know, though, is what level of deficiency would produce this effect in children; what is the cut-off point at which growth retardation would occur?

Dr. Guesry: May I first make a short comment: you focused in your chapter quite exclusively on absorption. I think we have also to consider fixation of minerals in bone. Low-birth-weight infants, when the phosphorus supply is insufficient, may absorb 50% of their calcium intake, but they don't fix it in the bone, and calcium is excreted in the urine. With the addition of phosphorus, hypercalciuria is reduced, and bone mineralization starts. All international bodies, such as the Committee of Nutrition of the American Academy of Pediatrics or the European Society of Pediatric Gastroenterology and Nutrition (ESPGAN), when they make recommendations for calcium intake, recommend at the same time that the calcium/phosphorus ratio should be between 1.2 and 1.8 or 2. You did not mention that ratio except that in rats when phosphorus intake increases, it has the same effect as providing a low-calcium diet. Could you comment and expand on the importance of phosphorus in the diet for calcium absorption?

Dr. Fraser: The importance of the calcium/phosphorus ratio goes a bit beyond the mere absorption of calcium from the diet. Again, the studies don't seem to have been done as thoroughly in man as they have in experimental and domestic animals. In most mammals and in birds, the calcium/phosphorus ratio is very important in optimizing the efficiency of utilization of both nutrients, and the variation of the ratio outside a fairly narrow range produces reduction in growth and possible bone abnormalities. Such studies haven't been done in man except in the case of premature children, so it would be difficult to predict exactly what is likely to happen in older children in the absence of this information. From the studies that have been done in experimental and domestic animals, it appears that if there is a large deviation from a narrow range, either with excessive phosphorus or with excessive calcium, then the absorption of the other nutrient will be impaired. An excess of phosphorus, for example, will tend to diminish the plasma calcium concentration, increase the excretion of calcium, and reduce the availability of calcium for its physiological functions in most cell types and certainly for the mineralization of bone. Thus, if there is an excess of phosphorus, one would predict that this would cause an impairment of the utilization of calcium. This does seem to apply, as you mentioned, in premature children. I would think that calcium deficiency is much less a problem than phosphorus deficiency in maintaining the growth of bone in that condition. The other circumstance, a high calcium supply, is very unlikely to occur. It can really occur only by excessive supplementation of calcium. I didn't, in fact, consider the possibility of phosphorus deficiency as being very significant in populations of children, but Dr. Michael Golden raised the possibility that phosphorus deficiency might be more common than has been reported. It doesn't seem to have been looked at very thoroughly even though the effect on growth is much more severe than any effect that calcium deficiency might have.

Dr. M. Golden: We find very low plasma phosphorus levels in Jamaican malnourished children, and they have very low urinary phosphorus excretion. At one stage we gave them magnesium supplements in the form of magnesium chloride, which we now know represents a massive acid load, and in the face of the massive acid load, there was no increase in phosphorus excretion. I take this to indicate that we have a low phosphorus status in our malnourished children. We have also been looking at stool silicon to try to get a measure of pica. Although we say that calcium intake is very low throughout much of the Third World, I think this is true if we just look only at the dietary calcium intake. Many children practice pica and significant geophagia, which I think has been underestimated to a great extent. What effect would geophagia by children in limestone areas potentially have on their phosphorus status? Would this really potentiate phosphorus deficiency? Much of the phosphorus in the diet may well be unavailable if it is present as phytate phosphorus.

Dr. Fraser: If I were to assume that the human child was the same as a young experimental animal, an increase in calcium would reduce the availability of phosphorus. However, it just doesn't seem to apply in adult humans, so whether or not this interaction occurs during growth I don't know. I could perhaps interpret your low plasma phosphorus and low urinary excretion of phosphorus in another way. Plasma phosphorus, unlike plasma calcium, is very susceptible to changes in the phosphorus flux, and if these children have stopped growing, then the amount of phosphorus that is coming from bone and from the diet may be very small, and so under the conditions of suppressed growth, I think plasma phosphorus could very well fall. Naturally then, urinary phosphorus would fall also; so I think that, apart from indicating phosphorus deficiency, which it could do, one would have to see whether or not growth itself was affected.

Dr. Martorell: You said that our notions about calcium requirements are really based on what we know from industrialized nations, and you were wondering to what extent these notions apply to developing countries. Bone loss, osteoporosis, for example, is a problem of great public importance in the United States and other Western nations where calcium intakes are high. The recommendations are such that, to meet them, people would have to drink a lot of milk or even take calcium supplements. In other regions of the world, bone demineralization and osteroporosis are much rarer, and yet populations exist on much lower calcium intakes. What are the physiological factors that can explain this? Nutrient interactions? Exercise? Genetic factors?

Dr. Fraser: I think that nutritionists in affluent societies have got calcium requirements completely wrong. They base their estimates of calcium requirements on two assumptions. One is that dietary calcium is very poorly absorbed: only 20 to 30% as measured by balance studies. That is true in the types of studies that are done. They also make the assumption that it is very important to supply lots of calcium in early life in order to protect against osteoporosis in later life, and this is an act of faith because there have been no studies that have actually demonstrated protection. The reasoning is that in cases of osteoporosis negative calcium balance occurs, i.e., a greater loss of mineral from bone than is actually introduced into bone during bone turnover. Thus, osteoporosis is regarded as a calcium balance problem, as a disease produced by inadequate supply of calcium. The whole concept is based on a nutritional approach, but it is possible to interpret osteoporosis in quite different ways. The point that you raised about exercise and the effect of mechanical stress on bone is probably of great importance, and it has not been considered widely in osteoporosis. The other possibility is that osteoporosis is really a change in the function of bone cells. If the bone cells are not actually incorporating mineral into bone at that time of life as effectively as they were in early life, then there isn't the same requirement for calcium and phosphorus obtained from the diet. Thus, the balance studies might merely reflect what those bone cells are doing. I suspect that if one were to reevaluate calcium requirements, one could quite easily look at what is happening in countries where calcium intakes are very low and see these people surviving perfectly well on low calcium intakes, with a very low incidence of osteoporosis. It would be necessary to reevaluate both problems: (a) whether or not calcium requirements need to be as high as the recommendations suggest when it is perhaps possible to increase the availability of calcium by adaptive mechanisms; and (b) whether or not the calcium supply at any stage in life is directly related to bone loss in the elderly.

Dr. Kraisid: Short-term studies in adults have shown that increased protein intakes tend to result in increased excretion of calcium in urine (2,3). Recently we have done a study in young children on the effects of different protein intakes on calcium and phosphorus excretion. Giving either a relatively low but adequate protein intake or double that amount had no effect, not like in adults. People in developing countries do not drink milk as they grow older; their calcium intake is low, and at the same time their protein intake is relatively low, adequate, or marginal. On the contrary, in industrialized countries protein intake usually is high, 1.5 to 1.6 times the recommended levels. This might cause some metabolic changes such as increased mobilization of calcium and phosphorus and increased excretion of calcium. Could this in the long run be an explanation for osteoporosis?

Dr. Fraser: I don't know if that is true, but it is an interesting area worth further investigation. The effect of a high-protein diet on calcium excretion is clear cut both in humans and in experimental animals—if you increase protein intake, calcium excretion by the kidney is increased also—but it is not well explained. There are various theoretical reasons why this may occur, but as far as I know, none has actually been proven. It is an interesting idea to think that a long-term intake of a high-protein diet, and perhaps the perpetuation of increased excretion of calcium by the kidney, may have some effect on the turnover of bone and the ability of bone to maintain its strength throughout total life-span. I think that those are points that should be considered and are much more interesting in fact than just the nutritional aspects of supplying adequate calcium and phosphorus in early life. This seems to be an obsession with people who have been working on osteoporosis, in that they have been unwilling to consider other possibilities even though they have been unable to solve the problem from the studies and the approaches that they have taken.

Dr. Barbara Golden: Undernourished children tend to get small bowel overgrowth, so they may radically alter their calcium availability through fermentation. Have there been studies done to show the differences in calcium availability in patients with small bowel overgrowth, and does it alter phosphate availability?

Dr. Fraser: You could have two processes that are acting against each other here. When you have small bowel overgrowth, you probably have an increased splitting of organic calcium complexes in the small intestine and theoretically an increased availability of that calcium for absorption. However, because in small bowel overgrowth you might have lower efficiency of the intestinal mucosa to absorb nutrients in general, and this seems to apply to calcium in particular under other conditions of malabsorption, then perhaps the enhanced availability of calcium is not an advantage because of the reduced absorption capacity. In studies on rats we tried to do an experiment to reduce the availability of calcium by feeding a high-cereal diet. If you do this in man, feeding a high intake of wheat bran, you can put adults into negative calcium balance within a few days (4). A sudden increase in the amount of cereal fiber in the diet has quite a marked effect on the availability of calcium. If you do the same study in rats, there is no effect whatsoever; calcium balance is maintained in the face of very high levels of these calcium complexes (5). The big difference between adult humans and rats is that rats are coprophagous and thus have a physiological overgrowth of bacteria in their small intestine, and it may well be that they are able to release this complex calcium whereas humans are unable to do this.

Dr. Mukherjee: Although protein–energy malnutrition is a deficiency disease, and although these patients sometimes have very low calcium intakes and low vitamin D levels, we do not see clinical signs of florid rickets in them, especially in severe cases like kwashiorkor and marasmus. I wonder if you could comment on this?

Dr. Fraser: I don't think that calcium deficiency alone or a marked reduction of the availability or supply of calcium is going to produce rickets. It will only do so, if the experiments in rats are relevant to humans, when the supply of vitamin D is also low. A clear example of this is the Asian immigrants in the U.K., particularly those that came from East Africa. When they were in East Africa, they had the same sort of diet that they were able to maintain when they reached Britain, and they showed no signs of vitamin-D-deficiency rickets. A few years after their arrival in Britain, vitamin-D-deficiency rickets became very common. The big difference between those two locations was in the supply of vitamin D, because in East Africa they had plenty of sunshine, there was an adequate amount of vitamin D, and there were no signs of rickets even though the low calcium availability or low calcium supply would have increased their requirements. When they arrived in Britain, because of the poor weather conditions, vitamin D supply was markedly reduced, the increased requirement for vitamin D was not being met, and they started showing signs of rickets. It is quite possible in your children that one of the protective factors is that they have enough sunshine to prevent the development of rickets. If their growth rate had been reduced because of the nutritional impairment, then that also would reduce their requirement for vitamin D. An increased requirement for vitamin D is only going to show up where there is rapid growth, inadequate calcium intake, and inadequate vitamin D status.

Dr. Milner: I don't understand why, when you have rats on a low calcium intake and with increased 1,25-dihydroxyvitamin D levels, this should stimulate an increased degradation of 25-hydroxyvitamin D. Is this a physiological adaptation or a pathological process? Teleologically, I would expect the body to wish to conserve the 25-hydroxy as a precursor for 1,25-dihydroxy synthesis, which the body needs. Could you explain this?

Dr. Fraser: I agree entirely. I cannot understand or explain it. How I interpret it at the moment is that it is not a purposeful destruction of vitamin D by the liver. I think this is a coincidental effect that has little importance except when there is a prolonged calcium deficiency and an inadequate supply of vitamin D. What I suspect is happening is that vitamin D is not, as was previously thought, a molecule that is active in only a few cells, the target tissues of the intestine, bone, and kidney. It is now apparent that most cell types in the body respond to 1,25-dihydroxyvitamin D, probably by modifying their ability to handle calcium. When there is a high plasma concentration of 1,25(OH)$_2$D, and because its half-life is exceedingly short in comparison to the other vitamin D metabolites, the liver takes up more 1,25(OH)$_2$D, and this may modify the liver's own ability to handle calcium. A secondary consequence of this may be an enhancement of the degradative pathways for vitamin D. One of the things that we hope to do in the near future is to study other degradative pathways and see whether they have also been stimulated, therefore indicating that this is a nonspecific effect, perhaps mediated by changes in cytoplasmic calcium affecting the degradative aspects of liver function.

Dr. Milner: As if it were a futile cycle?

Dr. Fraser: It would be a whole-body futile cycle, yes.

REFERENCES

1. Pettifor JM, Ross P, Wang J, Moodley G, Couper-Smith J. Rickets in children of rural origin in South Africa: is low dietary calcium a factor? *J Pediatr* 1978;92:320–4.
2. Johnson NE, Alcantara EN, Linkswiler HM. Effect of level of protein intake on urinary and fecal calcium and calcium retention of young adult males. *J Nutr* 1970;100:1425–30.
3. Hegsted M, Schuette SA. Urinary calcium and calcium balance in young men as affected by level of protein and phosphorus intake. *J Nutr* 1981;111:553–62.
4. Cummings JH, Hill MJ, Jivraj T, Houston H, Branch WJ, Jenkins DJA. The effect of meat protein and dietary fiber on colonic function and metabolism. 1. Changes in bowel habit, bile acid excretion, and calcium absorption. *Am J Clin Nutr* 1979;32:2086–93.
5. Fairweather-Tait SJ, Wright AJA. The effect of fibre-filler (F-plan diet) on iron, zinc and calcium absorption in rats. *Br J Nutr* 1985;54:585–92.

Linear Growth Retardation in Less Developed Countries, edited by John C. Waterlow. Nestlé Nutrition Workshop Series, Vol. 14. Nestec Ltd., Vevey/Raven Press, Ltd., New York © 1988.

The Role of Individual Nutrient Deficiencies in Growth Retardation of Children as Exemplified by Zinc and Protein

Michael H. N. Golden

Tropical Metabolism Research Unit, University of the West Indies, Kingston 7, Jamaica

When a wheat plant is grown in soil low in selenium, the result is a normally sized plant that has a low selenium concentration in its tissues. When a wheat plant is grown on a soil low in zinc, the result is a stunted plant that has a normal concentration of zinc in its tissues. If similar experiments are repeated with bacteria or laboratory animals, the same result is obtained. In each case, the deficit of the nutrient may be the same relative to a normal subject, but in one case this arises from a low tissue concentration within a normally grown subject, whereas in the other it arises from a small subject with a normal tissue concentration.

Thus, animals kept on a low selenium ration grow normally until they develop severe clinical disease; in the case of rats this is usually hepatic necrosis, and in other species it is cardiac or skeletal myopathy. After they get sick they may well demonstrate secondary growth failure because of the clinical disease, but this is not a primary phenomenon. Mild forms of selenium deficiency in animals are simply characterized by low tissue selenium concentrations and a resultant vulnerability to noxious stresses without a diminution in growth rate.

In marked contrast, rats placed on a low-zinc diet stop growing almost immediately: they can actually die from zinc deficiency without any reduction in the zinc concentration of their major tissues (1,2).

TYPES OF DEFICIENCY

There is clearly a fundamental and quite distinct difference between these two responses to a nutritional deficiency. I suggest that these two types of response should be clearly differentiated from one another, and nutrients classified according to whether they give rise to one response or to the other. The "type I" response is characterized by a reduction in tissue concentration; it first presents with a specific clinical deficiency and is without a primary effect on growth. The "type II" response presents with a primary cessation in growth without a reduction in tissue concentration and is not normally associated with specific signs and symptoms. It is probable that most nutrients can be classified according to whether the response to a deficiency is primarily of one type or the other, although they may not be so easily classified as selenium or zinc.

Nutrients with Body Stores

For those nutrients that have a body store that serves no immediate function, the picture is clearly more complicated. The prediction is that the first response, in every case, would be a consumption of the body store. Of necessity, in wholebody terms, the concentration of that nutrient would then fall; however, it would only fall in the storage tissues, not in the functional tissues. After the stores are consumed and a functional defect is impending, there may theoretically be either a type I or a type II response.

With a type I deficiency, one would expect to find both an absence of stores and a reduction in tissue concentration; it should first present as a clinical deficiency syndrome. I suggest that iron and iodine fall into this category.

In contrast, with a type II deficiency, although one would expect to find absent or greatly diminished tissue stores, there should be a normal concentration of the nutrient in the functional tissues and growth failure. There is no specific nutrient that seems to behave in this way. Indeed, absence of a body store in the healthy animal seems to be a characteristic of type II nutrients. However, this type of response is precisely what seems to happen with a fuel (energy) deficiency. Thus, the first response to a fuel deficiency is a consumption of the fat stores with no change in the energy content of lean tissue (total body energy concentration is reduced purely on the basis of loss of adipose tissue); at this stage there is no necessary change in the rate of longitudinal growth or lean tissue accretion. After the stores are consumed, the response is clearly a cessation of growth.

I have tentatively classified several nutrients in Table 1.

GENERAL CHARACTERISTICS OF THE DIFFERENT TYPES OF DEFICIENCY

From this starting point, we can predict certain characteristics of the different types of deficiency. With severe deficiency of a type I nutrient, there will be a negative balance for that specific nutrient until clinical signs become manifest, whereas, for a type II deficiency, whole tissue will be catabolized so that the individual will be in negative balance for all the components of lean tissue. Thus, energy, protein, zinc, or potassium deficiency will each lead to a negative balance of the other nutrients in proportion to their relative concentrations in the tissues that are being catabolized; it is only the deficient nutrient that will have a proportionately low excretion.

TABLE 1. *Tentative classification of nutrients into type I and type II*

Type I: initial normal growth, reduced tissue concentration, specific signs	Type II: primary growth failure, normal tissue concentration, no specific signs

IA. No identified stores
    Selenium
	IIA. No identified stores
	    Nitrogen
	    Essential amino acids
	    Zinc
	    Potassium
	    Sodium
	    Phosphorus

IB. Stored
    Iodine
    Iron
    Copper
    Calcium
    Thiamine
    Riboflavin
    Ascorbic acid
    Retinol
    Tocopherol
    Cobalamin
	IIB. Stored
	    Energy

IC. Specific defect in longitudinal growth, specific signs
    Manganese
    Vitamin D
	IIC.
	    None

Type I Deficiency

When one conceives of a specific nutritional deficiency, one automatically considers a type I deficiency. It results in a conceptually pleasing and easily envisaged chain of events. The diet is specifically low; this results in a reduced tissue concentration and an identifiable major defect in a metabolic pathway; this in turn gives rise to characteristic clinical signs and symptoms. The diagnosis is relatively straightforward: all that one has to do is measure the concentration of the nutrient in a tissue, measure the vulnerable pool of the nutrient, test the metabolic pathway where the defect lies, demonstrate an *in vitro* effect of adding the nutrient to some functional system, or recognize the specific clinical signs, whichever is most specific and/or convenient.

Type II Deficiency

The position with respect to type II nutrients (nitrogen, essential amino acids, zinc, potassium, sodium, phosphorus, energy) is quite different in many respects:

indeed, none of the maneuvers that can be used to diagnose a type I deficiency can be used unequivocally to diagnose deficiency of a type II nutrient. Thus, major difficulties, both conceptual and practical, arise when we try to understand, define, diagnose, and study these deficiencies. As growth failure, and hence stunting, is the major long-term characteristic of each of these deficiencies, I consider these difficulties and their implications in more detail.

First, the response to a deficiency—growth failure—is common to a deficiency of each nutrient; therefore, we cannot identify which nutrient is responsible when we observe growth failure.

Many thousands of experiements have been done in animals with diets deficient in one or another of these nutrients; in every case the primary response is a diminution or cessation of growth. As the deficiency progresses, the animal falls further and further behind the controls so that, with time, the animal becomes stunted. If the deficiency is more severe, there is loss of whole tissue, and the animal becomes wasted.

This response has been observed consistently and universally in all species studied, in both acute and chronic experiments, with each of the type II nutrients. So fundamental is this response that it is used to measure a growing animal's requirement for the nutrient with considerable precision and reproducibility. No other feature has been shown to correspond reliably with deficiency; indeed, there does not need to be any measurable "defect" in any of the animal's metabolic pathways that can be held responsible for the growth delay. Growth failure, and probably growth failure alone, is thus the *sine qua non* of protein, zinc, energy, etc. deficiency.

In the human context, one would predict that the response to a longstanding mild deficiency of any of these nutrients would be a diminutive person: progressive stunting (with the body in proportion). The extent of the stunting will be in relation to the integral of the degree of shortfall of the nutrient and time. Clearly, with a chronic mild deficiency there will be a corresponding progressive reduction in attained height relative to some acceptable standard through slowing of the growth rate. With an acute severe deficiency there will be loss of tissue leading to wasting, without necessarily time for stunting to occur. The balance between the severity of the deficiency and its duration will determine the relative amounts of stunting and wasting that are produced. Mild chronic deficiencies are expected to be more common than severe acute deficiencies, so stunting would be predicted to be more common than wasting; this is what is observed.

Second, there is a common repertoire of metabolic changes and reductive adaptations that take place in response to a deficiency. However, because whole tissue is being broken down, or at least there is no net synthesis, those nutrients that are in excess relative to the deficient nutrient have to be metabolized and excreted (or, in the case of fuel, put into storage). The balance among the various type II nutrients in the diet is thus very important. In the face of a deficiency of any one of them, we would predict a negative balance for them all.

Third, when a diet that is deficient in any one of these nutrients is given, the body has mechanisms to conserve that nutrient avidly. It is for this reason that it is extremely difficult to produce a deficiency of one of these nutrients in the non-growing animal by dietary means; there usually has to be a pathological loss of the nutrient from the body. Thus, urinary sodium and potassium can be reduced to remarkably low concentrations; even zinc losses can be reduced to almost zero (3). This leads, necessarily, to the next implication.

The appropriate rate of growth is the major determinant of the dietary requirement for the nutrient.

For example, children given a diet that supplied just enough energy for them to maintain their body weight without growing were able to remain in zinc balance and maintain their plasma zinc concentration with an intake of only 1.3 μmole/kg per day. When the same children were subsequently given sufficient energy to gain weight rapidly, their plasma zinc fell to very low concentrations; this fall in plasma zinc occurred despite a 10-fold increase in the amount of zinc consumed (14 μmole/kg per day) (4). Even with this relatively enormous zinc intake, zinc was limiting lean tissue synthesis (5–7): it is noteworthy that these children did not develop the signs classically ascribed to zinc deficiency; they simply did not synthesize tissue requiring more zinc than was supplied.

The implication of these observations is that no other sign, except for growth failure, is to be expected from a deficiency of one of these nutrients unless the deficiency is very profound.

There is a corollary of this observation that at first sight seems contradictory: it is that one would expect a diet that has a sufficiently low concentration of one of these nutrients to give clinical signs, other than growth failure, to produce signs in adults before children. This hypothesis is a direct consequence of the higher maintenance energy requirement of the child. The protein requirement of the child, for maintenance, is about the same as it is for the adult, 0.6 g/kg per day (8); however, the energy requirement for maintenance of the child is about 400 kJ/kg per day, whereas, that for the adult is about 160 kJ/kg per day. Hence, an adult taking his resting energy requirement must have 6% of the energy as protein, whereas, a child only requires about 2.4% of the energy as protein. Therefore, in a community, we should not expect to find anything other than growth failure in children: if the local diet is sufficiently deficient to give rise to other clinical signs, these should be manifested in adults before children. However, there is an extremely wide gap between the level that will give rise to growth failure and the level that will cause any other obvious feature of deficiency, so that even where growth failure is common, clinical signs should be very rare.

Because growth rate is the major determinant of the requirement for these nutrients, when we supply the missing nutrient there should be a catch-up growth response. We should be able to use this response as a test to diagnose that the growth failure was secondary to lack of a particular nutrient. However, even this, unfortunately, is not necessarily so. When the deficiency was developing, whole tissue was being catabolized. Consequently, there will be a deficit of all the components of that tissue irrespective of which nutrient was originally deficient. There will consequently be a greatly increased dietary requirement for all the nutrients during catch-up growth. This means that a catch-up response to giving the originally deficient nutrient may be short-lived, and the rate of catch-up may now be limited by another nutrient that, in the basic diet, was present in perfectly adequate amounts to sustain normal growth. The important variable will be the ratio of the requirement for normal growth and that for catch-up at an observable rate for each of the nutrients in the diet. A secondary catch-up response cannot then be taken as evidence of an original deficiency. The dietary requirements for catch-up growth are unknown. They are obviously of enormous importance.

Supplementation with the right nutrient should, of course, cause growth at at least the normal rate, unless more than one nutrient is deficient for normal growth rates: normal growth is sufficiently slow in man to make diagnosis by supplementation a correspondingly slow and difficult process.

Fourth, one response that seems to be common to a deficiency of each of these nutrients is anorexia; this is corrected if the nutrient is supplied. Thus, if a child with zinc deficiency is supplemented with zinc, he will regain his appetite and have an increased intake of protein, energy, potassium, and even nonsupplemental zinc in response to the specific supplement (9). Clearly, with these nutrients and this type of response, it is extremely difficult to interpret dietary intake data. The increase or decrease in the intake and utilization of the nutrient under consideration may be caused by a deficiency of a different nutrient altogether. There will clearly be complex interactions among these nutrients.

The etiology of the anorexia is unknown. It may be the deficiency itself; however, it may also be the relative surfeit of the other nutrients, which have to be metabolized and excreted to prevent them from being toxic (6,10). Since anorexia is not a consistent response, the latter may be more likely.

Because growth will be limited by the most deficient nutrient, it is only possible to have a "deficiency" in the classical sense with one type II nutrient at a time— the limiting one. Thus, even if a diet contains very reduced quantities of a particular nutrient—protein, for example—no response to supplementation and no specific consequences of that particular deficiency are to be expected if another type II nutrient is even more deficient.

Fifth, when a dietary supplement is given that does not contain all the nutrients required for new tissue synthesis, the rate of growth will be determined by the most limiting nutrient in the new diet (basic diet plus supplement), not in the original diet or in the supplement alone. Indeed, by diluting the original diet, an incomplete supplement can make a deficiency worse; there are probable examples of this in the literature (11).

Clearly, if an unbalanced supplement is given, the other nutrients in the supplement will be used inefficiently. The degree of inefficiency will be related directly to the magnitude of the discrepancy or imbalance between the actual limiting nutrient in the diet as a whole and the nutrient under consideration. If the supplement is almost devoid of any particular type II nutrient, then the supplement will be used with a zero efficiency unless that nutrient is in excess in the basal diet, in which case the efficiency of utilization will be related to the relative excess in the basal diet over the needs for accelerated growth. If we observe an inefficient use of nutrients (or, more commonly evaluated, energy), then we can infer that the diet is imbalanced and one of the type II ingredients is limiting growth and efficiency. Gross inefficiency is almost universal in reported supplementation trials: none of them have been formulated to contain all the type II nutrients in what is thought to be adequate amounts.

As yet a further complication, the response to the supplement and the required balance of nutrients in the supplement, will depend on the precise mix of tissues that should be laid down. This will depend, in turn, on the age of the subject, the degree of wasting and stunting that has to be made good, and the composition of the required new tissues. Clearly, the dietary requirement for skeletal growth, for muscle synthesis, for adipose tissue, and for skin synthesis will potentially differ, but by how much, in what way, and whether this is ever a major factor has not been explored.

Sixth, if conventional techniques are used to diagnose a deficiency of one of these type II nutrients, the results are likely to be totally misleading. Clearly, there is little point in doing a muscle biopsy and measuring the gross threonine or zinc concentration, for example, in that biopsy. Experience has shown that this approach simply does not work. If there is a change in the nutrient of concern in the biopsy, the change is just as likely to result from a deficiency of one of the other type II nutrients, from an alteration in metabolism consequent on a deficiency of a type I nutrient, or even from a metabolic alteration unrelated to nutrition as it is likely to be secondary to a deficiency of the specific nutrient under the spotlight. It should be noted that a small percentage of changes in type II nutrient tissue concentration can occur as the metabolic state alters; for example, structural protein to soluble protein ratios will affect the essential amino acid concentration, as will the intensity of protein synthesis. This would explain the small fall in tissue zinc concentration with an essential amino acid deficiency when there is none with zinc deficiency itself (12). In this way, a zinc deficiency, energy deficiency, or an infection is as likely a cause for a low albumin, prealbumin, or retinol-binding protein concentration in plasma as is a protein deficiency (13). Herein lies the difficulty: the response is not specific to any particular nutrient.

I tentatively suggest that much of the controversy that surrounds the definition of a deficiency, the signs and symptoms of deficiency, the diagnosis of deficiency, and the requirements of those nutrients that I have classified as type II nutrients stems from attempts to conceive of them as fulfilling the classical nutritional maxims that underlie, and have been so useful in evaluating, deficiencies of iron, iodine, the water-soluble vitamins, and other type I nutrients. The type II nutrients have to be considered together as fundamental cellular constituents.

NUTRIENTS THAT AFFECT GROWTH DIRECTLY

As with all schemes, there is a complication with this simple classification of nutrients into those that reduce their tissue concentration with continued growth and those for which the response is cessation of growth and avid conservation of the nutrient's tissue concentration. In the context of longitudinal growth, what happens if the specific metabolic defect of a type I nutritional deficiency itself interferes with longitudinal growth? Several nutrients, such as manganese, vitamin D, vitamin C, and copper, potentially fall into this category.

A manganese deficiency in animals leads to a specific defect in proteoglycan synthesis (probably on the basis of reduced activity of UDP-galactosidyl transferase I, a manganese metalloenzyme), leading to cartilage dysplasia and abnormal growth. However, not only is there a recognizable pathological lesion but also animals on a manganese deficient diet continue to gain weight, so that although they are stunted, they are not any lighter than the controls (14). This is in contrast to the stunting of zinc or protein deficiency, where the short animal is either in proportion or is, more usually, wasted.

Similarly, vitamin D deficiency gives rise to stunting—the classical cause of nutritional stunting—but is also associated with specific symptoms and signs and characteristic bone changes: the vitamin-D-deficient child is not simply diminutive. Vitamin D deficiency is associated with a clinical myopathy and muscle pain but not with wasting per se.

Interestingly, although copper deficiency is associated with gross osteopenia (secondary to a defect in lysyl oxidase, the enzyme necessary for cross linking the collagen molecules of bone matrix), it does not seem to be associated with stunting.

Again, vitamin C deficiency, which also leads to defective collagen synthesis, gives distinct pathological bone changes and specific signs in other systems that are relatively easily diagnosed; it does not seem to give rise to simple short stature.

The essential difference between these nutrient deficiencies and a type II nutrient deficiency is that these deficiencies all give rise to clearly pathological features in bone or cartilage that must be there before there is stunting. These nutrient deficiencies, therefore, may present a theoretical difficulty in anthropometric classification but are unlikely to present any difficulty clinically—they are not associated with simple diminutiveness.

ARE TYPE II DEFICIENCIES AN IMPORTANT CAUSE OF STUNTING?

Having laid the conceptual framework and considered some of its implications, we must ask ourselves if it is likely that deficiencies of any of the type II nutrients are, in practice, limiting growth in any substantial population group.

Because we do not yet know the precise requirements for normal growth of children for each of these nutrients, and we do not know the requirements for accelerated growth for any of them, the question of dietary adequacy, or inadequacy, cannot be decided at this time. It is thus not possible to say, from intake data, whether any type II nutrient limits growth, with the possible exception of fuel. We do have estimates of the energy requirements for both normal and accelerated gain in weight but not for gain in height.

It must be clear that the demonstration that a diet is adequate for only energy, protein, and the type I nutrients that have received attention is very far from addressing its adequacy as a diet. Assessment of the requirements for catch-up growth have not been seriously or systematically investigated.

I am unaware of any supplementation study in which even "informed guesses" of the requirements for catch-up of all nutrients known to be essential have been made and the response to giving such a supplement observed. Virtually all supplementation trials have either looked at the effect of a single nutrient alone or, more commonly, have tried to obtain a response from the cheapest available source of presumed adequate food without there being a clear idea of what nutrients are actually being given, what their availabilities are, how they relate to the requirements, and without an attempt to tailor the supplement to the nutrient composition of the basal diet. It is noteworthy that it is the mineral elements that have, by and large, been ignored despite the fact that most cultures place emphasis on minerals in culinary practice (*vide infra*). None of the field studies supplemented the diets with even a simple mineral mix. This situation is in marked contrast to the practice of virtually every agriculturalist and advisor in animal nutrition, where experience has led to an appreciation of the importance of the mineral content of the diet. We could learn from detailed attention and continuing research effort directed to preparing and refining the highly complex dietary supplements used for different aspects of commercial animal production.

Potential Catch-Up: What Should Be the Target?

What is the potential for catch-up in a stunted child? How far from this potential are the reported results of feeding trials? We do not know. In an attempt to get some idea of what could be achieved, the records of 417 children consecutively admitted to the Tropical Metabolism Research Unit (TMRU) with severe malnutrition were examined. The children were weighed daily and had height measured weekly to the nearest 0.5 cm. They were treated as previously described (15). The median age of the children was 12 months, and the median period of observation 9 weeks. The results are shown in Table 2. The range of height gain was from 0

TABLE 2. *Rate of gain in height of 417 children recovering from severe malnutrition in a metbolic ward[a]*

Height gain (mm/day)	Admission to discharge	Admission to > 90% wt. for ht.	> 90% wt. for ht. to discharge
< 0.1	5%	36%	14%
0.1–0.3	26%	20%	14%
0.4–0.8	59%	35%	46%
> 0.8	11%	8%	26%
Less than normal	31%	56%	28%
Greater than normal	70%	44%	72%

[a]From M. Golden and S. Walker (*unpublished data*).

to 9.5 cm during the 2 to 3 months of observation. Clearly, some of the children were capable of enormous height spurts.

The data were analyzed separately for the period of accelerated weight gain (from admission to 90% weight for height) and for the subsequent weeks, when their wasting had been corrected. Over 70% of the children gained height at more than the normal rate for this age; 44% gained significant height while they were gaining weight rapidly; after repletion of weight for height, 26% of the children gained height at more than twice the standard rate. This is despite the fact that the diets that the children receive are known not to be optimal. The children exhibit an abnormal body composition after they have recovered weight for height. (16). Significantly, they have a limitation of lean tissue synthesis, leading to abnormal muscle tissue (17) and, at this stage, very inefficient growth (5). Further, we have observed an acceleration of weight gain at an increased efficiency with zinc supplementation (5,6). When we gave children additional zinc throughout recovery, they synthesized much more lean tissue than fat tissue (7). It seems that our diets are still limiting in type II nutrients; we are certainly not achieving the full potential height gain.

Nevertheless, it is clear that a rapid, measurable, and substantial gain in height, of the order of 2.5 cm/month, can be achieved over a relatively short observation period in about a quarter of our children with what we know to be an inadequate intake. Clearly, with the proper supplementation, very prolonged studies with extremely precise measurements should not be required; the more inadequate our supplement, the harder it will be to show a difference. Perhaps this is why studies of height gain have a reputation for difficulty.

Against this background, we can examine the results of the various supplementation studies in third world populations. These have been reviewed by Beaton and Ghassemi (18). In these studies the supplement was usually dried skim milk, various combinations of wheat and soya, or local foods. The outstanding conclusion is that the supplements made very little difference, sometimes reaching statistical significance, sometimes not, but never achieving substantial gains. The harder it is to show a statistical difference, the less likely that difference is to be of biological significance. At some stage it is pointless to continue to pursue a statistical result, which can then be hailed as a ''success,'' when the difference is biologically trivial and clearly overshadowed by much more important variables, which are not being considered: the biological significance of all these studies is in doubt.

One way to examine the above mentioned data is to look at the efficiency of weight (or height) gain. The positive studies report an effect of the supplement of up to 1 kg/year. This implies that the supplement was responsible for an increased weight gain of 2.5 g/day. At an energy cost of tissue synthesis of 20 kJ/g (5 kcal/g), the energy needed to lay down this tissue amounts to only 50 kJ/day (12.5 kcal/day); this is a minute amount. The dietary supplements were usually substantial (16.6–33.6 MJ/day; 300–800 kcal/day); clearly the supplement was used very inefficiently. In most studies about one-third of the supplement actually is taken by the target subject because of ''leakage,'' food substitution, etc.; however, there is still a substantial difference between the supplement and the observed effect

(420–1,120 kJ/day versus 50 kJ/day; 4 to 12% efficiency). The poor efficiency is probably, in part, related to recurrent infection and malabsorption. However, it is precisely the result we would expect if insufficient attention was paid to one of the type II nutrients; we know that this was indeed the case in every study.

PROTEIN

Most of the studies that have reported a height gain with supplementation have used a milk- or soya-based supplement. Unfortunately, it is not possible to be certain whether this is an effect of the protein per se or whether it is caused by one of the "fellow travelers" added to these diets—phosphorus is an obvious contender in this respect. It has been said that these points are of little practical importance. That would be so if it were really only protein involved, but not if a "fellow traveler" proved responsible for the observed effect. Should we, then, be spending time, effort, and money to build fish farms on the basis of results obtained with milk supplements? Only if protein deficiency is in fact responsible.

The most important study is probably that of Malcolm (19,20). He studied a community of children living in an isolated boarding school in the New Guinea highlands. The whole community was fed exclusively on taro or sweet potato; the children were very stunted, even by local village standards. The children were divided into four groups: one received a supplement of 75 g skim milk powder daily; a second received 30 g margarine daily; the third had their intake of taro increased by a factor of 1.67; and the last group received no extra food. The results are shown in Table 3. The skim milk led to an incremental gain in height and weight

TABLE 3. *Effects of various supplements on the anthropometric increments of Bundi school children[a]*

Group	Control	Extra diet (1.67-fold)	Margarine (30 g)	Skim milk (75 g)
		Supplement for 13 weeks		
n	35	22	22	31
Age (years)	8.6	7.4	9.8	7.6
Height (cm)	1.10 ± 0.12	1.54 ± 0.13	0.96 ± 0.11	2.32 ± 0.11
Weight (kg)	0.50 ± 0.13	0.47 ± 0.14	1.05 ± 0.18	1.21 ± 0.10
Triceps skinfold (mm)	+ 0.17 ± 0.13	+ 0.77 ± 0.17	+ 2.28 ± 0.35	− 0.13 ± 0.14
		Supplement for 32 weeks		
			Skim milk	Skim milk
	Control		(10 g)	(20 g)
n	30		30	26
Height	1.75 ± 0.17		3.23 ± 0.13	3.45 ± 0.14
Weight	1.34 ± 0.18		1.98 ± 0.14	2.92 ± 0.13
Triceps skinfold	+ 0.78 ± 0.18		+ 0.26 ± 0.18	− 0.09 ± 0.15

[a]Data from Malcolm (19) and Lampl et al. (20). All results are expressed as mean ± SEM of increments over the study period.

with no change in skinfold thickness. Provision of energy, on the other hand, led to a substantial gain in skinfold thickness and no incremental gain in height.

It is clear that energy was not limiting height gain, for the additional margarine did not have any effect although it produced an increase in fat stores. The extra diet did not increase body weight, but it did increase both fat stores and height. Was there some nutrient in the diet in lower relative concentration than energy that permitted lean tissue to be converted to height gain? If so, it is clear, as could have been predicted, that the nutrient requirements for lean tissue and skeletal tissue growth are different. The additional milk produced the largest increment in height, with an actual reduction in fat stores. In effect, the additional milk contained some ingredient(s) that permitted conversion of soft tissue into skeletal tissue. This is despite the fact that the diet did not contain the additional energy required for accelerated height gain, and so endogenous sources had to be used, and skinfold declined. It is probably correct to say that energy deficiency does not lead to stunting in the presence of fat stores. Fat stores can be demonstrated in most stunted children. The result of this first study was confirmed, with a graded response to the two levels of supplementation, in the second study.

What were the components of the dried skim milk that produced this response? Certainly, total protein or one of its "fellow travelers" (particularly essential amino acids, zinc, phosphorus, or calcium) is a likely contender.

The question of what component of cow's milk is responsible cannot be answered. However, in a study of Finnish infants, Salmenpera et al. (21) compared the growth of exclusively breast-fed infants with those given formula. The breast-fed infants progressively fell behind the formula-fed infants, so that by 9 months of age 45% of them, versus 18% of the formula-fed infants, were more than 1 SD below the standard length. There was no difference in the children's weight. Skinfold measurements showed the breast-fed infants to have substantially more storage of fat. Obviously, energy or total breast milk intake was clearly not limiting height gain. Here again, as with the New Guinea children, the infants consuming cow's-milk-based formula were longer and thinner than the control group. However, in this study, cow's milk was compared to human milk, so that many of the confounding variables were different. Within the breast milk group itself, no correlation could be found between breast milk protein concentration, protein intake, or protein intake per unit body weight and either growth velocity or changes in relative length. As expected, the fat concentration of breast milk and the calculated fat intake were not related to gain in length. However, there were substantial differences in the protein intake of the two groups of infants. The increased protein supply was thus common to the two studies and must be the prime candidate nutrient for the effect. There will have been marked differences in other nutrients as well. For instance, the difference in phosphorus concentration of human and bovine milk is relatively greater than the difference in protein. Phosphorus intake was also much higher in Malcolm's supplemented children. Was protein, phosphorus, or some other nutrient altogether responsible?

However, it is equally clear that many of the supplementation studies that have used skim milk have not produced any increment in height, and in all the studies, including those of Malcolm, the actual increment in height was much less than the potential increment we think should be achieved if a "full supplement" had been given.

At present the question of whether substantial sections of the population have stunting secondary to protein deficiency must remain open. By analogy with animal studies and the responses to skim milk powder, it is likely that at least in some areas protein deficiency will transpire to be the limiting factor for longitudinal growth.

ZINC

The most carefully conducted studies of zinc supplementation have been done in the United States by Hambidge's group. They have shown unequivocally that additional zinc leads to increased rates of gain in length in stunted male infants and children in Denver.

In the first study (22), infants were randomly divided into two groups. One was given a proprietary infant formula (1.8 mg zinc per liter), the other the same formula with supplemental zinc (5.8 mg zinc per liter). The results of this study are shown in Table 4. After 6 months the male infants receiving the supplemented formula were over 2 cm longer and 500 g heavier than the unsupplemented infants. There was no difference in the female infants. It should be emphasized that these infants were all "normal" infants—they were not selected on the basis of having been short at birth.

Hambidge's next study (23) involved preschool children 38 to 60 months of age (mean age 50 months) who were selected on the basis of being below the 10th centile of the Iowa standards. The test subjects were calculated to receive an addi-

TABLE 4. *Growth increments and plasma zinc levels at 6 months of age in infants fed a proprietary formula with (5.8 mg Zn per liter) or without (1.8 mg Zn per liter) zinc*[a]

	Control	Supplemented	p value
Males *(n)*	8	14	—
Height (cm)	17.36 ± 0.88	19.46 ± 0.48	< 0.025
Weight (kg)	3.99 ± 0.27	4.53 ± 0.11	< 0.05
Head circumference (cm)	8.36 ± 0.42	8.85 ± 0.23	NS
Plasma zinc (µg/dl)	69.5 ± 3.2	80.5 ± 3.7	< 0.025
Females *(n)*	10	10	—
Height (cm)	16.73 ± 0.48	16.36 ± 0.52	NS
Weight (kg)	3.77 ± 0.20	3.94 ± 0.14	NS
Head circumference (cm)	8.33 ± 0.33	8.48 ± 0.24	NS
Plasma zinc (µg/dl)	73.9 ± 2.2	72.5 ± 4.1	NS

[a]Data from Walravens and Hambidge (22), expressed as mean ± SEM.

tional 4.2 mg zinc/day (0.3 mg/kg per day) based on estimated compliance; the control subjects were given placebo. The results are shown in Table 5. There was a highly significant increase in height velocity of the male children with an improvement in Z scores of height for age. Again, there were no significant changes in the female children.

There have been reports of growth responses in adolescents with delayed puberty in the Middle East given zinc supplements (see 12). However, in the only well-controlled study (24), there was no improvement with zinc supplementation. The other studies, although suggesting that zinc deficiency was responsible for stunting, were not well controlled and inconsistent, and much of the data were not presented.

Signs of severe zinc deficiency do occur in malnourished infants (25), and there is a suggestion that those with the worst zinc status are the most stunted (4).

Several conclusions are possible from these studies. First, zinc deficiency in man gives rise to limitation of longitudinal growth, as it does in experimental animals. Second, males are much more susceptible to zinc deficiency than females. If severe zinc deficiency is evident in children with malnutrition requiring admission to hospital, then, because of the large difference between the dietary intake necessary to cause growth retardation and that necessary to give clinical disease, it is likely that growth limitation caused by zinc deficiency is quite common.

On the other hand, there is a marked sex difference in the response to zinc supplements. If zinc was limiting growth, then one would expect boys to be much more stunted than girls; this is not the case.

As in the results of supplementation with protein-enriched sources, the increments in height with zinc supplementation were very modest. In certain circumstances zinc may well be the limiting nutrient, but clearly, if this is the case, when zinc is given, some other dietary constituent quickly becomes the limiting nutrient. Dried skim milk is not a particularly good source of zinc. One could speculate that in those studies in which there was a modest response to milk powder, zinc quickly became the second limiting nutrient for growth, whereas when zinc was given, protein or phosphorus became the limiting nutrient. This would explain

TABLE 5. Growth velocity and changes in Z scores for preschool stunted children given a zinc supplement (4.2 mg/day)[a]

	Control	Supplemented	p value
Males (n)	13	13	—
Height velocity (cm/year)	5.92 ± 0.19	6.66 ± 0.24	< 0.001
Weight velocity (kg/year)	1.67 ± 0.20	2.04 ± 0.26	NS
Change in height Z score	− 0.07 ± 0.05	+ 0.06 ± 0.05	< 0.001
Females (n)	7	7	—
Height velocity (cm/year)	6.48 ± 0.51	6.85 ± 0.36	NS
Weight velocity (kg/year)	2.04 ± 0.27	2.25 ± 0.23	NS
Change in height Z score	+ 0.19 ± 0.06	+ 0.18 ± 0.01	NS

why in each case the response was definite but modest. Of course, these arguments would apply with equal force to any of the other type II nutrients.

MINERAL NUTRITION

I am unaware of any trials of potassium or sodium supplementation or of attempts to measure the influence of potassium or sodium on growth. This may be because there are extremely effective physiological mechanisms to conserve these elements, so that an individual can remain in balance on a very low intake. But what of the requirements for growth? These are assumed to be met, but are they? It is worth remembering that large amounts of sodium can be lost in tropical climates from perspiration and that sodium and potassium losses are characteristic of diarrhea, a common complicating factor in these children. Much attention has been paid to the acute effects of electrolyte depletion. Could the chronic effects be growth failure? This question has not been seriously addressed. It may be significant that positive nutritional effects have been reported from giving oral rehydration fluid out of all proportion to the perceived nutritional contents of these solutions.

Mineral elements have received very little attention from those interested in child growth in the tropics; however, there are considerations, apart from the example of animal nutrition, that may indicate their importance.

Mineral Availability from Traditional Diets

There are strategies used by most traditional cultures to increase the mineral availability from their diets. Plant seeds and starchy roots contain metal-complexing compounds, principally phytic acid (inositol hexaphosphate). This is the phosphorus "store" of plant tissue. The phosphorus from phytate and the mineral elements it complexes are unavailable to man. Traditional culinary practices have evolved three general methods of improving the availability of minerals from vegetable diets.

First, many staples are fermented by the peoples who first used the staple. The Amerindians soak cassava in water troughs for days before it is eaten; the Polynesians bury breadfruit until it has almost liquefied before it is eaten; wheat flour is mixed with yeast and fermented; soy beans are ground and then fermented to make bean curd.

Second, the seed is allowed to germinate so that the endogenous phytase breaks down the phytic acid. An example of this would be the sprouting of beans widely used in Southeast Asia. Both of these techniques involve breaking down phytic acid, one with fungal phytase and the other with endogenous phytase.

The alternative third strategy is to increase the mineral content directly. The North American Indians burn certain plants (about 40 different species are used) and add the ash to maize meal (26). This tradition of adding plant ash to maize is common throughout all the tribes of North America (27). The practice of burning plants and adding the ash to food is also widespread among African tribes still living in their traditional way (28,29), South American Indians (30,31), and New Guinea natives (32). The ashes used are all rich in potassium, calcium, magnesium, phosphorus, iron, zinc, and the other trace elements; they may contain the "overlooked factor" that has been lost or made unavailable by modern methods.

Populations that are displaced have either changed from their traditional culture or have started to consume unfamiliar foods or both. They cease to prepare their staple foods in the traditional manner and give up the practice of adding plant ash to their foods. Thus, federal "aid" in the form of pure "unadulterated" maize meal that is supplied to the reservations may be far inferior to the traditionally prepared maize (33).

The net result of these changes will be mineral malnutrition. Many of these elements are type II nutrients, as I have defined them, and clearly magnesium, calcium, and phosphorus are central to skeletal growth.

CONCLUSION

We must conclude that the place of mineral elements, electrolytes, macroelements, and the trace elements, has been neglected for too long in the investigation of stunting. The place of protein deficiency as a cause of stunting has hardly been looked at because most investigators thought that protein deficiency gave rise to kwashiorkor, and it is well known that kwashiorkor children are not particularly stunted. Too much attention has been paid to diets and not enough to nutrients in studies of human growth (in contrast to the animal studies, where the exact opposite obtains). There has been almost no basic metabolic research into the nutritional determinants of longitudinal growth to give a sound nutritional basis to the field studies. Most of the field studies have been conducted because of inappropriate pressure to "do something quickly" about an enormous and highly complex problem. They have thus, for the most part, been naive and expedient and not posited on sound metabolic principles.

There is a requirement, in the investigation and treatment of stunting in the third world, for a series of physiological studies to be conducted so that we can increase our understanding before further large-scale, expensive, and difficult field studies are undertaken.

ACKNOWLEDGMENTS

This work was fully supported by the Wellcome Trust.

REFERENCES

1. Williams RB, Mills CF. The experimental production of zinc deficiency in the rat. *Br J Nutr* 1970;24:989–1003.
2. Aggett PJ, Crofton RW, Chapham M, Humphries WR, Mills CF. Plasma, leucocyte and tissue zinc concentrations in young zinc deficient pigs [Abstract]. *Pediatr Res* 1983;17:433.

3. Golden BE, Golden MHN. Dietary zinc and the output and composition of faeces. In: Howell JMcC, Gawthorne JM, White CL, eds. *Trace element metabolism in animals and man; vol 4.* Canberra: Australian Academy of Sciences, 1981:73–6.
4. Golden BE, Golden MHN. Plasma zinc and the clinical features of malnutrition. *Am J Clin Nutr* 1979;32:2490–4.
5. Golden BE, Golden MHN. Plasma zinc, rate of weight gain and the energy cost of tissue deposition in children recovering from severe malnutrition on a cow's milk or soya protein based diet. *Am J Clin Nutr* 1981;34:898–9.
6. Golden MHN, Golden BE. Effect of zinc supplementation on the dietary intake, rate of weight gain and energy cost of tissue deposition in children recovering from severe malnutrition. *Am J Clin Nutr* 1981;34:900–8.
7. Golden BE, Golden MHN. Effect of zinc supplementation on the composition of newly synthesized tissue in children recovering from malnutrition [Abstract]. *Proc Nutr Soc* 1985;44:110A.
8. Chan HC, Waterlow JC. The protein requirements of infants of about one year. *Br J Nutr* 1966;20:775–82.
9. Krebs NF, Hambidge KM, Walravens PA. Increased food intake of young children receiving a zinc supplement. *Am J Dis Child* 1984;138:270–3.
10. Chesters JK, Quarterman J. Effects of zinc deficiency on food intake and feeding patterns of rats. *Br J Nutr* 1970;24:1061–9.
11. Ronaghy HA, Reinhold JG, Mahloudji M, Ghavami P, Spivey-Fox MR, Halsted JA. Zinc supplementation of malnourished schoolboys in Iran: increased growth and other effects. *Am J Clin Nutr* 1974;27:112–21.
12. Golden MHN, Golden BE. Problems with the recognition of human zinc-responsive conditions. In: Mills CF, Bremner I, Chesters JK, eds. *Trace elements in man and animals; vol 5.* Slough: Commonwealth Agricultural Bureaux, 1985:933–8.
13. Golden MHN. Transport proteins as indices of protein status. *Am J Clin Nutr* 1982;35:1159–65.
14. Bell LT, Hurley LS. Ultrastructural effects of manganese deficiencies in liver, heart, kidney and pancreas of mice. *Lab Invest* 1973;29:723–36.
15. Jackson AA, Golden MHN. Protein energy malnutrition. In: Weatherall DJ, Ledingham JGG, Warrell DA, eds. *The Oxford textbook of medicine.* Oxford: Oxford University Press, 1983:8.12–8.21.
16. Brooke O, Wheeler EF. High energy feeding in protein–energy malnutrition. *Arch Dis Child* 1976;51:968–7.
17. Hansen-Smith FM, Picou D, Golden MHN. Growth of muscle fibers during recovery from severe malnutrition in Jamaican infants. *Br J Nutr* 1979;41:275–82.
18. Beaton GH, Ghassemi H. Supplementary feeding programs for young children in developing countries. *Am J Clin Nutr* 1982;35:864–916.
19. Malcolm LA. Growth retardation in a New Guinea boarding school and its response to supplementary feeding. *Br J Nutr* 1970;24:297–305.
20. Lampl M, Johnston FE, Malcolm LA. The effects of protein supplementation on the growth and skeletal maturation of New Guinean school children. *Ann Hum Biol* 1978;5:219–27.
21. Salmenpera L, Perheentupa J, Siimes MA. Exclusively breast fed healthy infants grow slower than reference infants. *Pediatr Res* 1985;19:307–12.
22. Walravens PA, Hambidge KM. Growth of infants fed a zinc supplemented formula. *Am J Clin Nutr* 1976;29:1114–21.
23. Walravens PA, Krebs NF, Hambidge KM. Linear growth of low income preschool children receiving a zinc supplement. *Am J Clin Nutr* 1983;38:195–201.
24. Carter JP, Grivetti LE, Davis JT, et al. Growth and sexual development of adolescent Egyptian village boys. *Am J Clin Nutr* 1969;22:59–78.
25. Golden MHN, Golden BE, Bennett FI. Relationship of trace element deficiencies to malnutrition. In: Chandra RK, ed. *Trace elements in nutrition of children.* New York: Raven Press, 1985:185–204. (Nestle Nutrition Workshop series; vol 8).
26. Kuhnlein HV, Calloway DH. Composition of traditional Hopi foods. *J Am Diet Assoc* 1979;75:37–41.
27. Kuhnlein HV. The trace element content of indigenous salts compared with commercially refined substitutes. *Ecol Food Nutr* 1980;10:113–21.
28. Junod HA. *The life of an African tribe; vol 2.* London: Macmillan, 1927.
29. Huntingford GWB. The economic life of the Dorobo. *Anthropos* 1955;5:602–34.
30. Roth WE. *An introductory study of the arts, crafts, and customs of the Guiana Indians.* Washington: Bureau of American Ethnology, 38th Annual report. 1924:223.

31. Levi-Strauss C. The use of wild plants in tropical South America. In: Stewart JS, ed. *Handbook of South American Indians; vol 6*. Washington: Bureau of American Ethnology, 1950; *Bulletin* 143:465–86.
32. Townsend PK, Liao S-C, Konlande JE. Nutritive contributions of sago ash used as a native salt in Papua New Guinea. *Ecol Food Nutr* 1973;2:91–7.
33. Calloway DH, Giauque RD, Costa FP. The superior mineral content of some American Indian foods in comparison to federally donated counterpart commodities. *Ecol Food Nutr* 1974;3:203–12.

DISCUSSION

Dr. Tomkins: Energy and protein intakes in zinc-supplemented children were about twice as high as in nonsupplemented children. The energy cost of tissue deposition in zinc-supplemented children was about 7 kcal/g versus about 11 kcal/g in the nonsupplemented children. Could we partition the amount of growth that is attributable to the increase of food intake as a result of the effect of zinc on appetite as opposed to the amount of growth that results from improved metabolic efficiency?

Dr. Golden: This is an extremely difficult question. We really don't have the data to answer it. In many of the children we do not see an appetite response to zinc, but we do see an increased metabolic efficiency. The balance of nutrients in the diet seems to be absolutely crucial. The most limiting nutrients in a diet will be used very efficiently; the rest of the nutrients will be used in proportion to the limiting nutrients. Any excess has then to be excreted, so there is a measure of inefficiency of use of all nutrients except for the limiting one. The degree of inefficiency of use for each nutrient seems to be related to this imbalance. In all the experiments carried out in rats, high-protein diets have been used. The protein, in the face of a zinc deficiency, is used very inefficiently and is broken down and excreted; the anorexia that is seen in rats seems to be related to this. If you take a rat and put it on a zinc-deficient diet, the rat becomes anorectic; if you then get the balance right by reducing the protein content of the diet, anorexia stops, and the rat uses its food very inefficiently and becomes slightly obese. The answer to whether you will get anorexia or inefficient use depends on the balance of nutrients in the diet. All these nutrients that I have called type II nutrients are very closely related to each other, and deficiency of one leads to loss or imbalance of them all. I think we have got to think in terms of the proportion of all these nutrients in the diet in relation to one another.

Dr. Mukherjee: What was the duration of the hospital stay of the 417 children whose rate of gain in length you presented? Since these children did not receive a zinc supplement, to what do you think their rapid linear growth can be attributed?

Dr. Golden: These children were unselected consecutive admissions to the ward. The median hospital stay was 9 weeks. We know that the diets that were given to these 417 children did not contain sufficient zinc. There were probably many other nutrients in the diet that were there in insufficient amounts. The children were growing at the rate, I presume, of the most limiting nutrient in our diet. The reason I presented these data was to show what can be achieved with a regular rehabilitation diet in a metabolic ward when treating malnourished babies: catch-up in height does occur; it occurs quite rapidly and is easily measurable. We are not talking about millimeters over weeks, we are talking about centimeters. I would suggest that if one does not see this type of response, one should analyze the diet given to the children and look for some other type of deficiency that remains uncorrected.

Dr. Waterlow: I like very much your distinction between type I and type II deficiencies.

This is a clarifying concept. The type II deficiencies seem to refer to structural components of the cell; one could think of potassium or magnesium as essential components of the cell. I wonder where you would put essential fatty acids. You surely remember the original work long ago by Kosterlitz and colleagues (5), who showed how the ratio of phospholipids to protein and RNA remains constant but is altered in relation to DNA. Secondly, you mentioned biopsies as being useless. I would like to suggest that they are not useless for these components if you relate them to DNA.

Dr. Golden: Essential fatty acids might be an example of nutrients that are stored, and when the store is depleted, they behave as type II nutrients. The reason I say biopsies are useless is that when you find that cell zinc or protein per DNA is low, you are immediately tempted to say that this is zinc or protein deficiency. What we are actually looking at is a metabolic change, which could be caused by a deficiency of any of these nutrients or of energy or by a metabolic aberration unrelated to nutrition, for example, infection.

Dr. Waterlow: I agree with that; I call it depletion, not deficiency. However, I was really trying to get back to what Dr. Milner said about hyperplasia and hypertrophy. You get a hypotrophy—small cells.

Dr. Golden: It is worth looking for, but not to diagnose a deficiency of that particular nutrient.

Dr. Kittima: In which type of nutrients do you classify calcium?

Dr. Golden: As you can see, my classification is incomplete. I haven't classified many of the nutrients. I have classified the ones I personally have thought about and looked at the literature on and don't have that much difficulty in deciding how to classify them. However, I have great difficulty in deciding where calcium and magnesium should go. Phosphorus we have heard should clearly be classified as a type II nutrient; calcium, I'm not sure about.

Dr. Martorell: You mentioned that supplementation trials have not shown much of an effect on growth. I think the basis for this view is the review article by Beaton and Ghassemi published in the *American Journal of Clinical Nutrition* (1), which everybody quotes. I think this article really underestimates the potential impact of nutrition because, first of all, it doesn't include all the trials that have been carried out. For example, it doesn't include the INCAP trial, which did show quite a pronounced effect on linear growth. On the other hand, it includes many so-called experiments that weren't experiments at all but evaluations of efforts to provide food to poor people, CARE programs and so on, with very poor research designs. As you mentioned, often the food was given to families and not directly to children; nobody knows whether the child actually ate any of the food. Sample size of some of these studies was very small, and many studies had no control group. It is dangerous to conclude from such studies that supplementation and dietary improvements will not have an impact on growth.

Another comment concerns Malcolm's study (2) in New Guinea, from which one would conclude that protein has a role. But the diet in that area is a very unusual diet based on root crops, which are very poor in protein. This conclusion may not apply to many regions in the world where the staple diet is made up of cereals, legumes, and so on. It may be a very different situation.

Dr. Golden: I agree with you entirely about the unusual diet in New Guinea and the fact that Malcolm's study is the only one really to show this type of effect so clearly. It may well be that protein is limiting in New Guinea and something else in most other places. The nature of the biological response in man to protein deficiency is one question; whether it actually occurs in practice is a totally different question, and I don't think we have addressed that question.

Your comments about Beaton's review are well taken; the Atole Fresco study (3) as well as a number of other studies have shown a statistically significant effect. However, I wonder how biologically significant it is to get a 1- or 2-cm difference in a population that is 12 cm short. When we look at what happens to patients with celiac disease or to what happens in the ward when we give what we now know to be a poor diet because we just don't know what the requirements for catch-up are for any of the nutrients, we should see a much better and biologically significant response than has been reported.

Dr. Tomkins: There are obviously different components in the impact of systemic infection on nutrition, whether it is weight or height gain. One of them is anorexia. Another is the increased energy cost of weight gain, which has been documented to a limited degree. In acute infection, plasma zinc goes down, but whole-body zinc status is not going to change. Could you give us your opinion on whether there is a role for zinc in the increased energy cost of growth in systemic infection, or is this just a transient decrease in plasma levels that has no physiological impact on weight gain?

Dr. Golden: The short answer is "yes." However, our ignorance is so vast on the requirements for normal growth of many of these nutrients in humans, let alone different requirements necessitated by accelerated growth, that we cannot judge the diets. I don't think we have sufficient information or even the correct concepts to study this properly. The reduction in plasma zinc in response to an infection is a redistribution within the body. The response to an infection is a change in metabolism. I think we will get similar changes in metabolism in response to deficiences of type II nutrients. I think there are common final pathways, and when we trace them back, quite arbitrarily we ascribe a metabolic aberration to what we consider may be the cause—deficiency, infection, etc.—without considering other possibilities.

Dr. Ousa: Did you find episodes of infection during recovery from malnutrition?

Dr. Golden: Children who had recovered on our diets, which we now know to contain insufficient zinc, had small thymuses and had a defect in cell-mediated immunity. We did not record an increase in infection in these children, however. The number of children we looked at was small, and they were housed under relatively hygienic conditions.

Dr. Valyasevi: Would you care to comment on the relationship between zinc and vitamin A, because in many areas there are good indicators of deficiency in both.

Dr. Golden: Clearly, there is a relationship between zinc and vitamin A. The progression and exacerbation of vitamin A deficiency despite quite large amounts of supplemental vitamin A may well be related to the sort of concepts I have considered. We put a child into an anabolic phase so that he had to make tissues and gain weight when we force fed him or put a tube down and gave him a lot of energy. In these circumstances we find exactly the sort of thing I have shown—acute depletion in zinc. Under these conditions we would expect there to be problems with epithelia, and we will undoubtedly find a synergism between preexisting vitamin A deficiency and an acutely induced zinc deficiency despite the fact that we have given a lot of zinc to the children. Yes, I think this is a very important point. On the contrary, I am not convinced about the value of retinaldehyde dehydrogenase measurements, because there seem to be very small changes in the dehydrogenase activity even in the face of severe zinc deficiency.

Dr. Colombo: A study is going on in Chile in which undernourished children are given a formula with zinc. The preliminary results show that they are growing better than the control group. However, the copper status of these children has also been evaluated, and it appears to be very low, which was related to the growth deficit. Do you have any comment on this?

Dr. Golden: Copper deficiency could give rise to stunting because of reduced lysyl oxidase activity and reduced desmosine formation. Whether it in fact does, I am not sure. Milk is exceptionally low in copper, particularly cow's milk, which is much lower than human milk. If we look at the difference in rates of growth of premature infants (who are born with low hepatic copper stores because they haven't laid down hepatic copper during the last trimester) on breast milk and on cow's milk, we see that their longitudinal growth is better on cow's milk than it is on breast milk. Shaw's balance studies (4) in these infants showed that they had good length growth despite very deficient copper intakes and despite the fact that they were in negative copper balance. Copper may fall into the same class as calcium. Longitudinal growth continues even though there is marked calcium deficiency, but the child ends up with thin bones. We certainly do not get any relationship in our children between longitudinal growth and changes in superoxide dismutase, which we are now using as a measure of copper status.

Dr. Rappaport: Zinc deficiency modifies immune tolerance and the immune system. How does this relate to the condition we are dealing with? Can it specifically be the cause of an increased incidence of infectious disease, or is the situation too complex to relate anything specifically to zinc deficiency?

Dr. Golden: Severe zinc deficiency creates problems with cell synthesis and cell turnover. All the rapidly dividing cells are affected, particularly in the gastrointestinal tract and the immune system. Zinc-deficient children do get an immunoincompetence. It seems to be particularly a T-cell immunoincompetence. The children who come in with low zinc have increased infection, particularly of the mucosae—candidiasis of the mouth, the stomach, and so on—but they have all sorts of other deficits as well, and it is very difficult to sort out specifically one problem from another.

REFERENCES

1. Beaton GH, Ghassemi H. Supplementary feeding programs for young children in developing countries. *Am J Clin Nutr* 1982;35:864–916.
2. Malcolm LA. Growth retardation in a New Guinea boarding school and its response to supplementary feeding. *Br J Nutr* 1970;24:297–305.
3. Habicht JP, Lechtig A, Yarbough C, Klein RE. The timing of the effect of supplementation feeding on the growth of rural preschool children. In: Arroyo S, Barta S, Bourges H, et al., eds. *Proceedings of the ninth international congress of nutrition, abstracts of short communications.* Mexico: 1972:149–56.
4. Dauncey MJ, Shaw JC, Urman J. The absorption and retention of magnesium, zinc, and copper by low birth weight infants fed pasteurized human breast milk. *Pediatr Res* 1977;11:1033–9.
5. Kosterlitz MW, Campbell RM. The relationship between ions in labile liver cytoplasm and urinary nitrogen excretion. *Biochem J* 1948;43:416–9.

Linear Growth Retardation in Less Developed Countries, edited by John C. Waterlow. Nestlé Nutrition Workshop Series, Vol. 14. Nestec Ltd., Vevey/Raven Press, Ltd., New York © 1988.

The Importance of Infections and Environmental Factors as Possible Determinants of Growth Retardation in Children

*David Nabarro, †Peter Howard, *Claudia Cassels, ‡Mahesh Pant, §Alet Wijga, and **Nigel Padfield

*Department of International Community Health, Liverpool School of Tropical Medicine, Liverpool L3 5QA, England (formerly of KHARDEP, Nepal); †Institute of Medical Research, Papua New Guinea) (formerly of KHARDEP, Nepal); ‡International Irrigation Management Institute, Kathmandu, Nepal; §KHARDEP Impact Studies of the Kosi Hill Area Rural Development Programme, Dhankuta, Nepal; and **East Street Health Centre, Thame, Oxford, England (formerly of Save the Children Fund Nepal Programme)*

In this chapter, we examine patterns of children's linear growth in Nepal and in Bangladesh. We then present an analysis of different variables associated with slowed linear growth; these include the child's sex, the place where the child lives, the season, the economic status of the household, the ethnic group to which the child belongs, and illnesses to which the child is exposed. We finally consider the relative importance of different factors in precipitating slowed linear growth.

Our review draws on a number of studies of children's growth and nutritional status undertaken in the Kingdom of Nepal between 1975 and 1985. Most of these studies were undertaken by or in partnership with His Majesty's Government of Nepal. They are summarized in Tables 1 and 2.

PATTERNS OF LINEAR GROWTH IN CHILDHOOD

Adult Nepalis are short in stature. One finding from the first round of the Kosi Hill Area Rural Development Programme (KHARDEP) Impact Studies is that in the seven sites studied, the mean height of adult men is 160 cm and that of adult women is 148 cm. The same studies reveal that adults from poorer families tend to be shorter than those from wealthier families (9,10).

The slowed linear growth of Nepalese children is noticeable even in infancy. Figures 1 and 2 show the mean values of children's weights and heights at different ages. The values are averaged from the data collected in Chuliban over 2.5 years.

TABLE 1. *Cross-sectional studies of children's nutritional status discussed in the text*[a]

Study title (ref.)	Date	Responsible agency	Purpose of study	Location	Details of sample	Number of children	Ages (months)	Season	Comments
Nepal Nutrition Survey (1)	1975	HMGN, CDC	Description of national situation	Nationwide	Random two-stage cluster	6,500	0–72	?	
Nepal Nutrition Survey (1)	1975	HMGN, CDC	Comparison group	Kathmandu Patan	Children from better-off families	486	0–72	?	Families could afford to provide adequate nutrition for their children
Surkhet District Nutrition Survey (2)	1977	SCF with HMGN	Description of district situation	Surkhet District (W. Nepal)	Random two-stage cluster	1,000	0–59	Premonsoon	
Baglung Nutrition Survey (3)	1979	SCF	Association of nutrition with HH wealth	Baglung District (W. Nepal)	All children in all HH from three Panchayats	1,490	0–71	?	Sufficiency of HH food production and milk buffalo as wealth indices
KHARDEP Baseline Survey (4)	1979	HMGN, (KHARDEP), SCF, BNMT	Base line for development program	Dhankuta Sankhuasabbha (E. Nepal)	Random two-stage; 40 sites; 457 HHs	907	0–95	Early monsoon	Total land area cultivated as HH wealth index

[a]All abbreviations are defined in Table 2.

TABLE 2. *Longitudinal studies of children's nutritional status discussed in this chapter*[a]

Study title (ref.)	Dates	Responsible agency	Purpose of study	Location	Details of sample	Number of children (midsurvey)	Ages (months)	Frequency of data collection	Extra data collected
Chuliban longitudinal study (5–7)	1977–82	SCF HMGN ODA	Influences of illness and season on child growth	Chuliban village, Dhankuta District	Children seen in a home visiting program	Approx. 200	0–71	Average 7 per year	Illness episodes; some detailed studies of individual HHs
KHARDEP Impact Studies (KIS) (8–10)	1980–85	HMGN (KHARDEP) ODA SCF	Impact of a rural development program	Dhankuta, Sankhuasabbha, Terathum, Bhojpur Districts	Stratified random at 7 sites; 760 HH	Approx. 450	0–71	2–3 per year	Socioeconomic; service use

[a]Notes for Tables 1 and 2: HH, household; KHARDEP, Kosi Hill Area Rural Development Programme; HMGN, His Majesty's Government of Nepal; CDC, Center for Disease Control, Atlanta, Georgia, U.S.A.; SCF, Save the Children Fund, U.K. (works under an agreement with HMGN Health Ministry); BNMT, Britain Nepal Medical Trust (works under an agreement with HMGN Health Ministry); ODA, British Government Overseas Development Administration.

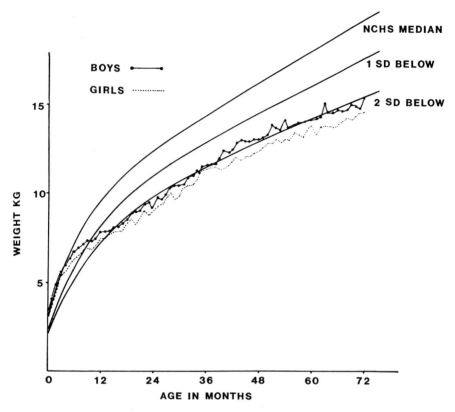

FIG. 1. Chuliban Longitudinal Study: mean weights of children compared to the NCHS reference.

The growth patterns of children studied in the Chuliban Longitudinal Study (6) and the KHARDEP Impact Studies (8,9) have been compared with the growth of children in the National Center for Health Statistics reference population (NCHS reference) (11). The average linear growth rate of the children (males and females combined) has been estimated from differences in their mean lengths or heights at different ages. These values, expressed as monthly linear growth rates (millimeter per month), are compared with the monthly growth rates derived from the NCHS figures. Weight gain figures, produced in a similar fashion, have been expressed in grams per month. They are compared with the reference-derived weight gain figures (Figs. 1 and 2).

Estimates for monthly linear growth rates and weight gains of children in the Chuliban longitudinal study and linear growth rates of children in the KHARDEP study are shown in Table 3.

The weight gain of children in Chuliban is far lower than reference values between the ages of 3 and 24 months; it increases between 24 and 36 months and then starts to fall off again between 36 and 72 months. Length increments are less than expected from birth onwards. The deficit is most marked between the ages

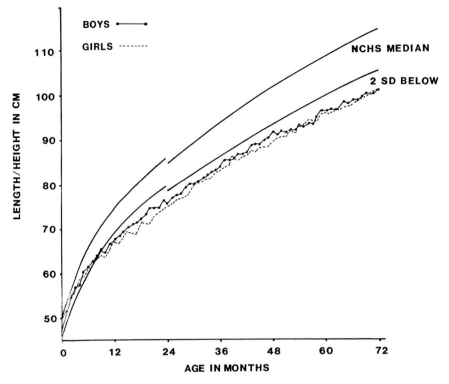

FIG. 2. Chuliban Longitudinal Study: mean lengths or heights of children compared to the NCHS reference.

of 3 and 12 months; linear growth rates improve (approaching 80% of the reference values) after the first year of life. Data from the KHARDEP Impact Study

TABLE 3. *Estimated monthly weight and length/height gain of children in Chuliban and length/height gain of children in KHARDEP Impact Studies compared with NCHS reference values*

Age (months)	Weight gain		Length/height gain				
			Reference ht. gain (mm/month)	Chuliban		KHARDEP	
	g/month	% ref.		mm/month	% ref.	mm/month	% ref.
0–3	780	117	30.0	26.7	89		
3–6	350	66	21.7	15.0	69	15.8	73
6–12	173	43	15.0	10.4	69	9.6	64
12–24	136	58	9.2	6.9	75	6.7	73
24–36	167	100	7.7	6.2	80	5.8	76
36–48	116	82	7.0	5.8	82	5.6	81
48–60	100	67	5.4	4.8	89	4.5	83
60–72	67	45	5.0	4.0	80	4.1	82

support the Chuliban results and reveal that slowing of linear growth is maxiumum between 6 and 12 months. Taken together (Fig. 3), the results confirm that slowed linear growth starts soon after birth and becomes pronounced during the first 12 months of life.

Cross-sectional studies reveal that in Nepal stunting (lengths or heights less than 90% of reference) is prevalent from an early age. The results of the Nepal Nutrition Status Survey showed that 48% of children in the 13- to 24-month age group were stunted; the prevalence rate rises to 63% in the 49- to 60-month age group.

ANALYSIS OF DIFFERENT VARIABLES ASSOCIATED WITH SLOWED LINEAR GROWTH

Stunting is widespread in South Asia, and workers in community health programs want to know its significance. Does it indicate that a child is in danger? If so, what can be done to reduce this danger? The risks associated with being stunted have been examined in Bangladesh (12,13): the stunted child does have a higher risk of mortality compared to the child whose height is close to the reference value. Hence, personnel working in health and development programs in East Nepal have been involved in analyzing factors associated with the high prevalence rate of stunting.

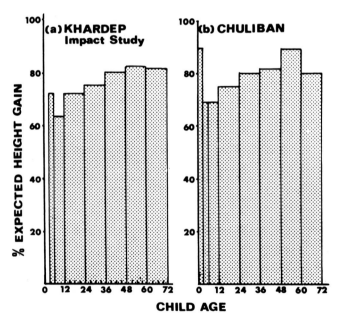

FIG. 3. KHARDEP Impact Study and Chuliban Longitudinal Study: estimated monthly length or height gain of children as a percentage of the expected gain (NCHS reference) by age group.

The Child's Sex

From the age of 3 months, female children in the Chuliban Longitudinal Study were an average of 1 cm shorter than males of similar ages. In the cross-sectional study of children under 5 years of age undertaken in Surkhet, the prevalence rate of severe stunting (height or length less than 85% of reference) was higher among girls (37%) than among boys (25%).

The Geographical Area

Results of the 1975 Nepal Nutrition Status Survey (1) revealed that 52% of children in rural Nepal aged less than 6 years were stunted. The prevalence rate of stunting in the hill terrain (55%) was higher than that in the lowland terrain (45%). Of all the geopolitical units in the country, the Eastern terrain had the highest prevalence rate of wasting and the lowest prevalence rate of stunting.

The Season

There is a pronounced seasonal variation in the climate in Nepal. Winters are cold; the early summer months (April and May) are hot and dry, though showers start toward the end of May. The late summer (July–September) is the monsoon season. The climate influences farming systems: harvests coincide with the end of the monsoon. The months before the harvest are associated with household food shortages, heavy demands on family members to undertake agricultural labor, and a high incidence of diarrheal disease.

Studies in rural Bangladesh have reported seasonal fluctuations in the nutritional status of preschool children; prevalence rates of wasting and stunting change with the seasons. The highest prevalence rates of mild and moderate wasting occur between July and December, the monsoon period that precedes the main rice harvest (14,15). There is a seasonal increase in prevalence rates of stunting between December and April, even though this is the period of maximum weight gain. Increased height gain and a fall in the prevalence rate of stunting occur about 3 months after the period of increased weight gain.

Data collected by several agencies reveal a similar seasonal variation in the prevalence rate of wasting among Nepalese children, with figures highest during the late monsoon months. The weight gain of children in the Chuliban study aged 12 to 35 months was greatest during the months from the middle of the monsoon, when the first cereal crops are harvested, until mid-January. Peak weight gains were recorded between mid-August and mid-October.

The length gain of children aged 12 to 23 months was greatest between mid-December and mid-April (Nepali months 9 to 12), 3 months after the period of maximum weight gain (Fig. 4).

Monthly prevalence rates for severe stunting in Chuliban (height or length less

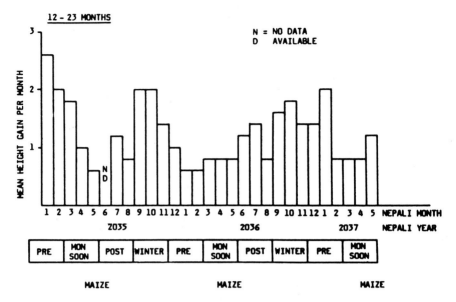

FIG. 4. Chuliban Longitudinal Study: monthly level of height gain in cm among children in the 12- to 23-month age group. The seasons and month of the maize harvest are also shown.

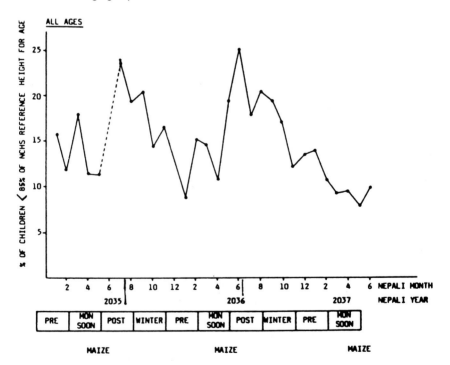

FIG. 5. Chuliban Longitudinal Study: prevalence of severe stunting (< 85% height for age) among children aged less than 6 years, by month. The seasons and month of the maize harvest are also shown.

TABLE 4. *Nutritional status (height/length for age) of children in SCF Baglung Nutrition Survey analyzed with respect to sufficiency of household food production during the previous year*[a]

Sufficiency of food production	Height/age < 90%			Height/age < 85%		
	No.	Total	%	No.	Total	%
No food	29	39	74	16	38	42
3 months	58	89	65	23	95	24
3–6 months	251	394	64	99	388	25
6–9 months	200	372	54	41	372	11
9–12 months	308	595	52	75	597	13
Total	846	1489	57	254	1490	17

[a]Chi squares: $x^2 = 9.79$, $df = 4$, $p < 0.05$; $x^2 = 44.55$, $df = 4$, $p < 0.0001$. Height/age 90% vs. food sufficiency 10.3, 4 df ($p < 0.05$). Height/age 85% vs. food sufficiency 48.1, 4 df ($p < 0.001$).

TABLE 5. *Nutritional status (height/length for age) of children in SCF Baglung Nutrition Survey analyzed with respect to household ownership of a milk-producing buffalo*[a]

Ownership of buffalo	Height/age < 90%			Height/age < 85%		
	No.	Total	%	No.	Total	%
No buffalo	413	683	61[b]	144	683	21[c*]
Buffalo	440	806	55	109	806	14*

[a]Asterisk indicates significant difference ($p < 0.01$).
[b]$x^2 = 4.98$, $df = 1$, $p < 0.05$.
[c]$x^2 = 14.45$, $df = 1$, $p < 0.001$.

than 85% of NCHS reference) are shown in Fig. 5. Between Nepali years 2035 and 2037 (1977–1979), the prevalence rates of severe stunting were highest between late August and mid-February (months 5–10, inclusive); this was the period of maximum weight gain.

The Economic Status of the Household

The association between growth patterns and household socioeconomic status was investigated in the Nepal Baglung Nutrition Survey in 1979 (Tables 4 and 5).

The results showed that the prevalence rates of both stunting and severe stunting among children from households classed as poorer was greater than those among children from wealthier households. Analysis of variance reveals that sufficiency of household food production is a highly significant predictor of height for age. This significance remains when the effects of age, sex, caste, and number of children aged less than 15 years in the family have been taken into account.

The 1979 KHARDEP Baseline Survey revealed that the prevalence rate of stunting varied both with the age of the child and with the socioeconomic status of the child's household (Table 6).

The prevalence rate of severe stunting among children aged less than 8 years from households cultivating less than half a hectare was significantly greater than that among children from households cultivating more than 1 ha. However, when the prevalence rate of severe stunting was studied among children in different age groups, the differential was evident in the 12- to 35-month and 60- to 95-month group but not in the 36- to 59-month group.

It seemed possible that children from households cultivating more than 1 ha showed catch-up in linear growth rates after the age of 59 months. The prevalence rate of stunting is lower among these households' children when they are aged 60 to 95 months than among children aged 36 to 59 months. This pattern, which suggests catch-up in linear growth, is not seen among children from the poorer households studied on the same occasion.

More recent results, obtained in the KHARDEP Impact Studies, show that it would be unwise to suggest that catch-up has occurred on the basis of cross-sectional data alone. Data obtained from approximately 400 children measured on seven occasions from year 2 (1982) to year 5 (1985) of the studies have been analyzed. Children were measured either in the dry winter season or in the monsoon. The prevalence rate of severe stunting at each visit shows considerable variation (Fig. 6) and is difficult to interpret, not least because the winter visits coincide with the likely period of maximum linear growth rates.

Food production data collected from the same households reveal that the harvest at the end of 1982 (year 2) was extremely bad. By the monsoon of 1983 (second visit, year 3), the prevalence rate of stunting in all age groups increased dramatically compared with the prevalence rate during the monsoon of 1982. The prevalence rate of wasting did not show a dramatic rise during the 1983 monsoon visit. Subsequent harvests were better, but the level of severe stunting in the 36- to 59-month age group remained high until 1985 (10).

Households were classified as poorer or wealthier on the basis of the area and type of land that they cultivated. Figure 7 shows that during all visits except 3.1,

TABLE 6. *KHARDEP Baseline Survey (Nepal 1979): prevalence of severe stunting (< 85% height for age) among children by age group and area of land cultivated by household*

Household land area (ha)	Age group of children (months)							
	12–35		36–59		60–95		0–95	
	No.	%	No.	%	No.	%	No.	%
0–0.5	25	24%	29	34%	40	52%	94	39%
0.51–1	42	19%	54	37%	74	45%	170	36%
Over 1.0	81	10%	71	32%	108	27%	260	23%
Total	148	15%	154	34%	222	37%	524	30%

the prevalence rate of severe stunting among poorer households' children was greater than that among the wealthy households' children. There was a marked increase in the prevalence rate of severe stunting among children from the poorer households following the bad harvest in 1982.

Taken together, the Nepal data suggest that the linear growth rates of Nepalese children are far slower than those of the children used to provide the NCHS refer-

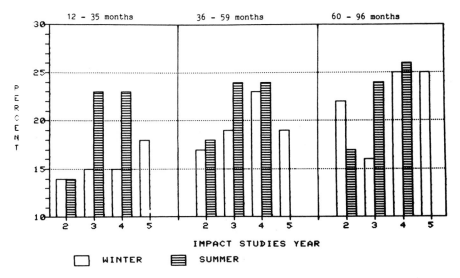

FIG. 6. KHARDEP Impact Studies: prevalence of severe stunting (< 85% height for age) during different visits by age group.

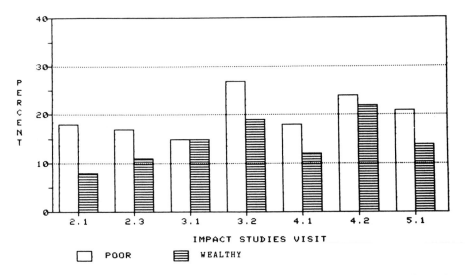

FIG. 7. KHARDEP Impact Studies: prevalence of severe stunting (< 85% height for age) among children aged 12–35 months by visit and household wealth.

ence figures. The difference is most marked in infancy. There is definite evidence of an association between linear growth rates in childhood and household poverty. This is exacerbated by the effects of harvest failure. The suggestion of seasonal variation in linear growth rates can complicate the interpretation of longitudinal data.

The Child's Ethnic Group

The people of Nepal are drawn from a number of different tribal and caste groups: some are of Indo-Aryan origin; others are of Tibeto-Burman origin. Physically the members of these two ethnic groups look very different: the Indo-Aryans tend to be slimmer, the Tibeto-Burmans stockier. There are clear genetic influences on the final height and physical shape of Nepali adults.

In the Surkhet District Nutritional Survey (2), the children of the Magars and Gurungs (Tibeto-Burmans) had a higher prevalence rate of stunting than did those of the Tharus (Indo-Aryans). The socioeconomic status of the two groups is broadly similar, though their habitat (hills versus plains) and feeding practices are different. Results from the KHARDEP Baseline Survey (4) revealed similar prevalence rates of stunting for Indo-Aryan and Tibeto-Burman children.

Studies of privileged households in Kathmandu, undertaken as part of the Nepal Nutrition Status Survey (1) in 1975, confirm that under favorable economic circumstances and environmental conditions, the linear growth of Nepalese children aged less than 5 years is similar to that of Western children. However, it is likely that the growth patterns of children in adverse economic and environmental circumstances will be determined to some extent by genetic factors.

Preliminary results suggest that when incidence of infections is high and nutrient intake is low, the linear growth rate of Tibeto-Burman children is less than that of the Indo-Aryan children. These associations will be studied further.

Infection

Childhood infections, particularly those affecting the intestinal and upper respiratory tract, are extremely common in East Nepal. They have an adverse effect on the nutritional status of preschool children. This may be a result of several different mechanisms.

Children who are ill lose their appetite; this anorexia will result in a reduction in food intake. Food may not be offered to the child for cultural or compassionate reasons, and food that is consumed may be lost through malabsorption or vomiting. The presence of fever may increase the child's energy needs above normal requirements. Of all these factors, anorexia and the mother's reluctance to feed the child are the most important in determining the nutritional response to an infection (16).

Data from the Chuliban Longitudinal Study reveal that children with diarrhea lose an average of 0.37 kg during the month after the episode compared with an average gain of 0.11 kg experienced by children who did not have diarrhea in the same month (6). Even greater differences are seen in children suffering from measles. This weight loss may be associated with a reduction in the rate of height gain. Preliminary results from the studies suggest that children who are less than 85% weight for height during the summer months gain less height than children whose weight is greater than 85% of the reference weight for height at this time.

The influence of infections on growth has been observed in many other parts of the world (17–19). Results suggest that frequent episodes of infection, particularly diarrhea, lead to acute weight loss and impaired linear growth. In one study in Bangladesh, each episode of prolonged diarrhea was associated with a 0.56-cm reduction in linear growth (20). Studies in northeast Brazil reveal that among children aged 1 to 2 years, the average increase in height of those with diarrhea during a 3-month period was 41% less than in children with no diarrhea during the same period (21).

Until recently, most investigators had been unable to determine the precise effect of infection on the growth of children. They needed to separate the effects of infection from other factors usually associated with the presence of both infection and malnutrition—lack of adequate food, sanitation, clean water, time for child care, access to health services, in other words, a poor social and economic environment. However, the group working in northeast Brazil has demonstrated that diarrhea remained a significant contributory cause of stunting even when age, socioeconomic status, and initial nutritional status were taken into account (21). Thus, though children may quickly regain weight lost during an episode of diarrhea, the long-term effect of the infection on linear growth persists.

THE ASSOCIATIONS AMONG INFECTIONS, ENVIRONMENTAL FACTORS, AND SLOWED LINEAR GROWTH

We have identified several factors that together account for the slowed linear growth of children in developing countries. We suspect that in young children there is an association between weight for height and the potential for subsequent linear growth. During the period of maximum height increment in seasonal environments, children who have been thin for long periods in the preceding months probably grow less in height than children who have been fatter.

Children are likely to have low weight for height as a result of infection and diminished food intake. The length of time for which a child remains below the expected weight for his height is likely to determine his linear growth during the succeeding months. The duration of low weight for height may be a more important determinant than the incidence rate of low weight for height. If this hypothesis is true, children who gain weight rapidly after an episode of infection will subsequently gain in height at the expected rate. Children whose catch-up growth is less satisfactory will, in turn, gain less in height.

Such a hypothesis explains the association between poverty and height gain rates, as poor families are less able to ensure rapid catch-up after their children's infections. It also explains why conditions that worsen the position of the poorest in a community may result in increased stunting prevalence rates with only a transient, if any, effect on wasting prevalence rates.

These hypotheses need to be examined further in order that the linkages among poverty, illness, food intake, wasting, catch-up growth, height gain rates, and stunting can better be elaborated in the children of the developing world.

ACKNOWLEDGMENTS

We quote results obtained from studies undertaken by His Majesty's Government, Ministry of Health, Kathmandu, Nepal; His Majesty's Government Ministry of Panchayat and Local Development, Kathmandu, Nepal; Save the Children Fund (SCF), UK; and Overseas Development Administration (ODA), UK Government.

We acknowledge financial assistance from the Overseas Development Administration Nutrition and Health Research Funds (Grant No. R3625, Child Nutrition in Nepal; Grant No: R4143, Assistance with data collection in Nepal), and from the Save the Children Fund. Some of the data quoted were collected while D.N, C.C., M.P., and A.W. were contracted to assess the impact of the Kosi Hills Area Rural Development Programme.

REFERENCES

1. His Majesty's Government of Nepal, Office of Nutrition, Development Support Bureau. *Nepal Nutrition Status Survey*. Washington: United States Agency for International Development, 1975.
2. Black N. Surkhet District Nutritional Status Survey. *J Inst Med Nepal* 1979;1:1–26.
3. Howard P. *Nutritional and socio-economic status of children in Western Nepal—a baseline survey as a guide to planning*. London: University of London, London School of Hygiene and Tropical Medicine, 1984.
4. Thompson B. *Preliminary findings of a Nutrition Status Survey conducted in the Kosi Hills, Nepal in June 1979*. London: University of London, London School of Hygiene and Tropical Medicine, 1979.
5. Nabarro DN. Influences on child nutrition in Eastern Nepal. *J. Inst Med Nepal* 1982;4:47–66.
6. Nabarro DN. Influences on the growth of children: observations from Nepal. *J Nepal Paediatr Assoc* 1985;2:137–205.
7. Roberts NCE. *Programmes and studies*. Reading: University of Reading, 1981.
8. Nabarro DN, Innes J. *Monitoring and evaluation of the Kosi Hill Area Rural Development Programme—methods and procedures used in the study of programme impact*. Kathmandu: Co-ordinator's Office, KHARDEP, 1982; KHARDEP Impact Report Number 1, CNLRDCP-361/Nepal-03-148/82.
9. Nabarro DN, Innes J. *Monitoring and evaluation of the Kosi Hill Area Rural Development Programme—the impact of the Kosi Hill Area Rural Development Programme: description of data collected in the first year of the KHARDEP Impact Studies*. Kathmandu: Co-ordinator's Office, KHARDEP, 1982; KHARDEP Impact Report Number 2, CNLRDCP-363/Nepal-03-149/82.
10. Nabarro DN, Cassels C, Pant M, Wijga A. *Monitoring and evaluation of the Kosi Hill Area Rural Development Programme—results of the KHARDEP Impact Studies (1980–1985)*. Liverpool: KHARDEP Impact Report Number 7, 1986.
11. Hamill PVV. *NCHS growth curves for children*. Hyattsville, MD: National Center for Health Statistics, 1979; DHEW publication no. (PHS) 78-1650 (Vital and health statistics; series 11:165).

12. Chen LC, Chowdhury AKMA, Huffman S. Anthropometric assessment of energy–protein malnutrition and subsequent risk of mortality. *Am J Clin Nutr* 1980;33:1836–45.
13. Bairagi R, Chowdhury MK, Kim YJ, Curlin GT. Alternative anthropometric indicators of mortality. *Am J Clin Nutr* 1985;42:296–306.
14. Chen LC, Chowdhury AKMA, Huffman SL. Seasonal dimensions of energy protein malnutrition
in rural Bangladesh: the role of agriculture, dietary practices, and infection. *Ecol Food Nutr*
1979;8:175–87.
15. Brown KH, Black RE, Becker S. Seasonal changes in nutritional status and the prevalence of
malnutrition in a longitudinal study of young children in rural Bangladesh. *Am J Clin Nutr*
1982;36:303–13.
16. Mata LJ, Kromal RA, Urrutia JJ, Garcia B. Effect of infection on food intake and the nutritional
state: perspectives as viewed from the village. *Am J Clin Nutr* 1977;30:1215–27.
17. Rowland MGM, Cole TJ, Whitehead RG. A quantitative study into the role of infection in determining nutritional status in Gambian village children. *Br J Nutr* 1977;37:441–50.
18. Black RE, Brown KH, Becker S. Longitudinal studies of infectious diseases and physical growth
of children in rural Bangladesh—patterns of morbidity. *Am J Epidemiol* 1982;115(3):305–15.
19. Mata LJ. *The children of Santa Maria Cauque: a prospective field study of health and growth.*
Cambridge, MA: MIT Press, 1978.
20. Black RE, Brown KH, Becker S. Effects of diarrhea associated with specific enteropathogens on
the growth of children in rural Bangladesh. *Pediatrics* 1984;73:799–805.
21. Guerrant RL, Kirchoff LV, Shields DS, et al. Prospective study of diarrheal illnesses in north-
eastern Brazil: patterns of disease, nutritional impact, etiologies, and risk factors. *J Infect Dis*
1983;148:986–97.

DISCUSSION

Dr. Tanner: You are absolutely right in saying that the rate of growth, not only now but
also in the last century during the course of industrialization, has been used by economic
historians as an indicator of the living conditions of the working class and that around the
world the correlation between height and social conditions, for means of populations, is
very close. I would just like to add a professional auxologist's warning about getting far
away from the data, turning it into percentages, using references, etc. For example, people
sometimes forget that the NCHS has a big break at 3 years old: the first 3 years are from
a totally different group than the rest. The reason that your children appeared smaller in
the first 3 years is that they were being compared to a highly privileged Northwest European Caucasian stock measured at the Fels Institute. At 3 years old the NCHS shifts gear
totally, and it is then a proportionate sample, theoretically at least, of all children in the
United States.

There is another problem; I don't know if it would affect your data, but I think it may
have done. If you take a percentage of the median, the coefficient of variation isn't the
same as the child gets older. So 85% of median at one age gives you lots more children
undernourished than 85% at another age.

Dr. Rappaport: Dr. Tanner, how would you express the results in this type of study?

Dr. Tanner: I would quite simply look at the means and variances of the heights in the
various groups.

Dr. Nabarro: Would you compare the heights that we have obtained with the reference
values and express them as standard deviation units, or would you be particularly interested
in the means and variances of the actual heights?

Dr. Tanner: I'd be particularly interested in the means and variances of your heights,
but if I were then going to put them in relation to any reference value, which is a very
popular thing to do, then indeed I would do that in terms of SDs.

Dr. Nabarro: We would very much like to have data from a reference population showing means and variances of length and height increments. That was what we were really after when doing that work, but we couldn't find any data.

Dr. Tanner: That is exactly what our present paper is about. There is a paper (1), again from the Fels Institute, on 6-month increments only. However, 6 months is perhaps too long. You would prefer 3 months; Prof. Waterlow wanted 1 month. So we have gone down to 1 month or 2.

Dr. Waterlow: Dr. Nabarro, referring to Bangladesh you said they calculated that if the children had no diarrhea, they would have grown an extra 0.4 cm each year, and if worm-free, 1.2 cm. That is in children of what age? How do those figures relate to the expected annual increment?

Dr. Nabarro: The first data were obtained by Black and colleagues in Matlab, Bangladesh (2). They studied 177 children aged between 2 and 48 months over 12 months. The second set were obtained by Evans and colleagues in Jamalpur as part of a collaborative project involving the Save the Children Fund (3). They studied 467 children aged 2 to 5 years over 12 months. Examination of the NCHS reference figure reveals that children aged between 12 and 24 months would be expected to gain about 9 cm a year.

Dr. Waterlow: The impression I get is that the differences are not very great, and I have been arguing for some time that the effects of infection are often exaggerated. When you compare the growth in either weight or height between highly infected children and much less infected children, the differences are not very large (4). The problem is to relate the duration as well as the prevalence of illness over fairly long periods, say a year, to the growth during that year. I don't believe there's going to be a uniform pattern everywhere.

Dr. Nabarro: Our evidence suggests very strongly that there are 3 or 4 months in the year in Nepal when children aged between 12 and 23 months gain on average about 1.5 to 2 cm in length. For the rest of the year, they appear to gain very little. This suggests that, just as with weight gain, there are circumstances under which length increment can be extremely "good." It seems very unlikely to us that the poor linear growth during the other 9 months of the year can be accounted for on the grounds of infection alone. I think that the processes are more complex and that we have insufficient information to permit us to suggest causes of retardation in linear growth. There are only certain months in the year when both weight gain and length increment are sufficient for children to achieve their maximum growth potential.

Perhaps the relative importance of infection or inadequate nutrient intake in retarding linear growth will not be of great relevance to national development policy makers in Nepal. The most important finding is that households that cultivate less than half a hectare of land are most likely to have children who are severely stunted; these same households are also likely to have children who are suffering from a wide variety of disabilities and risks to their health.

Dr. Tanner: To follow up what Professor Waterlow was saying, if you lose a centimeter every year, then it becomes a lot. One of the good ways to end up very small is to grow not at the 50th centile but consistently at the 40th. A one-time response to deparasitization would be fine, but if it's something that continues, even that centimeter can be very important.

Dr. Tomkins: You've made a very interesting observation, that there was a dramatic increase in stunting and not in wasting at a certain period in the year. You also observed that there were two genetic groups in your population and that there may be genetically different responses to an infection. Were the increases in stunting and wasting the same in both ethnic groups?

Dr. Nabarro: No. It's still difficult for us to give consistent answers. If we analyze children from households with broadly similar economic status but belonging to these two ethnic groups, we find in some of our studies that there are substantial differences in the prevalence rates of both stunting and wasting between the groups. We have not yet been able to demonstrate differences in the linear growth rates of children belonging to the two groups. Perhaps we should do more than consider the maximum potential growth of children belonging to different ethnic groups. We should also consider how genetic factors influence the way in which children respond to deprivation.

Dr. Rappaport: Is there any other model in which you could sort out genetic factors that might control catch-up growth?

Dr. Nabarro: It would be possible, I am sure, in parts of northern India. However, it may be that disaggregated data are not yet available to make this kind of comparison possible.

Dr. Kraisid: Do you find any difference in terms of feeding practices, especially in supplementary feeding, among these different ethnic groups? In Indian populations, complementary feed usually starts at 6 to 12 months. Among Burmese or people in southeast Asian countries, supplementary foods are given earlier. This may have some effect.

Dr. Nabarro: There are certainly differences in feeding practices; there may also be differences in rates of infection. As you say, these may be relevant.

Dr. Waterlow: Dr. Nabarro made a point that I think is extremely important, that the increase in length when things improve in the course of the seasonal effects follows the increase in weight. From a physiological point of view, this seems to be most interesting. I wonder whether Dr. Golden has similar information about the way children behave when they are being rehabilitated in hospital. I certainly have the impression that gain in length in our recovering children followed gain in weight. I would like Dr. Nabarro and Dr. Golden to comment on this.

Dr. Nabarro: We observed this 3 years ago when we compared children who had shown good height gain and children who had shown poor height increment over an interval of 6 months. We looked at the weight for height of these children at the start of the 6-month interval. We found that the amount of height gained was highest in the children with the greatest weight for height values. We did not follow this up. However, in view of Dr. Rappaport's report, it seems to be highly relevant. Similarly, our observation made some years ago that seasonal differences in weight gains and height increments came 3 to 4 months apart now appears to be highly relevant too. We would like to reexamine some of our longitudinal data to study these observations in more detail.

One possibility will be a study of the very high prevalence rate for stunting in the third year of the KHARDEP Impact Studies in 1983. Was there a detectable decrease in the rate of weight gain of the children who became stunted during the 3 or 4 months before they should have increased in height?

Dr. Golden: We have only started to look at the question of what happens during recovery from malnutrition. About 8% of the children start to gain height as soon as they enter the ward; about 15 to 20% don't gain any height at all while they're in the ward, and we don't know what differentiates them. The vast majority of children suddenly begin to gain height when they have reached a median of 85% weight for height; then, they get their first half-centimeter increment in height. At the moment we are trying to look at the variance of their weight per height at the time when they get their first height spurt. It seems at first sight to be quite narrow and certainly centered around 85% weight for height. It also seems at the same time to be that their somatomedin-C levels show a sharp increase, but this is very preliminary data based on a small number of children.

Dr. Nabarro: Perhaps the different timing of weight gain and height increment in the children we studied would be reflected in their growth hormone and somatomedin-C levels. A careful study of the associations between seasonal growth and hormone levels might explain these differences. Clearly, such a study would not be easy to undertake under field conditons.

Dr. Rappaport: That should probably be interesting, but it is a difficult approach. Dr. Golden, could you tell us what is more important? Is it the amount of weight that is gained when the child is in the ward or the percentage of weight for height reached during the same period?

Dr. Golden: We don't have body composition studies, but I think it's much more important to know the lean tissue mass in relation to height rather than the total weight for height. The absolute amount of weight gain by the children does not seem to be very important. The children who start off very low in weight for height will fill out, and when they reach 85% then they start to gain height. The children who come in much less stunted, or the children with kwashiorkor who just lose their edema and then gain up to 85% weight for height, will then have a reasonable height. Thus, the absolute amount of gain does not seem to be related, nor does the absolute amount of height deficit that the children come in with. The age of the children, however, is related to the height gain. The younger children show this height spurt at reaching 85% weight for height very much more regularly than the older children.

Dr. Martorell: It's an interesting finding that when the situation improves, children first put on weight for height and afterwards grow in length. To me, this suggests that stunting and wasting are caused by the same factors and that a child, when faced with a nutrient deficiency that is not severe, may cope simply by slowing down in growth; we don't know much about effects of physical activity. If the deficiency is severe, cessation of growth alone is not enough, and in addition the child has to subsist on his own tissues. When the situation improves, the child first puts on weight for height and then starts growing in length. Could stunting and wasting be caused by the same factors, the difference simply being a reflection of the severity, acuteness, or suddenness of the causal factors?

Dr. Nabarro: This is our explanation for what we have seen, with the proviso that children from different ethnic groups do not respond to the causal factors in the same way. Thresholds at which they slow their growth and start to become wasted may vary in the different ethnic groups. This hypothesis needs to be tested.

Dr. Colombo: First a short comment. A 6-year follow-up study of about 400 malnourished children has been conducted in Chile; a very good correlation was found between weight for height after discharge—these children were hospitalized for about 5 months—and subsequent growth. I have also a question. Have you done any psychomotor studies in the children you were working with?

Dr. Nabarro: No, we have not done this.

Dr. Ousa: Our experience in treating children with severe protein–calorie malnutrition (PCM) is that those who come in with severe PCM gain weight and height more quickly than the ones who come in with less severe PCM. Wasted children with similar intakes, e.g., 4 g of protein and 175 kcal/kg, gain weight better than stunted children. Some children may appear very healthy although their weight is far below their expected weight for age, down to 60%. For that reason, we always rely on the weight for height. The cut-off point for discharge is 85%; when the children leave the hospital earlier, the relapse rate increases substantially.

Dr. Nabarro: Do you have any length or height increment figures for these children?

Dr. Ousa: Yes, we do.

Dr. Nabarro: It would be interesting to examine the height increment of children less than, say, 85% weight for height during succeeding months and then their height gain once they pass that particular cut-off figure. Of course, it may not be 85% in your situation.

Dr. Tanner: It seems to me important to know the family structure, the number of children in the family, the interval between pregnancies, and also when these children between 6 and 12 years old actually go out to work and the sort of work they do. Have you gone into that?

Dr. Nabarro: Yes, we have. What I was showing here were three indicators that we finally identified to disaggregate the children we studied into meaningful socioeconomic groups. We looked at very large numbers of variables before deciding to use the area of land cultivated by the household, the number of months for which food production is sufficient, and the presence or absence of a milk-producing buffalo. I agree that if we were to require a more precise indication of the actual wealth of a household, we would need much more detailed information about household assets and to relate it to household size (dividing the assets by the number of "adult consumption units" in the household). We should also take into account the amount of "off-farm" income coming into the household. The methods we used to indicate household wealth will inevitably have led us to misclassify certain households. However, it has enabled us to draw some broad conclusions about associations between household wealth and child nutritional status.

Dr. Waterlow: I don't want to see the point made by Dr. Martorell—that he regarded stunting and wasting, if I may still use these words, as the same condition—to go unchallenged. I totally disagree with him, even more after the previous chapters. That does not, of course, mean that I am right and that he is wrong. But, first of all, I disagree with him on the statistical evidence that was produced by Dr. Keller, and, second, I think we should bear the physiological points in mind that have been raised by Dr. Rappaport and Dr Milner: the body consists of different kinds of tissues—very roughly, let us say, the visceral tissues, peripheral or muscle tissue, and the skeleton. There is no question that these tissues respond to malnutrition and to rehabilitation in different ways: albumin and liver regenerate quickly, muscle less quickly, and bone, from what we have heard, perhaps still less quickly. It seems to me a very unphysiological attitude to look on these tissues as the same. However, it is probably wrong to open such a discussion at this point; it may come up again in the general discussion.

Dr. Nabarro: The kind of observations that we are producing suggest that the two processes—slowed weight gain and linear growth—are not necessarily caused by the same factors. They also suggest that children will only show a substantial increment in linear growth if they have had satisfactory weight gain during the preceding months. Retardation in weight gain and linear growth are not necessarily results of the same process, but there appears to be a definite permissive relationship between the two processes. The annual increase in a Nepalese child's length or height may well depend on postharvest weight gain.

REFERENCES

1. Roche AF, Himes JH. Incremental growth charts. *Am J Clin Nutr* 1980;33:2041–52.
2. Black RE, Brown KH, Becker S. Effects of diarrhea associated with specific enteropathogens on the growth of children in rural Bangladesh. *Pediatrics* 1984;73:799–805.
3. Evans J, Martin J, Mascie Taylor N. *The effects of periodic deworming with pyrantel pamoate on the growth of pre-school children in Northern Bangladesh.* Cambridge: Maltano Institute, 1984.
4. Waterlow JC. Observations on the suckling's dilemma—a personal view. *J Hum Nutr* 1981; 35:85–98.

Linear Growth Retardation in Less Developed Countries, edited by John C. Waterlow. Nestlé Nutrition Workshop Series, Vol. 14. Nestec Ltd., Vevey/Raven Press, Ltd., New York © 1988.

The Risk of Morbidity in a Stunted Child

Andrew Tomkins

Department of Human Nutrition and Department of Clinical Tropical Medicine, London School of Hygiene and Tropical Medicine, London WC1E 7HT, England

The general relationships between malnutrition and infection have been recognized for centuries, but the details of the links have been defined considerably only during the last few decades. Many of the studies examining the effect of malnutrition on the response to infection have been reviewed (1,2). However, most of the clinical, epidemiological, and experimental reports have emphasized the importance of severe protein–energy malnutrition (PEM), underweight, and thinness rather than shortness of stature or slow rates of height gain. It is the purpose of this chapter to review what is known about the relationship between short stature and subsequent risk of disease and death. The classification and causes of short stature are reviewed elsewhere (3), but for the purpose of this review the term "short" will be used for those children who are significantly different from standard height/age. Children who are less than 90% height/age will be called "stunted," as proposed by Waterlow and co-workers (4).

There are considerable differences of opinion among experts about the significance of malnutrition. Gopalan maintains that "to plead the virtues of 'smallness' is to acquiesce in the preservation of the status quo of poverty, ill health, undernutrition, and socioeconomic status" (5), whereas Seckler and Sukhatme (6) maintain that "small is healthy." In recent years there has been considerable use of the term "nutritional adaptation" to describe some of the factors contributing to the slow growth rates of children in less developed countries compared with richer countries. A timely review of the topic (7) has clarified some of the confusion that surrounds the use of the term "adaptation."

A FRAMEWORK FOR ANALYSIS

Before infection can develop, the pathogen, whether bacteria, parasite, or virus, must first broach the body's immune system (Fig. 1). The nature of the impact of nutrition on the individual components of the immune response are comprehensively reviewed by Chandra (8). In general we are concerned with nonspecific host defenses, antibody formation, and the cellular immune system. Once the infection invades the superficial tissues or infiltrates into deep organs, there are various host

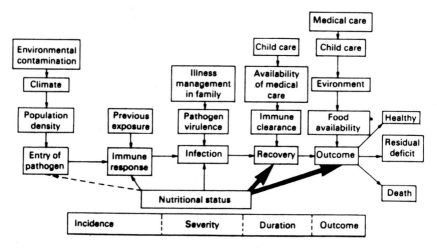

FIG. 1. A framework for analysis of risk factors for morbidity and malnutrition.

factors determining whether an abscess becomes a septicemia, a few intestinal parasites start to replicate prolifically, or whether a bacterial colonization syndrome develops.

The physiological response to infection may vary; intestinal secretion to an enterotoxin-producing enteric pathogen differs according to the nutritional state. Duration of the infection depends on a competent immune mechanism and adequate repair of damaged tissues. The outcome of the infection may be variable. Rapid recovery without residual deficit or complication is what we hope for, but persistent pathology such as the blinding malnutrition following precipitation of deficiency of vitamin A by severe measles is a lifelong complication of a transient infection and disorder of nutrition.

Death itself is more frequent among the severely malnourished, but community-based studies in developing countries have usually experienced difficulties in accurately ascribing a single cause of death in their analyses. Indeed, in all stages of the development and evolution of an infection, we have to consider the result of infection in an individual child to be influenced, to a greater or lesser degree, by the social and physical environment as well as by biological responses to pathogens. Thus, the availability of food and of somebody to prepare and feed it, perceptions of appropriate foods to be given for particular illnesses, and access to medical resources will all have an influence on the outcome of an infection.

IMMUNE DEFENSE SYSTEM

Previous studies in children with severe PEM (marasmus or kwashiorkor) showed a variety of disturbances of cellular immunity (CMI) with atrophy of the thymus and thymus-dependent lymphoid tissues (9). These could be detected by *in vivo* tests of responsiveness to antigens injected into the skin or *in vitro* tests on a range of cell types. These findings have been implicated as the major reason why severely malnourished children have such a high incidence of tuberculosis and monilial infections.

There were also several studies of CMI in children with milder grades of PEM (10,11). Most of them showed intermediate responses in CMI among children with moderate PEM (weight/age 60–75%) and normal responses in those with mild PEM (weight/age 75–90%) compared with results in well-nourished children. However, the authors did not report the length or height of these children.

Studies of the humoral responses in severe PEM have shown relatively little evidence of impaired function. Several reports described lower levels of IgA in tears, intestinal secretions, and jejunal mucosa (12). However, seroconversion to measles vaccine appears to be satisfactory, albeit delayed, in some children (13). Again, none of these reports included information on height or length.

The nonspecific immune functions such as integrity of mucosal surfaces and gastric acidity (14) are all abnormal in severe PEM, but there is no information on gastric acidity in moderate or mild PEM and no data on the relationship between gastric acidity and height/age.

In view of the absence of any data on the impact of stunting on the immune response, it might be valuable to inspect the literature on immune response in fetal malnutrition. There are problems of interpretation in that neonates who are born with a low birth weight and shorter length have been exposed to different nutritional and nonnutritional stresses than those experienced by a child who becomes stunted postnatally. It is necessary to distinguish those neonates whose physical development is appropriate for the gestational age (AGA) from those that are small for gestational age (SGA). The latter group might have been born small as a result of maternal undernutrition, hypertension, preeclamptic toxemia, maternal infection, or placental insufficiency (8).

Studies of rosette-forming T lymphocytes and hypersensitivity reactions to skin antigens show abnormal results that persist for as long as 5 years after birth among SGA children, whereas the immune system of AGA children is either normal from birth or improves rapidly within a few weeks of delivery (8).

There is some deficit in transplacental transfer of antibodies to tetanus toxoid in SGA infants together with generally lower levels of serum IgA and IgG and a slight decrease in titers of antibody to polio vaccine following immunization (15), but, in general, most immunization responses are equally effective in SGA and AGA infants.

Neutrophil function, migration of polymorphonuclear leucocytes, neutrophil bactericidal activity, and opsonic activity are also decreased in SGA infants. Studies in Guatemala showed an increased mortality for SGA babies compared with AGA babies (16). An interesting feature of SGA babies is that many of them develop circulatory antibodies to food antigens (17). This may well set the scene for persistent diarrhea in which food intolerance is thought to play an important role.

INCIDENCE OF INFECTION

There is no doubt that infection rates among children are higher in those countries where malnutrition is also prevalent, whether the malnutrition is categorized as underweight (low weight/age), short stature (low height/age), or thinness (low weight/height). A crude global estimate suggests that only 6% of children less than 5 years of age in more developed countries (where stunting is rare) have an episode of diarrhea during a year, whereas the majority of children in less developed countries have more than two episodes annually (18). Thus, on international comparison, there is a link between stunting and incidence of infection.

However, longitudinal studies of nutritional status of individual children within a single community and their subsequent morbidity do not show a clear relationship between stunting and incidence of infection (19,20).

A total of 2,019 children aged 12 to 23 months were weighed, and their height was measured, in a rural area of Bangladesh. Their attack rate for diarrhea was then assessed by recording the number of visits to a diarrhea treatment center during the following 24 months (21). Frequency of visits was similar among taller and shorter children. Neither was there any greater frequency among those who were underweight or thin. A more recent study in the same area in Bangladesh (22) examined the relationship between nutritional status among 197 children less than 4 years of age and their attack rate for diarrhea as assessed by regular home visits by trained field workers in the subsequent 60 days. Again, there was no greater attack rate among the underweight, short, or thin than among the better nourished.

Three hundred forty-three children aged 6 to 36 months living in a rural area of Malumfashi District, northern Nigeria, were measured, and diarrhea morbidity was assessed by weekly home visits (23). As in the Bangladesh studies, there was no greater frequency of diarrhea in those who were shorter or more underweight, although there was a slight but significant increase in frequency among those who were wasted (<80% weight/height). Subsequent analysis showed that there was a bias in this group because many of the wasted children were just recovering from measles, and they may well have been more susceptible to the postmeasles diarrhea syndrome.

The factors affecting the incidence of diarrhea in an individual or community are reviewed in more detail elsewhere (24) and summarized in Table 1. The main

TABLE 1. *Possible risk factors for high incidence of infection*

Prevalence of pathogen in food and water
Behavioral factors encouraging transmission
Poor sanitation
Climatic
Numbers of pathogens ingested
Adhesion characteristics of pathogens
Intestinal immunity
Gastric acidity

point is that only two of these (gastric acidity and intestinal immunity) are likely to be influenced directly by nutritional status, and even then the data on gastric acidity (14) and intestinal immunity (12) are only available from severely malnourished children.

The complexity of biological, behavioral, and environmental factors affecting the frequency of episodes of diarrhea is such that they may well override any effect of malnutrition on incidence. In a recent longitudinal study of children aged 6 to 36 months in Bakau, an urban community in the Gambia, West Africa, there was a high attack rate for diarrhea among the community as a whole, but a quarter of the children managed to survive the rainy season, an unpleasant time with high humidity, environmental temperature, and contamination of food, without any diarrhea at all (25). When 38 variables, including style of house, water supply, sanitation, and education of parents were analyzed, there were only two that correlated significantly with attack rate. This may seem surprising at first, but a walk through the township soon reveals that young children do not stay within the social and environmental groups of their parents. Play activities in the streets, visits to a variety of other compounds, and snack eating are all major opportunities for the acquisition of enteropathogens that may not exist in their own homes. Thus, the data available do not eliminate the possibility that stunting has an important effect on disease incidence, but in the face of overwhelming environmental stress affecting the whole community, well nourished as well as undernourished, the hypothesis that stunting increases the incidence of infection is not yet proven.

SEVERITY OF INFECTION

Many studies have emphasized the severity of illnesses such as measles, watery diarrhea, dysentery, and pneumonia among the severely malnourished (26). However, recent studies have shown that measles infection may be very severe, even among the well nourished, if it develops during the first year of life. Studies in South Africa (27) and Guinea-Bissau (28) showed that mortality rates were very high among urban children in whom severe measles occurred during infancy and early childhood. It seems possible that the severity may be caused by the poor host response in the younger child, whatever the nutritional status. The high-density living conditions for poor blacks in the slums of South Africa and Guinea-Bissau and for poor whites in the slums of Scotland earlier this century (29) may encourage a large inoculating dose of infection, which may account for the severe clinical picture (27). Unfortunately, there are no data on the attack rate or clinical severity of measles according to height/age.

DURATION OF INFECTION

There is more convincing evidence that stunting is associated with prolonged illness (Table 2). In the study of children in Malumfashi, northern Nigeria (23), episodes of diarrhea lasted 30% longer among the stunted than in the taller chil-

TABLE 2. *Possible risk factors for prolonged duration of infection*

Delayed immune clearance of pathogen
Delayed repair of damaged tissues (e.g., PEM, folate or zinc deficiency)
Persistent mucosal damage (e.g., food intolerance)
Carbohydrate malabsorption (e.g., lactase deficiency)

dren. A similar finding was noted in the nutrition/diarrhea study in Bangladesh (22), where, overall, there was a 26% longer duration in the shorter than in the taller children. A particularly valuable aspect of this study is that microbiological investigations were performed in a high proportion of diarrheal episodes. When those episodes attributable to enterotoxin-producing *Escherichia coli* only were analyzed, the diarrhea lasted about three times longer among the shorter than among the taller children. There was a similar threefold increase in duration of *E. coli* diarrhea among the most underweight and the thinnest compared with the better nourished in each category. In addition, there was a similar though less striking pattern in cases attributable to *Shigella*. In both the Nigerian and Bangladesh studies, the greatest association was between wasting and subsequent duration of diarrhea. It is interesting that such a relationship has also been found in Indonesian children (30), but unfortunately no data are available on the relationship between stunting and diarrhea incidence or duration in that country.

A more recent study has examined the relationship between anthropometric indices and subsequent disease patterns among children in Bakau, an urban community in the Gambia, West Africa (31). Although this study examined a wide range of illnesses (fever, respiratory infections, skin infections, and accidents as well as diarrhea), the data on morbidity were not collected as frequently as in the Nigerian or Bangladesh studies. Nevertheless, it was possible to calculate the prevalence of illness. For all the disease categories except diarrhea, prevalence was similar among the undernourished (whether more underweight, shorter, or thinner) and better nourished (32). The differences in prevalence of diarrhea between stunted and taller children were especially marked in the second year of life.

There are several possible biological reasons for prolonged symptoms in infection. Cellular immunity and hormonal immunity (especially secretory lgA) may be less active, thus limiting the speed at which a pathogen is cleared from the host. There is an abundant literature on the effect of dietary deficiency (nearly always severe by any standards) on the immune status and clearance of experimental pathogens in animals, but data on milder nutritional deficits are minimal, and the hypothesis that a stunted child has more persistent symptoms because of delayed clearance of intestinal pathogens is neither proven nor disproven.

Several studies have concentrated on the effect of nutritional status on function of the intestinal mucosa. Studies in protein–energy malnutrition (33), folate deficiency (34), and zinc deficiency (35) all show mucosal atrophy as a result of decreased rates of production of enterocytes in the crypts of the intestinal villi. This may have a direct effect by decreasing surface area for intestinal absorption. It may also affect the type of cell that lines the intestinal villi; in nutritional deficiency the cells covering the villi are predominantly immature, cuboidal enterocytes with poorly developed microvilli and low levels of digestive enzymes (36). This may be especially important among children receiving milk (either human or cow's), where secondary hypolactasia may contribute to the prolongation of diarrhea (37). A further nutritional factor affecting the gut is the secretory characteristics of immature enterocytes; they have high levels of Na^+ ATPase. This may well explain why there is a particularly increased secretory response of water and electrolytes when cholera toxin is perfused in the small intestine of animals with experimental zinc deficiency (35).

There are also important social factors affecting the relationship between duration of disease and stunting. It is frequently observed that within a region or community, those children who are stunted are often from poorer socioeconomic environments (31) not only with respect to type and availability of food but also housing, sanitation, parental education, and access to health services.

The importance of obtaining treatment at an early stage of infection for diarrhea (especially dysentery, where antibiotics may be indicated) is obvious. Delays in initiation of treatment may result in prolonged illness. Despite the many evaluations of the utilization of health services by communities, none has examined whether stunted children obtain effective treatment at a later stage than better-nourished children. Thus, the suggestion that the increased duration of morbidity in stunted children is caused by delays in therapy is, although perfectly logical, unproven.

MORTALITY

Prospective studies in India (38) and Bangladesh (39) have demonstrated an important relationship between weight/age and subsequent risk of death. Other studies demonstrated a relationship between thinness, whether by midarm circumference (40) or by weight/height as in Bangladesh (39) and Papua New Guinea (41), and subsequent mortality. The detailed study in Bangladesh in which deaths were recorded during the 2 years following anthropometry showed an increase in mortality in relation to weight/age, weight/height, and height/age, but only among the severest by each anthropometric category (39). This threshold relationship has been highlighted by reviewers who have emphasized that high-risk children can be identified by anthropometric screening. However, a more recent analysis of these data, in which only deaths occurring in the 12 months after anthropometry were computed, suggests a more cautious interpretation (42). It appears that the relationship between anthropometry and risk of death varies considerably according to the season in which the measurement is made. If children are measured in June (at the beginning of the rains), the subsequent risk of death for the thinnest (assessed by weight/height) is eight times greater than that for the fattest. If, however, the children are measured in October (at the beginning of the dry season), the thinnest have the same risk of death as the fattest. The predictive value of height/age is also much less if the child is measured in October compared with measurements in June or August.

Mortality during the 18 months following anthropometry among children aged 6 to 60 months in Papua New Guinea was almost twice as high in the thin (less than 90% weight/height) than in the better nourished (41). Among the thin children, mortality rates were nearly three times higher in the stunted children. A study in Africa showed no relationship between anthropometry and death in the 100 days after measurement among children aged 6 to 59 months (43). It is interesting that a high proportion (54%) of the children in this urban community in Zaire died of measles. It could be informative to analyze the nonmeasles deaths separately.

Considerable problems exist in drawing a unifying conclusion from these studies because they differ with respect to age of children, duration of follow-up for assessment of mortality risk, environment, climatic season, and cause of death. Nevertheless, the data indicate that under certain circumstances height/age is a strong predictor of subsequent mortality. The report from Narangwal, India, which only described weight/age, showed a stronger relationship during the first 6 months compared with the second 6 months after anthropometry (38). The data from Bangladesh (42) show a strong, graded mortality rate in relation to anthropometry for the first year, but the relationship with mortality showed a threshold pattern if children were followed for a further year (39).

COFACTORS

Any study of malnutrition and risk of infection or death should recognize that children who are malnourished usually come from underprivileged families with greatest difficulties in obtaining employment, food, potable water, decent housing and sanitation, or even access to the most basic medical care facilities (Table 3). Short stature often relates closely to social and economic deprivation. A recent study in urban Gambia (Bakau) showed a close relationship between stunting and variables such as type of housing, sanitation, water supply, and maternal education, each of which could have a major impact on the risk of infection and mortality (31). It seems likely that the severity of an infection, whether it be measles,

TABLE 3. *Factors coexisting with stunting that may increase risk of morbidity and mortality*

Poverty
Poor housing and climatic stress
Inadequate water supply and sanitation
Inadequate parental education and health knowledge
Inappropriate feeding practices
Poor access to health facilities

malaria, or diarrhea, is the end result of much more than a balance between host immunity and pathogen virulence. The management of the child by parents or guardians may be markedly affected by any of the above cofactors, which affect childcare. Thus, withholding breast milk, avoidance of certain nutritious foods, purging, and delays in obtaining medical assistance such as sound advice or drugs can all contribute to increases in severity, duration, and complicated outcomes of the illness (44). Some of these variables, particularly withholding of breast milk or food, seem more important in certain Asian communities than African communities and may contribute to variations in disease-specific mortality rates. Again, the lower socioeconomic status of families with stunted children suggests that parents may have less time and/or money to take a child for medical treatment.

In the Bangladesh study analyzed by Bairagi (42), the greater mortality associated with stunting when the children were measured at the beginning (June) or middle (August) of the rains could be accounted for by the greater prevalence of infection and scarcity of food at this time of the year. Admittedly, there is no information on the months in which death was most frequent throughout the year, but from previous studies in this area, most occur during or immediately after the rains. The age of the cohort is such that mortality would be maximal during the months immediately after the anthropometry, thereafter declining as the children enter their third year of life. Perhaps a stunted child who becomes infected during the rains receives less food, parental time, and medicine than a stunted child who becomes infected during the dry season, when there is more food and less pressure on parents' time.

CONCLUSION

At the present time, there are many reports about the numbers of stunted children in less developed countries and how these numbers differ with respect to age, dietary patterns, previous illness, and the season of measurement. There is also reasonable evidence that stunted chidlren have more prolonged infection and have a higher mortality from infection in certain communities. That the rate of linear growth is related to the type and amount of diet is incontrovertible, even though a concise, integrated, biological account of the nature of the deficits responsible for stunting is not yet available. It may be that the same nutritional inadequacy that limits the achievement of genetic potential for linear growth is also responsible for dysfunctions of host immunity and tissue repair. However, it is also clear that stunted children often come from homes with social, economic, and environmental deprivation. Those factors that may well explain why the dietary intake was not adequate to achieve the potential for linear growth in the first place may also influence the outcome of an infection in a stunted child.

REFERENCES

1. Scrimshaw NS, Taylor CE, Gordon JE. *Interactions of nutrition and infection*. WHO Monograph no. 57. Geneva: World Health Organization, 1968.

2. Chandra RK. Nutrition, immunity and infection: present knowledge and future directions. *Lancet* 1983;1:688–91.
3. Martorell R. Child growth retardation; a discussion of its causes and its relationship to health. In: Blaxter K, Waterlow JC, eds. *Nutritional adaptation in man*. London, Paris: John Libbey, 1985:13–29.
4. Waterlow JC, Buzina R, Keller W, Lane JM, Nickaman MZ, Tanner JM. The presentation and use of height and weight data for comparing the nutritional status of groups of children under the age of 10 years. *Bull WHO* 1977;55:489–98.
5. Gopalan C. "Small is healthy?" For the poor, not for the rich! *Bull Nutr Found India* 1983:October.
6. Seckler D, Sukhatme PV. In: Sukhatme PV, ed. *Newer concepts in nutrition and their implications for policy*. Puna, India: Maharashtra Association for the Cultivation of Science Research Institute, 1982:127–48.
7. Blaxter K, Waterlow JC. *Nutritional adaptation in man*. London, Paris: John Libbey, 1985.
8. Chandra RK. *Immunology of Nutritional Disorders*. London: Edward Arnold, 1980.
9. Suskind RM. *Malnutrition and the immune response*. New York: Raven Press, 1977 (Kroc Foundation series vol 7).
10. Kielmann AA, Uberoi IS, Chandra RK, Mehta VL. The effect of nutritional status on immune capacity and immune responses in pre-school children in a rural community in India. *Bull WHO* 1976;54:477–84.
11. Reddy V, Jagadeesan V, Ragharamulu N, Bhaskaram C, Srikantia SG. Functional significance of growth retardation in malnutrition. *Am J Clin Nutr* 1976;29:2–7.
12. Green F, Heyworth D. Immunoglobulin containing cells in jejunal mucosa of children with protein energy malnutrition and gastroenteritis. *Arch Dis Child* 1980;55:380–3.
13. Wesley A, Coovadia HM, Watson AR. Immunization against measles in children at risk for severe disease. *Tran R Soc Trop Med Hyg* 1979;73:710–5.
14. Gracey M, Cullity GJ, Suharjono S. The stomach in malnutrition. *Arch Dis Child* 1977;52: 325–7.
15. Chandra RK. Levels of IgG subclasses, IgG, IgM and tetanus antitoxin in paired maternal and foetal sera. Findings in healthy pregnancy and placental insufficiency. In: Hemmings WA, ed. *Materno-foetal transmission of immunoglobulins*. London: Cambridge University Press, 1975:77–90.
16. Mata LJ. Malnutrition–infection interactions in the tropics. *Am J Trop Med Hyg* 1975;24:564–74.
17. Chandra RK. Food antibodies in malnutrition. *Arch Dis Child* 1975;50:532–7.
18. Chen LC, Scrimshaw N. *Diarrhea and malnutrition. Interactions, mechanisms, and interventions*. New York: Plenum Press, 1983.
19. Delgado HS, Valverde V, Belizan JM, Klein RE. Diarrheal diseases, nutritional status and health care; analysis of their interrelationships. *Ecol Food Nutr* 1983;12:229–34.
20. James JW. Longitudinal study of the morbidity of diarrheal and respiratory infections in malnourished children. *Am J Clin Nutr* 1972;25:690–4.
21. Chen LC, Huq E, Huffman SL. A prospective study of the risk of diarrheal diseases according to the nutritional status of children. *Am J Epidemiol* 1981;114:284–92.
22. Black RE, Brown KH, Becker S. Malnutrition is a determining factor in diarrheal duration but not incidence among young children in a longitudinal study in rural Bangladesh. *Am J Clin Nutr* 1984;39:87–94.
23. Tomkins AM. Nutritional status and severity of diarrhoea among preschool children in rural Nigeria. *Lancet* 1981;1:860–2.
24. Manuel PD, Walker-Smith JA, Tomkins A. *Infections of the gastrointestinal tract*. Edinburgh, London: Churchill Livingstone, 1986.
25. Pickering H, Hayes RJ, Tomkins AM, Carson D. Alternative measures of diarrhoeal morbidity and their association with social and environmental factors in urban children in the Gambia. *Trans R Soc Trop Med Hyg* (*in press*).
26. Morley D, Woodland M, Martin WJ. Measles in Nigerian children. *J Hyg (Lond)* 1963;61:115–34.
27. Coovadia HM, Wesley A, Brain P. Immunological events in acute measles influencing outcome. *Arch Dis Child* 1978;53:861–7.
28. Aaby P, Bukha J, Lisse IM, Smits AJ. Measles mortality, state of nutrition and family structure. A community study from Guinea-Buissau. *J. Infect Dis* 1983;147:693–701.
29. Morley D. "Severe" measles. In: *Paediatric priorities in the developing world*. London: Butterworths, 1974:207–30.

30. Sommer A, Katz J, Tarwotjo I. Increased risk of respiratory disease and diarrhea in children with pre-existing mild vitamin A deficiency. *Am J Clin Nutr* 1984;40:1090–5.
31. Tomkins AM, Hayes RJ, Dunn DT, Pickering H. Socio economic factors associated with child growth in two seasons in an urban Gambian community. *Ecol Food Nutr* 1986;18:107–16.
32. Tomkins AM, Dunn D, Hayes R. How important is protein energy malnutrition as a risk factor for morbidity among young children in an urban Gambian community? In: *Abstracts of XIII International Congress of Nutrition*. Brighton, UK: 1985:162.
33. Brunser O, Reid A, Monckeberg F, Maccioni A, Contreras I. Jejunal mucosa in infant malnutrition. *Am J Clin Nutr* 1968;21:976–83.
34. Tomkins AM. Folate malnutrition in tropical diarrhea. *Trans R Soc Trop Med Hyg* 1979;73:498–502.
35. Roy SK, Drasar BS, Tomkins AM. The impact of zinc deficiency on the intestinal response to cholera toxin. *Proc Nutr Soc* 1986;45:39A.
36. Tomkins AM. Tropical malabsorption; recent concepts in pathogenesis and nutritional significance. *Clin Sci* 1981;60:131–7.
37. Brown KH, Parry L, Khatun M, Ahmed MG. Lactose malabsorption in Bangladeshi village children: relation with age, history of recent diarrhea, nutritional status and breast feeding. *Am J Clin Nutr* 1979;32:1962–9.
38. Kielmann AA, McCord C. Weight for age as an indicator of risk of death in children. *Lancet* 1978;1:1247–50.
39. Chen LC, Chowdhury AKMA, Huffman SL. Anthropometric assessment of energy–protein malnutrition and subsequent risk of mortality among pre-school aged children. *Am J Clin Nutr* 1980;33:1836–45.
40. Sommer A, Loewenstein MS. Nutritional status and mortality: a prospective validation of the QUAC stick. *Am J Clin Nutr* 1975;28:287–92.
41. Heywood PF. Growth and nutrition in Papua New Guinea. *J Hum Evol* 1983;12:133–43.
42. Bairagi R, Chowdhury MK, Kim YJ, Curlin GT. Alternative anthropometric indicators of mortality. *Am J Clin Nutr* 1985;42:296–306.
43. Kasongo Project Team. Anthropometric assessment of young children's nutritional status as an indicator of subsequent risk of dying. *J Trop Pediatr* 1983;29:69–76.
44. Tomkins AM. Protein–energy malnutrition and risk of infection. *Proc Nutr Soc* 1986;45:289–304.

DISCUSSION

Dr. Martorell: I am not sure I understood you: which of the two is more related to duration of diarrhea, stunting or wasting?

Dr. Tomkins: The relationship between wasting and duration of diarrhea may differ considerably from one community to another. In the Nigerian study I showed, you may have noticed that there was an increased incidence of diarrhea among wasted children. This has not been corroborated by the Bangladesh study. I made an analysis of why the Nigerian children were wasted. For a very high proportion of them, it was because they had developed measles in the month before measurement. Anthropometric measurement was made at the end of the dry season, and postmeasles diarrhea (certainly in many parts of Africa and apparently in Bangladesh too) is a major feature and confounding variable in these studies. I don't know whether measles epidemiology was tested for in the analysis of the Bangladesh study. So, one can say that in the Nigerian study diarrhea lasted 30% longer in stunted children but nearly 100% longer in wasted children. There was no association, however, between wasting and the prevalence of diarrhea in our Gambian study. The answer is therefore that there may well be differences in the relationship between wasting and risk of infection according to where you are.

Dr. Martorell: Do you think, in looking at the relationship between height for age, for example, and either the duration or attack rate of infection, that it is important to control for socioeconomic status? Could it be that shorter children are ill more often simply because they are poor and that it is a third factor, poverty, that is causing the association?

Dr. Tomkins: Is there perhaps a confounding variable whereby a child who is stunted is a child who is living in poor socioenvironmental conditions and therefore has a higher attack rate? I agree with you that it is what one would expect, but it doesn't seem to be the case. That is why I spent some time in reviewing the studies. Neither the Chen and Black study nor ours has shown an increased incidence of infection in stunted children. With reference to the Gambian study, we have examined 36 variables; many of them were related to hygiene and feeding practices, and of the 36, we found only two that related to the incidence of diarrhea. Diarrhea, particularly in an urban community, is ubiquitous. Feces are indiscriminately excreted. Children are always running in and out of the compounds; they all live together. I think this explains why in certain societies this kind of study has not picked up these variables, because children don't stay in their familial socioenvironmental background. It means that when we are looking at risk factors, we need to consider at least two variables: the first is the one that Dr. Nabarro referred to, which is a "family income and poverty index"; the second is a "microlevel family or mother–child behavioral index." We have not gone into that in this analysis, but I think differences between the two may explain the failure for there to be an impact of height for age on incidence of diarrhea.

Dr. Guesry: As there is apparently a direct relationship between stunting and wasting on the one hand and duration and frequency of diarrheal episodes on the other, I thought both could be attributed to the same socioeconomic factors and that the apparent relationship between the two was only artifactual.

Dr. Tomkins: All I can say is that in the studies that I have reviewed, perhaps surprisingly, I have found very little evidence that malnutrition in its broadest terms, whether it be height for age or weight for age, is associated with an increased attack rate. I think the reason is that most of these studies have been done within relatively homogeneous communities with respect to the environment. In other words, the environment may be very dirty regardless of whether it is in a wealthy compound or in a poorer one. It is interesting that the rate of malaria, for instance, has no relationship whatsoever to socioenvironmental status in our community; indeed, one could postulate that a mosquito does not care how wealthy you may be before biting. Therefore, the relationships that I have put forward are predominantly on the duration of diarrhea. I have suggested that previous measles infection is one possible biological reason for the fact that wasting is associated with an increased duration of diarrhea. The question is: Why does a child who is shorter suffer longer episodes of diarrhea? I think the reason that the question has not been answered so far is that we have concentrated too much on one sector of the child–environment interaction with time. Shortness of stature is associated with increase in duration, but we don't necessarily know why in each situation.

Dr. Valyasevi: Do you have data on the etiology of the diarrhea in the studies that you reviewed?

Dr. Tomkins: Black's study, which showed a very interesting linear correlation between duration of diarrhea and height for age, concerned only enterotoxin-producing *Escherichia coli*. When he looked at all diarrheas in which the pathogen was not identified, the relationship was not so strong. One factor that emerges from this kind of study is that one has to be much clearer in defining what is actually causing the diarrhea biologically.

Dr. Aponso: I agree with you. Prevalence of diarrhea, I believe, depends on the etiological and environmental factors, which are the same whether you are short or tall.

However, at present we know that duration of diarrhea is related to early preventive treatment. That is the story of oral rehydration. I don't know whether your study was carried out in the pre-ORT era or afterwards. We all remember that in 1978 the *Lancet* hailed the discovery of oral rehydration. This was reported to be one of the most significant medical discoveries of the century. Maybe the mothers whose children were taller were also more educated, more motivated, and therefore able to make use of the services that were made available and accessible. Those variables should, I think, be considered. Were these mothers using ORT, and, if so, was it related to the duration of diarrhea?

Dr. Tomkins: These are very valuable points. To give you exact information on the Gambian study, the whole community had been very closely involved in promotion of oral rehydration therapy for about 2 years prior to the study; 88% of diarrhea episodes were treated with sugar–salt solutions made up in the home. There was no evidence that the management of diarrhea by better-educated mothers—we were using the criterion of how many years they had been to school, although I am not sure that that is necessarily an indication of education—was any different from the management by those who were less educated. In this community, early use of oral rehydration was incredibly popular; it was widely used at an early stage; but in general your point is a very valid one.

Dr. Nabarro: You were showing us, from your Bakau data, material mostly on diarrhea. Do you have anything on measles?

Dr. Tomkins: We had about 89% coverage with measles vaccination. We saw no cases of measles.

Dr. Nabarro: You studied six variables that you have not shown. You have discussed only diarrhea. Were there any interesting differences in any of the others? Accidents probably are not too relevant, but what about illness, fever, rash?

Dr. Tomkins: In fact, those six variables were the variables that related to stunting, not to the diarrheal epidemiology. When we look at the 36 in relation to diarrheal attack rate, which is a slightly separate study, only two of the variables actually related to diarrheal attack rate. One was referred to by Professor Aponso—maternal education, how many years she had been to school; the other was what the field workers felt the mother knew about feeding during illness and the cause of diarrhea. We have analyzed the variables in relationship to fever. There was no association.

Dr. Nabarro: So there was no association between the degree of stunting and the number or duration of episodes of fever, for example?

Dr. Tomkins: No, the only association that I mentioned briefly was respiratory infection. During the dry season, there was a higher prevalence of respiratory infection among those who were short. That was the only other nutrition–infection relation to be found.

Dr. Waterlow: I would like to explore the same line a bit further. The theme of the last few papers is the functional accompaniments, if any, of environmentally determined shortness in height or deficit in linear growth. What we are interested in, at this stage, is not so much what causes children to be stunted but whether that condition of the body has an effect on infection. You have shown rather small and not very consistent effects. You have also made the point of a very uniform environment for these children. Are the environmental factors totally swamping any possible effect of the state of the host?

Dr. Tomkins: You have raised a very interesting point regarding what is actually going on in this society, which is a relatively affluent one. It is an urban African situation where we do not see marasmus or kwashiorkor but where there is a very high prevalence of diarrhea and fever and quite a marked seasonal change in nutritional status. In this chapter we are not dealing with anything to do with the origins of the acquired height of those children. Your question was: Are environmental factors so strong in this area that they override any immunity? In this society I think they do, because there was no relationship between these variables and the diarrheal incidence.

Dr. Waterlow: Not in Bangladesh?

Dr. Tomkins: Neither in Bangladesh. In Black's and in Chen's study, incidence was not increased in those who were short or even in those who were thin, but duration was. That is the point I am making.

Dr. Waterlow: This shows, then, that everybody is open to infection but that the under-privileged body is less able to get rid of it.

Dr. Tomkins: That is a very reasonable assumption. The point that I am making is that it is very easy to take a biological perspective and talk about clearance of enteropathogens, and it may well be right. We would really like to know what the diarrheal pathogen was, for how many days it was excreted in a short child, and for how many days it was excreted in a taller child. This would be a very interesting study to do. There are virtually no data that have rigorously analyzed this. However, children who are short are also short because they come from families with a variety of forms of social deprivation; often a child is not treated for dysentery with antibiotics because the mother has no time. We cannot assume that because a child is short, there is an immunological reason why he has got persistent diarrhea. We need a bigger framework in which the social interactions of the management of disease processes are addressed. I wish it were simple enough to think in pure biological terms. It would be so easy if we could just explain it in terms of shortness, immunity, and clearing of enteropathogens. However, it does not seem logical to do so in the face of the other confounding variables such as access to health services, use of antibiotics, etc.

Dr. Waterlow: My conclusion is that you need to find somewhere to carry out such a study, where there are perhaps fewer confounding varibles. I don't remember exactly what Trowbridge found in his Haiti study.

Dr. Tomkins: I think you are referring to the analysis that was published in the *American Journal of Clinical Nutrition* (1) on the relationship between anthropometry and diarrheal prevalence. It is difficult to use that study as a reference point because he used retrospective morbidity data. He asked the children's mothers if they had been ill in the 1, 2, and 3 months before the measurement. All the studies emphasize the need for very regular and reliable morbidity measurements. In the study you referred to there was no account of the social constraints on maternal management of illness, and this is important. When one re-views the literature, one may see either some very clear biological explanation or some rather loose anthropological explanation but never an analysis of the interactions between the two. Your question is absolutely valid. However, I do not believe that these variables have been adequately controlled in any study that has been carried out. What you are asking for is an incredibly difficult study because you need to control about 30-odd variables of social behavior.

Dr. Waterlow: I would have thought that you and Dr. Nabarro could have answered that question from your seasonal data, if analyzed in the appropriate way.

Dr. Nabarro: It seems that there would be enormous problems to be faced if the outcome of the stunting and illness association were to be examined using cohort studies. An alterna-tive approach is to use case-control methods, to examine children with infections of varying degrees of severity, and to study their antecedent weight-for-height status. We have used this when trying to study relationships between severe measles and nutritional status in Nepalese children.

Dr. Tomkins: A case-control study is extremely valuable. I didn't give you the results of the case-control study we did of mortality in relation to preceeding nutrition and social vari-ables. It does help with the numerous problems that one has. The sample size, for instance, to be able to do these things would otherwise be quite enormous.

Dr. Mukherjee: What was the incidence of tuberculosis in the group that you studied?

Dr. Tomkins: Three children had tuberculosis on clinical diagnosis. Tuberculosis is not something that you can look at in relationship to stunting, as the prevalence is too low in a population of this size. It is an important public health problem, but the group in which it was diagnosed was too small to show any relationship between nutrition and tuberculosis.

To me, a short child is not only a child who is a different immunological subject but is also a child who is at increased risk of some of the variables affecting the outcome. That was why I analyzed the data in such a way.

Dr. Tanner: Just to give you some data about adults that appeared in a supplement of the *Acta Medica Scandinavica* last year (2), in 1954, 2 million Norwegians compulsorily had a mass mini-X-ray, and somebody had the bright idea of taking their heights and weights. Since then some 150,000 have died, and so now we have mortality rates for a substantial population. There is a close relationship between height and the incidence of death in the 30s, 40s, and 50s, and 60s; it gets less at 70, and it disappears at 80 because then you die however tall you are.

This is the only study I know of that indicates that in the long run taller people survive longer. It doesn't, however, sort out the factors concerned, and I agree totally with what you said along those lines. But in the long run, height does seem to affect health. Growth is perhaps the sole and best bioassay of health.

Dr. Tomkins: Was there any control for the socioenvironmental background of those people who were shorter as opposed to taller?

Dr. Tanner: No, not in the publication, but I think there is a lot more to come.

REFERENCES

1. Trowbridge FL, Staehling N. Sensitivity and specificity of arm circumference indicators in identifying malnourished children. *Am J Clin Nutr* 1980;33:687–96.
2. Waaler HT. Height, weight and mortality: the Norwegian experience. *Acta Med Scand [Suppl]* 1984;679:1–56.

Linear Growth Retardation in Less Developed Countries, edited by John C. Waterlow. Nestlé Nutrition Workshop Series, Vol. 14. Nestec Ltd., Vevey/Raven Press, Ltd., New York © 1988.

Mental Development and Stunting

M. Colombo, I. de Andraca, and I. López

Unidad de Neuropsicologia, Instituto de Nutrición y Tecnologia de los Alimentos (INTA), Universidad de Chile, Santiago 11, Chile

Mental development is a product of the interaction between hereditary and environmental factors. If one assumes that the brain is the organ for intellectual functioning, it is important to point out that its development extends over a very long period of time, the longest of all organs in the body, and is therefore susceptible to the influence of a great variety of events that might interfere with its normal evolution: traumas, infections, deprivations, nutritional deficits, etc.

The concept of the vulnerability of the brain is based on the observation that during its prolonged period of development, the brain follows a definite pattern of growth in a certain period of time and that lesions or deficiencies produced at any specific stage may lead to irrecoverable sequelae. Thus, nutritional deprivations seem to affect brain development from the last trimester of gestation until the second year of postnatal life (1).

Environment is also essential for mental development. Innumerable environmental factors exist that act on the psychological development of the child: sensory stimulation, affection, language, and the mother–child relationship. Absence of these factors by themselves may negatively influence the mental development of the child (2,3).

Stunting (deficit in height for age) has been used as an indicator of nutritional status over a prolonged period of time (4). It has generally been associated with protein–energy malnutrition (PEM) in its different forms, but especially with marasmus (5).

In developing countries, infantile undernutrition is a very frequent phenomenon; it always occurs in a context of poverty and misery, with lack of adequate environmental stimulation. Nutritional deprivation in this highly unfavorable environment, prevailing during the greater part of the individual's life and in the majority of cases over generations, affects the physical and mental development of the child.

However, whether there is an association between stunting, supposedly caused by nutritional deficits, and mental development remains a controversial issue.

In this chapter, which is based on our experience, we successively consider the child's development at different ages, (a) the first 2 years of life, (b) preschool age, and (c) school age, in relation to nutritional status.

FIRST 2 YEARS OF LIFE

A retrospective study including 228 marasmic infants aged 261.2 ± 13.03 days, hospitalized in Closed Nutritional Recovery Centers (CNRC) in Santiago, Chile, showed that their growth and psychomotor development were markedly affected (6). Weight/age (W/A) was the most affected parameter, followed by height/age (H/A) and head circumference/age (HC/A) (Table 1).

The psychomotor development of these infants was evaluated using a Chilean scale (7). Average developmental quotient (DQ) of these infants was 0.59 ± 0.17 (normal 0.85 ± 1.15). Developmental quotient was normal in 7% of these infants, and 24% presented with mild retardation (Table 2). The nutritional status of these two groups of infants did not differ significantly from the group as a whole.

Multivariate analysis demonstrated that the anthropometric parameters weight/height (W/H), H/A, and HC/A conjointly could only explain 23.6% of the variance of DQ.

No significant correlation was found between the degree of stunting and psychomotor development.

TABLE 1. *Anthropometric and psychomotor evolution after rehabilitation of 228 undernourished infants*

	Admission (mean ± SD)	Discharge (mean ± SD)	t	p
Weight/age (%)	58.6 ± 8.8	83.4 ± 9.1	37.6	<0.001
Height/age (%)	86.3 ± 4.9	89.7 ± 3.4	12.2	<0.001
Weight/height (%)	83.5 ± 8.1	103.4 ± 9.6	26.1	<0.001
Head circumference/age (%)	91.4 ± 3.4	95.9 ± 2.4	22.2	<0.001
Developmental quotient	0.59 ± 0.17	0.79 ± 0.14	15.2	<0.001

TABLE 2. *Distribution of severely undernourished infants according to their developmental quotient*

	Developmental quotient	Number	Percentage
Normal	1.15–0.85	16	7.0
Mild retardation	0.84–0.70	51	22.4
Moderate retardation	0.69–0.55	72	31.6
Severe retardation	0.54 or less	89	39.0
Total		228	100.0

TABLE 3. *Variations in developmental quotient after rehabilitation in 228 undernourished infants*

Developmental quotient	Admission (mean ± SD)	Discharge (mean ± SD)	Variation	N
Normal (1.15–0.85)	0.91 ± 0.07	0.89 ± 0.12	− 0.02 ± 0.12	16
Mild retardation (0.84–0.70)	0.76 ± 0.04	0.83 ± 0.11	0.07 ± 0.10	51
Moderate retardation (0.69–0.55)	0.62 ± 0.04	0.78 ± 0.14	0.16 ± 0.15	72
Severe retardation (0.54 or less)	0.42 ± 0.10	0.75 ± 0.15	0.33 ± 0.17	89

These children received nutritional care and psychomotor stimulation for a period of 4 to 5 months, at the end of which a very significant improvement in growth and DQ could be observed (Table 1).

The improvement of DQ was dependent on the DQ on admission (Table 3). Infants presented with more severe retardation improved their performance more markedly. Since all these children came from very deprived environments, those who were admitted with normal DQ or only mild retardation, and who did not improve their performance significantly, probably had better personal interactions and received more adequate stimulation at home. This points out the importance of environment as a fundamental determinant of a child's DQ.

No significant correlation could be found between stunting and recovery of the DQ. These findings are in disagreement with those published by Grantham McGregor (8), who, in a study done on 39 children recently recovered from severe PEM, showed a significant correlation between stunting and DQ ($p < 0.005$).

PRESCHOOL AGE

Our data are based on a follow-up study carried out with 42 preschool children (average age 57.7 ± 7 months) who received nutritional care and psychomotor stimulation in CNRC during infancy. The anthropometry of these children is shown in Table 4. Percentage H/A in children with antecedents of undernutrition was only 92 ± 4.8.

The intellectual capacity of these children was evaluated using the Wechsler Intelligence Scale for Preschool Children, and compared to a control group of similar sex, age, and socioeconomic level but without antecedents of undernutrition (Table 5).

The performance of children with antecedents of undernutrition was significantly less than that of controls. Only 26% of the infants with antecedents of undernutrition had a normal IQ compared to 52% in the control group (Table 6). On

TABLE 4. *Anthropometry of preschool children with and without antecedents of early undernutrition*

Anthropometry	With antecedents of early undernutrition (N = 42) (mean ± SD)	Control group (N = 29) (mean ± SD)	t	p
Weight/age (%)	85.6 ± 11.1	103.6 ± 8.21	7.74	<0.001
Height/age (%)	92.2 ± 4.8	99.43 ± 4.61	6.30	<0.001
Weight/height (%)	99.4 ± 9.6	103.5 ± 6.4	2.13	<0.05
Head circumference/age (%)	94.9 ± 2.8	98.8 ± 2.6	5.93	<0.001

TABLE 5. *Intelligence quotient of preschool children with and without antecedents of early undernutrition*

Intelligence quotient	With antecedents of early undernutrition (N = 42) (mean ± SD)	Control group (N = 29) (mean ± SD)	t	p
Verbal	83.6 ± 15.8	90.4 ± 10.4	2.16	<0.05
Performance	80.9 ± 12.9	90.83 ± 12.6	3.18	<0.01
Full Scale	80.7 ± 14.0	90.0 ± 11.5	3.02	<0.01

TABLE 6. *Distribution of intelligence quotient among preschool children with and without antecedents of undernutrition*

Intelligence quotient	With antecedents of early undernutrition (percentage)	Control group (percentage)
Normal (IQ ≥ 90)	26.19 (N = 11)	51.72 (N = 15)
Normal–slow (IQ = 80–89)	30.95 (N = 13)	31.04 (N = 9)
Borderline (IQ = 70–79)	19.05 (N = 8)	13.80 (N = 4)
Mental retardation (IQ ≤ 69)	23.81 (N = 10)	3.44 (N = 1)

the other hand, 24% of the previously undernourished children presented with mental retardation.

No correlation was found at this age between intellectual performance and present nutritional status. The correlation coefficient between percentage H/A and IQ was only 0.07. The results show that no correlation exists between mental development at preschool age and stunting in children with antecedents of malnutrition in infancy (9).

However, many authors have reported positive correlations between nutritional status and intellectual development. Freeman and collaborators (10), in Guatema-

TABLE 7. *Familial characteristics and intellectual capacity of preschool children with antecedents of undernutrition*

Familial characteristic	Intelligence quotient (mean ± SD)		
Presence of both parents ($N = 30$)	83.7	±	15.3
Absence of one or both parents ($N = 11$)	74.2	±	6.8
t =	2.67	, $p<$	0.02
Psychiatric pathology and/or alcoholism			
Absent ($N = 32$)	84.3	±	13.0
Present ($N = 9$)	69.7	±	13.5
t =	2.74	, $p<$	0.01

lan children aged between 3 and 4 years, found a significant correlation between cognitive measures (language, memory, and perception) and height and also between cognitive performance and social factors. Multivariate analysis of their data showed that the amount of variance explained by the social factor index was generally less than by the nutritional measure, whereas in our study, although the nutritional status did not correlate with mental development, significant correlations could be found between some social factors and the IQ (Table 7).

SCHOOL AGE

We studied four groups of children aged between 7 and 10 years, all belonging to very low socioeconomic strata. Two of these groups included stunted children (percentage H/A 95, according to the standards of the National Center for Health Statistics), and the two others eutrophic children.

The first group of stunted children had been followed up since infancy, when they were treated in CNRC for an acute episode of protein–energy malnutrition. These children were compared to eutrophic children of the same age and socioeconomic level; significant differences were observed for all growth parameters (Table 8).

The intellectual capacity of these two groups of children evaluated with the Wechsler Intelligence Scale for Children (WISC) was significantly different (Table 9).

Among the stunted children with antecedents of undernutrition, 57% presented with an IQ below normal and 13% with mental retardation (Table 10). When IQ was correlated with anthropometrical parameters within this group (simple correlation coefficient of Pearson), a significant positive correlation was found only between head circumference/age and IQ. No significant correlation was found between percentage H/A and IQ (Table 11).

These data suggest that although early undernutrition affects growth and mental

TABLE 8. *Anthropometry of school children with and without antecedents of early undernutrition*

Anthropometry	With antecedents of early undernutrition (mean ± SD)		Control group (mean ± SD)		t	p
Height/age (%)	82.62 ±	11.93	102.73 ±	11.12	7.125	< 0.001
	N = 30		N = 37			
Weight/age (%)	90.16 ±	4.65	98.35 ±	3.49	8.24	< 0.001
	N = 30		N = 37			
Weight/height (%)	100.73 ±	7.54	105.34 ±	7.75	2.435	< 0.001
	N = 30		N = 36			
Head circumference/age (%)	95.39 ±	2.39	98.85 ±	2.84	4.748	< 0.001
	N = 29		N = 34			

TABLE 9. *Intelligence quotient of school children with and without antecedents of early undernutrition*

Intelligence quotient	With antecedents of early undernutrition (mean ± SD)	Control group (mean ± SD)	t	p
N	30	38		
Verbal	85.80 ± 12.39	98.39 ± 12.39	4.16	< 0.001
Performance	85.93 ± 14.51	101.28 ± 11.82	4.18	< 0.001
Full scale	84.30 ± 13.72	99.60 ± 11.25	5.06	< 0.001

TABLE 10. *Distribution of intelligence quotient among school children with and without antecedents of early undernutrition*

Intelligence quotient	With antecedents of early undernutrition (percentage)	Control group (percentage)
Normal (IQ ≥ 90)	30 (N = 9)	84.21 (N = 32)
Normal–slow (IQ = 80–89)	30 (N = 9)	10.52 (N = 4)
Borderline (IQ = 70–79)	26.66 (N = 8)	5.26 (N = 2)
Mental retardation (IQ ≤ 69)	13.33 (N = 4)	—

development, no positive correlation exists between them: the smallest child is not the one with the lowest IQ.

Environment seems to influence the mental development of children considerably. Nurturing styles and maternal expectancies, as part of the microenvironment, contributed most to the variance in intellectual performance (Table 12) (11). The same conclusion can be drawn from the correlation matrix among IQ, anthropometry, and socioeconomic level (Table 13).

TABLE 11. *Correlation between intelligence quotient and anthropometrical parameters in school children with antecedents of undernutrition*

Variables	Regression equation	r	p
IQ, % weight/height	$y = 103.82 - 0.04\ x$	− 0.0666	0.7316
IQ, % weight/age	$y = 83.95 - 0.02\ x$	− 0.0182	0.441
IQ, % height/age	$y = 86.63 - 0.04\ x$	0.1234	0.260
IQ, head circumference/age	$y = 87.33 + 0.09\ x$	0.431	0.0186

TABLE 12. *Multiple correlation among intellectual performance, anthropometry, and microenvironment in school children with antecedents of undernutrition*

Variables	r^2	Percentage contribution
Nurturing style	0.144	14.4
Maternal expectancies	0.247	10.3
Weight/age (%)	0.315	6.8
Weight/height (%)	0.338	2.3
Head circumference/age (%)	0.353	1.5
Height/age (%)	0.335	− 2.3

The other group of stunted school children had no antecedents of early undernutrition. They were compared with eutrophic school mates. Average intelligence quotients, evaluated with WISC, were not significantly different (Table 14). Within these groups, no correlation could be found between percentage H/A and IQ.

The following conclusions were drawn from these data in school children:

1. When stunting is prevalent in a poor and deprived population, and infants suffer from early and severe undernutrition, mental development is affected in the long term. However, because of characteristics of brain growth, its particular needs, and its dependence on environmental stimulation in early life, one does not observe a direct correlation between deficits in physical growth and deficits in intellectual capacities in this population.

2. Mental development seems to be preserved in stunted children without antecedents of acute and severe undernutrition in infancy, although they probably suffered from prolonged and persistent nutritional restrictions. Intelligence quotient is within the normal range, albeit at the lower limit. No direct correlation exists between the degree of growth deficit and intellectual capacity.

Different authors have described the effects of early and severe undernutrition on growth and intellectual performance of school-age children (12–18). In all these studies, family environment has always been considered to be a fundamental determinant of the children's performance, but no significant correlation could be demonstrated between height and mental development.

TABLE 13. *Correlation matrix among intelligence quotient, anthropometry and socioeconomic level (SEL) in school children with antecedents of undernutrition[a]*

	IQ	H/A (%)	HC/A (%)	SEL
IQ	1	0.117	0.417*	0.455*
Height/age (%)		1	0.331	0.18
Head circumference/age (%)			1	0.292
SEL				1

[a]$r^2 = 0.298$; $r = 0.546$; *$p < 0.05$.

TABLE 14. *Intelligence quotient and anthropometry of stunted children without antecedents of acute undernutrition and eutrophic school children*

	Eutrophic ($N = 37$) (mean ± SD)		Stunted ($N = 27$) (mean ± SD)	
Weight/age (%)	96.19	10.38	79.41	7.37
Height/age (%)	98.66	10.01	90.83	2.49
Weight/height (%)	101.31	5.79	104.08	8.34
IQ				
Full scale	96.90	10.59	97.74	8.21
Verbal scale	96.11	8.94	95.89	6.83
Performance	98.27	12.69	100.26	12.02

Severe malnutrition in infancy, small stature, and disadvantageous social background were examined separately by Richardson (14) for their association with IQ. He found that the largest contributor to the variance was social background. He concluded that under the most favorable conditions of being tall and having an advantageous social history, malnutrition has little effect on IQ. But under the most unfavorable conditions of short stature and a disadvantageous social background, there is a clear correlation between malnutrition and low IQ. However, these conclusions could be biased because the children examined in this investigation presented different types of malnutrition in infancy—marasmus, kwashiorkor, and marasmic kwashiorkor; their effects could be different.

CONCLUSIONS

Our data seem to indicate that stunting and impaired mental development have no causal link but are both associated effects of poverty and deprivation.

One should point out that in humans mental development is highly dependent on the biological and environmental events occurring during the first 2 years of life. Thus, any nutritional restriction influencing intellectual performance should not be considered a variable of the continuous type, as could be the case for growth. Early and severe undernutrition is a risk factor of mental retardation, especially in poor socioeconomical conditions in which the child is subjected to multiple deprivations. This is not directly related to stunting.

When nutritional deprivation is the only risk factor, and other determinants such as socioaffective interaction with the family are adequate, cognitive functions and development of children living in poor socioeconomic conditions would not be substantially affected. In this case, the environment would have the capacity to compensate for the potentially adverse effects of nutritional restrictions. On the contrary, the simultaneous and persistent occurrence of multiple adverse variables implies a very high risk of altering the normal course of mental development independently of growth.

ACKNOWLEDGMENTS

We are indebted to all the personnel of the Closed Nutritional Recovery Centers from CONIN, the children, and their parents for their invaluable collaboration in the research presented here. We want to thank Mrs. Irene Truffello for the statistical analysis and Mrs. Viola Lyon for her secretarial work.

REFERENCES

1. Dobbing J, Sands J. The later development of brain and its vulnerability. In: Davis SA, Dobbing J, eds. *Scientific foundation of pediatrics*. London: Heinemann, 1974;565–77.
2. Haskins R, Finkelstein NW, Stedman DJ. Infant stimulation programs and their effects. *Pediatr Ann* 1978;7:123–43.
3. Cravioto J, Arrieta P. Desnutricion y desarrollo mental. *Cuad Nutr* 1984;7:17–32.
4. Waterlow JC. Note on the assessment and classification of protein energy malnutrition in children. *Lancet* 1973;2:87–9.
5. Branko Z. Height, weight and head circumference in survivors of marasmus and kwashiorkor. *Am J Clin Nutr* 1979;32:1719–27.
6. Colombo M, de Andraca I, López I. Desnutrición severa en el niño desarrollo psicomotor, neurológico y conducta. In: Celedón JM, ed. *Nutrición et Inteligencia en el niño*. Santiago: Ediciones de la Universidad de Chile, 1983;73–121.
7. Rodriguez S, Arancibia U, Undurraga C. *Escala de evaluación del desarrollo psicomotor 0–24 meses*. Santiago: Pontificia Universidad Católica de Chile, 1976.
8. Grantham McGregor S. The relationship between developmental level and different types of malnutrition in children. *Hum Nutr Clin Nutr* 1982;36C:319–20.
9. Carrasco MI, Marshall B, Poblete M. *Rendimiento intelectual de preescolares con antecedentes de desnutrición severa*. Santiago: Pontificia Universidad Catolica de Chile, 1982.
10. Freeman HE, Klein RE, Kagan J, Yarbrough C. Relations between nutrition and cognition in rural Guatemala. *Am J Public Health* 1977;67:233–9.
11. González M, Venegas MS. *Capacidad intelectual de niños en edad escolar con antecedentes de desnutrición precoz grave*. Santiago: Universidad de Chile, 1984.
12. Monckeberg F. Effects of nutrition on brain and intellectual development. In: Richardson F, ed. *Brain and intelligence. The ecology of child development*. Hyattsville, MD: National Educational Press, 1973:207–34.
13. Hertzig ME, Birch HG, Richardson SA, Tizard J. Intellectual levels of school age children severely malnourished during the first two years of life. *Pediatrics* 1972;49:814–24.
14. Richardson SA. The relation of severe malnutrition in infancy to the intelligence of school children with differing life histories. *Pediatr Res* 1976;10:57–61.

15. Richardson SA, Koller H, Katz M, Albert K. The contribution of differing degrees of acute and chronic malnutrition to the intellectual development of Jamaican boys. *Early Hum Dev* 1978;2:163–70.
16. McLaren DS, Yaktin US, Kanawati AA, Sabagh S, Kadi Z. The subsequent mental and physical development of rehabilitated marasmic infants. *J Ment Defic Res* 1973;17:273–81.
17. Stoch MB, Smythe PM, Moodie AD, Bradshaw D. Psychosocial outcome and CT finding after gross undernourishment during infancy: a 20 year developmental study. *Dev Med Child Neurol* 1982;24:419–36.
18. Cabak V, Najdanvic R. Effects of undernutrition in early life on physical and mental development. *Arch Dis Child* 1965;40:532–4.

DISCUSSION

Dr. Valyasevi: Does the appearance of the network of dendrites in malnourished subjects depend only on stimulation, or does its development also require adequate nutrition?

Dr. Colombo: We have made this study in rats, not in children. Results depend on the age at which you stimulate the animals. If, in rats, it is done before 30 days of life, there is very good rehabilitation and appearance of these dendrites. If this is done after 30 days of life, there is no change.

Dr. Guesry: You showed that the prevalence of severe retardation increased between the time of discharge from the rehabilitation center and early school age. Do you think that this was because of alterations in the development of the brain during the period of malnutrition or of other phenomena occurring after rehabilitation?

Dr. Colombo: First of all, I want to make clear that there is no correlation between psychomotor development and intellectual capacity. Very good mental rehabilitation was obtained by the intensive stimulation of these children during their stay at the recovery center. One should notice, however, that they were stimulated with material that was used afterwards in the different tests, so the good results could be somewhat artificial. Nevertheless, it is important to point out that the children with the lowest developmental quotient (DQ) present with the best improvements; they probably also come from the worst environments. Thus, although severe undernutrition affects brain growth and brain development, the environment is very important. It has now been shown by many authors that if you stimulate a rat or a rabbit, there is hypertrophy of the dendrites; the dentritic tree grows. So stimulation could, in a way, make up for the negative effects of malnutrition. The concept of the plasticity of the central nervous system is very important.

Dr. Waterlow: Richardson (1) attempted an analysis of the contributions to the variance in IQ, and it turned out that having a previous episode of severe malnutrition accounted for about 25%, the presence of stunting, which he considered a general measure of the nutritional status of the child between infancy and school age when they were tested, another 25%, and social stimulation in the home, about 50%. If I understand correctly, this is in line with your opinion.

Dr. Colombo: Broadly speaking, yes; but what he found, and we did not, is that the shorter child of low socioeconomic status was the worst.

Dr. Waterlow: I have the impression that there are considerable cultural differences in this respect. To follow up your previous point, Dr. MacGregor (2) in Jamaica found that the IQ of malnourished children in hospital, with good stimulation, automatically goes up, and when they are discharged, it goes down again. If, however, there was intervention with monthly visits to the mother, teaching her and training her in playing with the children, then this drop after discharge was prevented. That would again fit in with your data.

Dr. Colombo: Yes, that is true. Dr. MacGregor has very important data. For example, in a group of undernourished children that she has followed up for 36 months without specific stimulation, she found that the most stunted children at admission were the ones that had the best developmental quotient at 36 months, although they were also the ones with the lowest DQ scores initially (3).

Dr. Milner: Those who were the most disadvantaged before admission to hospital may be the ones most likely not to return to the nuclear family. Action is taken to prevent that happening, and a foster home is found. Have you studied a subgroup of that nature, and what is the outcome when they go into a neutral or "more advantageous" environment subsequently?

Dr. Colombo: We are trying to do that now with institutionalized children, whose environment, in fact, is also bad, and with adopted children in good sociocultural environments. We want to compare the effects of these different environments: poor families, institutions, and families from higher socioeconomic levels. However, this is a difficult study, because most children who do not return home are adopted by people in the United States or in Sweden.

Dr. Davies: At one time the long-term follow-up studies of children who had been malnourished prenatally indicated that they didn't do quite as well as controls, and people wondered whether this could be explained by Dobbing's hypothesis of early vulnerability of brain growth to undernutrition. However, when the perinatal histories of these children are examined in detail, it appears that if intrapartum asphyxia, to which prenatally malnourished babies are especially prone, is allowed for, these children have normal mental function. I was wondering, especially in your group of severely handicapped children with an IQ below 65, whether there were any abnormal neurological accompaniments that might perhaps point to an episode of asphyxia during the birth process and that might have indicated that these disadvantaged children could also have been disadvantaged before birth?

Dr. Colombo: These children were scrutinized very precisely. They all had a birth weight above 2,500 g. Neurological examination of these children, at every age, reveals only very discrete abnormalities; the clinical picture at school age is very similar to what has been called the "syndrome of attention deficit." The neurological examination was never suggestive of prenatal or perinatal brain damage.

Dr. Mukherjee: We examined the amino acidogram in the cerebrospinal fluid of severely malnourished children, either kwashiorkor or marasmus, and we observed that there was a shift from the essential to the nonessential amino acids and that this shift was reversed during recovery (4). Have you done similar studies?

Dr. Colombo: No, we have not.

Dr. Mukherjee: Nature always tries to protect the brain and supply it with nutrients in priority. Nevertheless, severe malnutrution causes mental retardation. Does nature in this case fail to protect the brain efficiently, or is this a sort of adaptation?

Dr. Colombo: I think mental retardation in this case is a consequence of many factors. Severe malnutrition at the time when the brain is developing very rapidly is certainly very important, but afterwards there are many environmental factors that play a role. Mental retardation results from many things, but one should always consider that an episode of undernutrition entails a risk of mental retardation.

Dr. Davies: You referred to one study (5) that indicated, in an African population, that there was good correlation between head circumference and later ability. Two recent studies in Oxford (6) and Hong Kong (7) have shown that accompanying secular changes in weight and length, there are also definite secular changes in head circumference. Oxford children show a difference of about 1.5 cm over 25 years (6). We might speculate perhaps that children from Oxford would also be the equivalent of 1.5 cm more clever than they were 25 years ago, but there is no indication of this. How do you view these secular changes in head circumference growth? Do you think that it is related to a bigger brain, a better brain, a bigger skull?

Dr. Colombo: In the development of man's intelligence, the brain has been growing. This is probably an adaptation to the environment. We see that we can accomplish much more than our ancestors. The concept of the plasticity of the brain implies that the brain is growing, and therefore the skull. Whether the size of the brain is related to intelligence, I don't know.

Dr. Davies: Are you actually postulating work hypertrophy? In other words, if the brain works harder, its growth rate will increase just as muscles increase in size when they work more. Is this your hypothesis?

Dr. Colombo: Yes, maybe. You cannot observe that phenomenon as much as in the muscle, but dendritic trees, during a particular period of life, grow when they are stimulated.

Dr. Waterlow: You said that about 70% of IQ was hereditary, and one could easily visualize the vicious circle of less intelligent people getting worse jobs, becoming poor, etc. Has anybody controlled for the variable of parental intelligence in these studies?

Dr. Colombo: We have not, but a long time ago, Dr. Monckeberg (8) showed the correlations existing between the IQs of mothers and their children as well as the height of these children. There was a direct relationship between the height of the children and the IQ of the mothers.

Dr. Waterlow: But then if you remove the genetic or hereditary factors, would there be any relationships left of the kind that you showed?

Dr. Colombo: Yes, I think so.

Dr. Milner: I want to comment on the idea that there is a vulnerable period of brain development that culminates at the age of 2 years. When one reflects, again clinically, about the acquisition of language, the critical period takes us up to about 4 years. If we fail to teach a child with a speech delay beyond the age of 4 years, he has lost the opportunity to learn. That probably interacts with the postintervention period in a very important way.

Dr. Colombo: Yes, you are right.

Dr. Nabarro: Is there any information on what happens to the siblings of these children?

Dr. Colombo: No. We have not done that study.

Dr. Nabarro: Have you any idea whether the interaction between the mother and the child was affected by the mother's attitude to the child following malnutrition? Did the child's malnutrition have a distancing effect on the mother's relationship with the child?

Dr. Colombo: We investigated the mothers' expectancy regarding their children at school age: what they expected their children to be, what they thought their children would become later, etc. We found that children of mothers with better expectancies had a higher intellectual capacity. It is generally well known that when the expectancies of the parents are better, children tend to have a higher IQ. We didn't, however, verify that point in the undernourished population and, more particularly, during recovery after an acute episode of malnutrition. That could be very interesting.

Dr. Martorelli: From your chapter it was very clear that within this group of children with an episode of severe malnutrition, height was not related to IQ. There are many studies such as those from Monckeberg's group and from Guatemala, which you mentioned, that show associations between height and IQ. I would be inclined to think that there is an association between stunting and IQ, but we have problems in interpreting this relationship. Do you think your study is unusual in not showing this association? Is it because the sample is restricted to children who had had malnutrition?

Dr. Colombo: In the whole group of children who suffered an episode of extreme undernutrition, we find a relationship between IQ and stunting, but we do not always find that relationship when we investigate the children individually. Linear growth seems to be affected by nutritional deficits and inappropriate environmental conditions in a different way from brain growth. The timing of the insult could be important here.

Dr. Tanner: I would like to join forces with Dr. Martorell on this particular point, as somebody who has had the occasion to review world literature on normal children, not divided into normal and "stunted" groups. There is an absolute universality in these data. The relationship between stature and, at first, academic ability in schools and, later, IQ tests of one sort or another was first described in Russia and simultaneously in St. Louis in the 1880s. A great debate then developed as to whether this was a coadvancement of stature and "IQ" or whether this was going to persist when the child finally became an adult (see ref. 9 for discussion). The data on reaching adulthood are apparently fairly clear. The best are from Husen in Stockholm (10): the correlation of the army-type IQ test and stature for all Swedish young males called up for conscription was 0.24; in Belgium very similar, and in Holland also. It is a very low correlation and tells you absolutely nothing about an individual, but it does tell you something about either the genetic or the social system or both.

The other thing one has to say is that there is very strong evidence that short people migrate, in Western countries at least, down the social scale: tall people migrate up the social scale (see ref. 11 for discussion). Naturally, in due course that produces a social stratification, presumably both in stature and in IQ. So it is very complex.

REFERENCES

1. Richardson SA. The relation of severe malnutrition in infancy to the intelligence of school children with differing life histories. *Pediatr Res* 1976;10:57–61.
2. Grantham McGregor S, Schofield W, Harris L. Effect of psychosocial stimulation on mental development of severely malnourished children: an interim report. *Pediatrics* 1983;72:239–43.
3. Grantham McGregor S, Powell C, Stewart M. Schofield W. Longitudinal study of growth and development of young Jamaican children recovering from severe protein energy malnutrition. *Dev Med Child Neurol* 1982;24:321–31.
4. Mukherjee DK, Gazder Ad, Chatterjee A, Mukherjee KL. Polyacrylamide gel electrophoresis of serum and CSF protein in classical cases of kwashiorkor and marasmus, on admission and at recovery. In: Ghai OP, ed. *Proceedings of the fifteenth International Congress of Pediatrics.* New Delhi: 1977.
5. Stoch MB, Smythe PM, Moodie AD, Bradshaw D. Psychosocial outcome and CT findings after gross undernourishment during infancy: a 20 year developmental study. *Dev Med Child Neurol* 1982;24:419–36.
6. Ounsted M, Moor VA, Scott A. Head circumference charts updated. *Arch Dis Child* 1985;60:936–9.
7. Davies DP, Leungh SF, Lau SP. Secular trends in head growth. *Arch Dis Child* 1986;61:623–4.
8. Monckeberg F, Tisler S. Toro S, Gattas U, Vega L. Malnutrition and mental development. *Am J Clin Nutr* 1972;25:766–72.
9. Tanner JM. *A history of the study of human growth.* Cambridge: Cambridge University Press, 1981:217–9,240–1.
10. Husén T. Undersökningar rörande sambanden mellan somatiska förhållanden och intellektuell prestationsförmåga. *Militür Hälsovård* 1951;76:41–74.
11. Tanner JM. *Foetus into man.* Cambridge, MA: Harvard University Press, 1978:148–9.

Linear Growth Retardation in Less Developed Countries, edited by John C. Waterlow. Nestlé Nutrition Workshop Series, Vol. 14. Nestec Ltd., Vevey/Raven Press, Ltd., New York © 1988.

Body Size, Physical Work Capacity, and Productivity in Hard Work: Is Bigger Better?

G. B. Spurr

Department of Physiology, Medical College of Wisconsin and Zablocki VA Medical Center, Milwaukee, Wisconsin 53295; and Department of Physiological Sciences, Universidad del Valle, Cali, Colombia

The relationship in poorer, developing nations of the world between small body size of the adult population and nutritional deprivation during the period of growth has been discussed at length in previous chapters. Some of the functional consequences have also been discussed. It is my task to address the results of chronic undernutrition and associated small body size on physical work capacity (PWC) and productivity in work that can be classified as heavy. I attempt to demonstrate that, within limits, larger individuals have an advantage in this kind of work over their smaller counterparts in the same population. It has been suggested that in mild or moderate states of malnutrition, where individuals may be "small but healthy," there is little or no functional deprivation, and that when assessing the incidence of malnutrition, different standards than those used for more advantaged groups ought to be applied to populations where smallness is common (1). Gopalan (2) has rejected this double standard for rich and poor. Furthermore, Margen (3) has stated that although it is obvious that a larger individual can perform heavier work than a small one, this may not be the proper interpretation since, if expressed per unit of lean body mass (LBM), the work that can be performed by a small person is as great as that of a large one. This chapter attempts to show that mild to moderate malnutrition is accompanied by functional decrements in work capacity that have particular importance when it occurs during the period of growth and that it is the total work capacity that matters, not the PWC normalized for weight or LBM.

The concern with PWC and its relationship to hard physical work is valid only if both hard physical work and malnutrition are associated. In the less developed areas of the world, where the incidence of protein–calorie undernutrition is high and mechanization is at a minimum, human labor provides much of the power for economic productivity (4). For example, using data published by the United Nations (5), it is possible to estimate for six South American countries that about

54% of the actively employed male population is engaged in work that can be classified as moderate to heavy (agriculture, forestry, mining, construction, etc.). Arteaga (6), using the same source of data for 1972, concluded that in all of Latin America, about 54% of employed men were engaged in heavy work, 20% in medium-intensity work, and 26% in sedentary occupations. Consequently, hard physical work is a reality for the majority of adult males in the work force of poor countries, and factors that affect it will have bearing on economic development (7).

DEFINITIONS

Malnutrition is used here as a convenient synonym for undernutrition and, in the present context, refers to chronic undernutrition in which the subjects' daily struggle to obtain sufficient nutrient intake may be a losing one, lasting over many years or a lifetime where the food supply is precarious.

The definitions of physical fitness and physical work capactity (PWC) are difficult to formulate (8). An expert committee of the World Health Organization was able only to relate one to the other: "Physical fitness is the ability to perform muscular work satisfactorily" (9). Physical fitness is frequently confused with physical performance as measured by tests representing basic performance demands (skill, flexibility, strength, etc.). These tests are related to special gymnastic or athletic performance and consequently are not suitable for evaluation of basic physiological functions (10). Where gymnasia are few or unknown, subject populations are handicapped, and even in more developed areas, previous motor learning is an important factor (8). Consequently, in this discussion physical performance is limited to measures of productivity (where these exist) in actual work situations and to a few measures of performance in relation to load carrying. Productivity is also an elusive concept, but in some types of industrial and agricultural work, payment is based on piecework, and so productivity in terms of the manufactured or harvested goods or pay received can be measured. Work is a complex entity and involves, in addition to the biologic component, psychological (motivational), type-of-work, and work-setting components (11). The effects of malnutrition on work and productivity deal only with the biological component.

The overall physical fitness of an individual is best determined by the maximal work capacity (physical work capacity) as measured by the maximal oxygen consumption ($\dot{V}o_2$ max). The PWC of a person is the result of a number of contributing factors: natural endowment (genes), physical condition (training), sex, age, and, as will be discussed, nutritional status, to mention the most important. Measurement of the $\dot{V}o_2$ max provides information on the maximal output of aerobic energy-liberating processes in the skeletal muscles involved in the work as well as the functional capacity of the circulation, since there is a high correlation between $\dot{V}o_2$ and cardiac output in both submaximal and maximal work (10). Consequently, the $\dot{V}o_2$ max as an assessment of physical work capacity is a measure of functional (physiological) capacity and has particular importance when related to nutritional status with its implications for the developing world (12–14). The $\dot{V}_{O_2}$ max, then, can be defined as the highest oxygen uptake an individual attains during physical work while breathing air at sea level (10). $\dot{V}_{O_2}$ max, aerobic capacity, and maximal aerobic power are terms that are frequently employed interchangeably, but because of the emphasis in this chapter on the absolute oxygen cost (liters/min) of submaximal work tasks in comparison to the maximum $\dot{V}_{O_2}$ (liters/min), a distinction will be made. Thus, the term $\dot{V}_{O_2}$ max is limited to this measurement in units of liters per minute, whereas the term maximal aerobic power or capacity is retained for the maximal oxygen consumption as a function of body weight (milliliters/min/kg) or one of the compartments of body weight such as the lean body mass (LBM), muscle cell mass (MCM), etc. Endurance, in the present context, means the maximum time an individual can continuously sustain a given submaximal work load.

Mechanical efficiency is the ratio of work accomplished to the energy required to do the work. In terms of the intact organism, it has been measured using the oxygen cost of performing work on the bicycle ergometer or treadmill and expressed as a percentage with or without the subtraction of various base lines (15–17). It appears that Δ efficiency [(change in work accomplished/change in energy expended) $\times$ 100] represents the most accurate estimate of muscular efficiency (16). However, even this has been questioned, since values obtained by the subtraction of various base lines yield unreasonably high efficiencies when compared to those found for isolated muscle preparations. Furthermore, considerations of elastic energy storage and eccentric contractions further complicate the picture (18). Stainsby et al. have suggested that although exercise efficiencies using base line subtractions may be useful, they do not indicate muscle efficiency, and that studies of exercise (work) metabolism might be more profitably directed at quantifying the determinants of energy expenditure (18). Thus, the energy expenditure (oxygen uptake) at various tasks might better be termed the economy of submaximal work (exercise) expressed per unit of body weight (19).

STUDIES IN ADULTS

Because short adult stature is largely the result of chronic undernutrition during growth, the results of studies of acute starvation and semistarvation under laboratory conditions, which have been reviewed (13,14), are not treated here. Attention is directed to the few studies available in the literature on the relationships among nutritional status, PWC as measured by the $\dot{V}_{O_2}$ max, and productivity in some work situations with comments on endurance as a component of productivity in chronically undernourished subjects. Since the malnourished individual is usually not working (a reason for his malnourished state), particularly in moderate or heavy work tasks, it has not been possible to relate malnourished states directly to productivity. Rather, the attempt has been made to relate both nutritional status and productivity (measured in nutritionally normal, employed subjects) to a common measurement ($\dot{V}_{O_2}$ max) and from these relationships to infer the association between nutritional status and productivity in moderate to heavy work. Most reports in the literature are the result of measurements in male subjects.

Malnutrition and $\dot{V}O_2$ max

Viteri (20,21) compared the PWC of several groups of young Guatemalan adults, one of which, their subjects from San Antonio La Paz (SAP), can probably be considered at least marginally malnourished on the basis of the adiposity, LBM, and muscle cell mass (MCM, calculated from daily creatinine excretion). The SAP group, another group of recent inductees into the army who were from a similar rural socioeconomic background, and 10 nutritionally supplemented agricultural workers all had significantly lower $\dot{V}O_2$ max and maximal aerobic power (expressed per kilogram of body weight and of LBM) than army cadets from middle or upper socioeconomic levels who had never been exposed to nutritional deprivation. When compared on the basis of "cell residue" (body weight less fat, water, and bone mineral), all differences in maximal aerobic power between groups disappeared. Viteri (20) observed that the differences in maximal aerobic power were associated with differences in body composition and not with differences in cell function.

We have studied three groups of chronically malnourished adult males who were selected for their existing degree of undernutrition (22). The most severely malnourished of these subjects were also studied during a 45-day basal period in the hospital and during 79 days of a dietary repletion regimen (23). Subjects were classified into those with mild (M), intermediate (I), and severe (S) malnutrition based on their weight/height (W/H) ratio, serum albumin concentrations, and daily creatinine excretions per meter of height (Cr/H) as detailed in Table 1. Each group was significantly different ($p<0.001$) from the other two in regard to each variable used in the classification. Detailed body composition and biochemical measurements on the three groups were made shortly after admission to the metabolic ward (24) and during the dietary repletion regimen of group S (25). On entry into the

TABLE 1. *Selection criteria (A) and observed values (B) of mild (M), intermediate (I), and severely (S) malnourished adult males (means ± SD)*

Subject groups		Weight/height (kg/m)	Serum albumin (g/dl)	Daily creatinine/height (mg/day per m)
M (n = 11)	A	> 32	> 3.5	> 600
	B	33.3 ± 2.1	3.8 ± 0.5	660 ± 67
I (n = 18)	A	29–32	2.5–3.5	450–600
	B	30.8 ± 2.0	3.0 ± 0.7	559 ± 75
S (n = 18)	A	< 29	< 2.5	< 450
	B	27.4 ± 2.1	2.1 ± 0.5	391 ± 76

From Spurr (13).

hospital, the subjects were placed on an energy intake (2,240 kcal/day, 9.4 MJ/day) adequate for the sedentary conditions of the metabolic ward but were maintained on the same protein intake (27 g/day) they were ingesting prior to entry.

Studies of work capacity and endurance in the severely malnourished men were made at the beginning and end of the 45-day basal period on this diet. The protein intake was then increased to 100 g/day for the 79-day repletion regimen; the increased caloric intake from protein was balanced by reducing carbohydrate intake to maintain the diets isocaloric. Measurements of $\dot{V}O_2$ max and endurance were repeated after 90 and 124 hospital days. The results for the three groups and the changes in the severely malnourished men during dietary repletion are presented in Figs. 1 and 2 and compared with data on 107 nutritionally normal control subjects who were sugar cane cutters (26), loaders (27), or general farm laborers (28). There were progressive differences in body weight, W/H ratio, serum albumin, and total proteins in the control (C), M, I, and S groups (Fig. 1). Groups C and M were not significantly different in regard to hematocrit and blood hemoglobin, but I and S were significantly and progressively depressed in these measurements. There was a slight gain in body weight of group S during the basal period, but otherwise the variables did not change. Weight, W/H ratio, and the serum proteins showed progressive improvement during the repletion regimen, but the hematological values did not show improvement until the final round of measurements (Fig. 1).

Figure 2 presents the results for maximal heart rate (f_H max), maximal aerobic power ($\dot{V}O_2$, ml/min/kg body weight), and $\dot{V}O_2$ max (liters/min) for the control and malnourished subjects. Average f_H max values were not different in the various groups, nor did they change during dietary repletion. However, $\dot{V}O_2$ max and max-

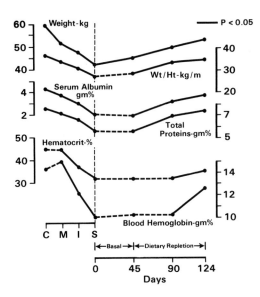

FIG. 1. Average values of some anthropometric and blood variables in nutritionally normal (C) subjects and men with mild (M), intermediate (I), and severe (S) malnutrition. The severely undernourished were studied during a basal period on adequate calories and low protein followed by a dietary repletion period on an isocaloric but high-protein diet. *Solid lines* connect points that are significantly different from each other. (From Spurr, ref. 13.)

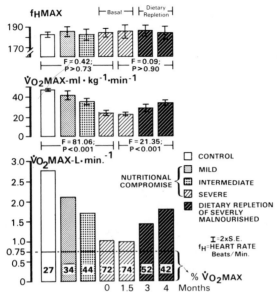

FIG. 2. Maximum heart rates (f_H), aerobic power, and $\dot{V}O_2$ max in control, undernourished, and severely malnourished subjects and during dietary repletion of the latter. **Lower panel** shows a fixed submaximal work load (0.75 liter/min) in terms of percentage $\dot{V}O_2$ max. (From Spurr, ref. 13.)

imal aerobic power were progressively less in C, M, I, and S subjects, did not change in the latter during the basal period, and then progressively improved during dietary repletion, although they did not return to even the level of group M during the period of study. Figure 2 also expresses a theoretical submaximal work load of 0.75 liters/min $\dot{V}O_2$ in terms of percent $\dot{V}O_2$ max for each of the groups. From Fig. 2, it is clear that $\dot{V}O_2$ max and maximal aerobic power are markedly depressed in chronic malnutrition and that the degree of reduction is related to the severity of depression in nutritional status. Among the three groups of malnourished subjects, a stepwise multiple regression analysis (22) revealed that the W/H ratio, log of the sum of triceps and subscapular skinfolds in millimeters (SK), total body Hb (TotHb) obtained as the product of blood Hb and blood volume (grams per kilogram body weight), and daily creatinine (Cr) excretion (grams per day per kilogram) contributed significantly to the variation in $\dot{V}O_2$ max (liters/min):

$$\dot{V}O_2 \text{ max} = 0.095 \text{ W/H} - 0.152 \text{ SK} + 0.087 \text{ TotHb} + 0.031 \text{ Cr} - 2.550 \quad (1)$$

$$r = 0.931; \text{ SEE} = 0.21$$

All of the variables in the equation are related to nutritional status.

Figure 3 expresses the data for the three malnourished groups and for group S during recovery in terms of various body compartments. It was not possible to do detailed body composition studies on the control subjects. The salient feature of Fig. 3 is that over 80% of the difference in $\dot{V}O_2$ max between M and S subjects is accounted for by difference in MCM. The remaining difference might be ascribed to reduced capacity for oxygen transport either because of low blood Hb (Fig. 1) or reduced maximum cardiac output. There do not seem to be any reports of studies on maximum cardiac output in malnourished subjects. Another possibility is

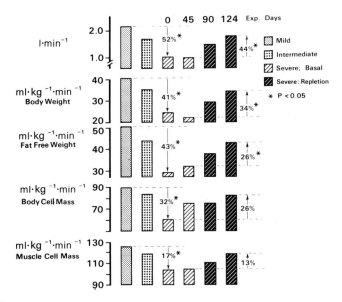

FIG. 3. $\dot{V}_{O_2}$ max expressed in terms of various body compartments for the undernourished subjects and during dietary repletion of the most severely malnourished. (From Spurr, ref. 13.)

that the skeletal muscle cells have reduced maximal aerobic power because of reduced oxidative enzyme content. Tasker and Tulpule (29) found a marked decrease in the activities of oxidative enzymes in skeletal muscle of protein-deficient rats, and Raju (30) reported that after recovery from 13 weeks of reduced protein intake, rat skeletal muscle had an increase in glycolytic and a decrease in oxidative enzymes and activity. However, there appear to be no studies that have measured similar biochemical changes in humans, although Lopes et al. (31) have recently shown that malnourished patients exhibited marked impairment in muscle function. There were both an increased muscle fatigability in static muscular contraction and a changed pattern of muscle contraction and relaxation, which were reversed in patients undergoing nutritional supplementation. Their data indicate the possibility of a decreased content of ATP and phosphocreatine in the skeletal muscle tissue of malnourished subjects.

The data of Heymsfield et al. (32) indicate changes in the biochemical composition of skeletal muscle in both acute and chronic semistarvation, particularly in glycogen and total energy contents. In any event, it should be emphasized that the $\dot{V}_{O_2}$ max not accounted for by differences in MCM is small (Fig 3). After 2.5 months of recovery, the $\dot{V}_{O_2}$ max increased significantly in liters per minute when expressed in terms of body weight and LBM, but, although mean values were elevated in terms of body cell mass (BCM) and MCM, the increases were not statistically significant. However, at the termination of the experiment, PWC had not returned to values comparable to those seen in mild malnutrition (Figs. 2 and 3), which indicates that the recovery process is a long one, particularly under the sedentary conditions of the hospital metabolic ward. It is interesting to note that the $\dot{V}O_2$ max was increased 45 days after beginning the repletion diet (90 hospital days), when blood Hb concentration had not yet increased (Fig. 1) but MCM was significantly increased over basal values (25). This also points to a primary dependence of $\dot{V}O_2$ max on MCM (Fig. 3). Furthermore, it appears that supplying adequate calories alone was not sufficient to bring about an increase in $\dot{V}O_2$ max or MCM and that only after increasing the protein intake to 100 g/day was there improvement in these two variables (23,25).

Endurance

An endurance test is carried out on a treadmill or bicycle ergometer at a work load ($\dot{V}O_2$) of 70 to 80% of the subject's maximum until exhaustion supervenes, usually with the f_H within about 5 beats of f_H max. Because of the difficulty in performing this test, only a few laboratories have attempted measurement of endurance times in normal individuals and, to our knowledge, none except our own in malnourished subjects.

From a number of sources, it is known that the maximum relative work load that can be sustained for an 8-hr work day usually does not exceed about 35 to 40% $\dot{V}O_2$ max. Thus, Michael et al. (33) found in laboratory treadmill work that 8 hr could be tolerated without undue fatigue when the relative load did not exceed 35% $\dot{V}O_2$ max. In the building industry, Åstrand (34) reported that about 40% $\dot{V}O_2$ max was the upper limit that could be tolerated for an 8-hr work day, and we have estimated that sugar cane cutters worked at about 35% of their $\dot{V}O_2$ max during an 8-hr day (26). These studies were performed in physically fit subjects. Sedentary individuals can be expected to have lower upper limits for 8 hr of work (10, p. 292).

We have measured maximum endurance times at 80% $\dot{V}O_2$ max (T_{80}) in the groups of malnourished subjects described above (22,23). We did not find any significant differences among the groups (M, I, and S) of malnourished men; T_{80} averaged $97 + 12$ min (mean $\pm$ SE) in all subjects (22). However, it might be assumed that the $\dot{V}O_2$ max of group S subjects would be about 2.4 liters/min had they not been malnourished, and that about 35% (0.84 liter/min) could be sustained for an 8-hr work day. The value of 0.84 liter/min is 80% of the $\dot{V}O_2$ max (1.05 liters/min) for these subjects, who had maximum endurance times at this relative work load of a little over 1.5 hr, a loss of about 6.5 hr of daily working time or about an 80% reduction in productive potential (22). Using a similar method of estimation, Barac-Nieto (35) has calculated a 16% reduction in work output of the M subjects, a 35% decrease in I, and a 78% reduction in S men.

In the case of group S during dietary repletion, an interesting change in T_{80} was observed. Endurance times were significantly reduced from 113 min at the first measurement of the basal period to 42 min at the final determination at the end of the dietary repletion (23). The explanation for this surprising reduction is still not clear. Hanson-Smith et al. (36) reported decreased work endurance times in rats on high-protein diets compared to animals ingesting an isocaloric carbohydrate diet, and Bergstrom et al. (37) and Gollnick et al. (38) have shown that diets in which the energy value of carbohydrate has been replaced with fat and/or protein lead to reduced stores of muscle glycogen. Furthermore, Bergstrom et al. (37) demonstrated that the maximum endurance time in humans is directly related to the initial glycogen content of skeletal muscle. During the dietary repletion period of the group S subjects, carbohydrate intake was reduced from 64% to 50% of calories. In a normal individual this amount of carbohydrate should be sufficient to maintain muscle glycogen stores, but definitive studies seem not to have been done (39). The rebuilt muscle tissue of group S subjects may not store glycogen normally and, together with the lack of regular exercise in the protracted sedentary existence in the metabolic ward, may lead to reduced muscle glycogen and shorter endurance times. Heymsfield et al. (32) found reduced muscle glycogen in subjects who had undergone acute or chronic semistarvation prior to death. Muscle nutritive supply and the metabolic and endocrine responses that regulate it during both short-term and prolonged exercise have not been investigated in malnourished individuals. Even though there is little reason at the moment to suspect abnormal muscle function in acute exercise testing to maximum levels, the responses to prolonged exercise may be worth investigating.

Productivity and Physical Work Capacity

With a direct relationship established between nutritional status and physical work capacity in undernourished men, attention can now be directed towards the association between $\dot{V}o_2$ max and productivity. The amount of work done in terms of output of a product is usually difficult to measure, particularly in the lighter work tasks in which the intellectual component may have as much or more to do with "productivity" as the physical use of one's body. In moderate and heavy work, it has sometimes been possible to estimate productivity by measuring the quantity of product or income where piecework is the basis for payment of the worker. Sugar cane cutting and loading are heavy work tasks, and the weight of cane cut or loaded is measured carefully since workers are usually paid by the tonnage cut. Because the pay scale in many sugar-harvesting operations is very low, one might expect that the motivation factor would be fairly similar in different groups of workers and that they would work close to the limit of their physical capacities. Also, logging is heavy physical work (40) and has been used to relate productivity to worker characteristics. The time to accomplish standard work tasks is another method that has been utilized to estimate productivity (21).

Hansson (41) measured submaximal work and estimated $\dot{V}o_2$ max in a group of "top" producing lumberjacks and a group of average producers and found that the former had a higher estimated $\dot{V}o_2$ max than the latter. Davies (42) studied sugar cane cutters in East Africa, dividing them into high, medium, and low producers based on the daily tonnage cut. He found no difference in the three groups in height, weight, summed skinfolds, LBM, leg volume, or the circumferences of biceps and calf but did encounter a significant correlation between daily productivity and $\dot{V}O_2$ max ($r=0.46$; $p<0.001$). Davies et al. (43) also measured productivity in Sudanese cane cutters during a 3-hr period of continuous cutting and reported a significant correlation between $\dot{V}O_2$ max and rate (kilograms per minute) of cane cutting ($r=0.26$; $p<0.01$).

We have studied nutritionally normal sugar cane workers in Colombia, where the tasks of cutting and loading the cane are performed by separate gangs of men. The former is a self-paced and continuous task, whereas the loading of cane is discontinuous, depending on the availability of wagons. The cutters were divided into good (group I), average (group II), and poor (group III) producers, depending on the daily tonnage cut. The cutters worked at about 35% of their $\dot{V}O_2$ max during the 8-hr day (26), which is close to the maximum that can be sustained for this period of time (33,34). In relating various anthropometric measurements and age to productivity, there were statistically significant positive correlations of height, weight, and LBM with productivity (44). The correlations with age and body fat were not significant. Figure 4 summarizes the relationship of $\dot{V}O_2$ max and maximal aerobic power with productivity, both of which were significantly correlated. A stepwise multiple regression analysis revealed that $\dot{V}O_2$ max, percentage body fat (F), and height contributed significantly to the variation in productivity (tons/day) such that

$$\text{Productivity} = 0.81 \, \dot{V}O_2 \, \text{max} - 0.14 \, F + 0.03 \, H - 1.962 \qquad (2)$$

$$r = 0.685; \, p < 0.001$$

The $\dot{V}O_2$ max and body fat are influenced by present nutritional status (20,22),

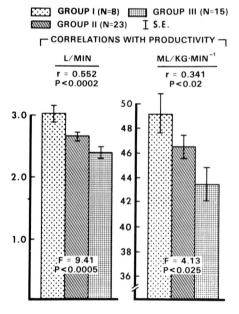

FIG. 4. $\dot{V}O_2$ max and maximal aerobic power of good (group I), average (group II), and poor (group III) sugar cane cutters, ages 18–34 years. F ratio values are from a one-way analysis of variance. (From Spurr et al., ref. 44.)

and adult height by past nutritional status during the period of growth (45). Equation 2 states simply that those who are presently in poor physical condition or malnourished (low $\dot{V}O_2$ max) or whose height is stunted because of past undernutrition are at a disadvantage in terms of ability to produce in cutting sugar cane. The negative coefficient for percentage body fat indicates that there is some advantage to low body fat content. The relatively low correlation coefficients between productivity and $\dot{V}O_2$ max obtained in our studies (Fig. 4) and those of others (43,44) preclude the use of regression equations in the prediction of productivity and bring into question the homogeneity of motivation alluded to above. The results shown in Fig. 4 indicate that the more physically fit subjects were better producers. Also, since malnutrition reduces $\dot{V}O_2$ max, one can predict that it will have proportional effects on productivity in hard work.

Even in the case of the sugar cane loaders, who do not work continuously, productivity was positively correlated with maximal aerobic power and negatively with resting and working f_H, demonstrating again the relationship of productivity to the physical condition of the worker (27).

In the case of sugar cane cutting, which at an average expenditure of 5 kcal/min per 65 kg of body weight during the 8-hr day (26) can be classified as moderate industrial work (40), the worker productivity is related to his body size, height, weight, and LBM (44). This has also been demonstrated by Satyanarayana et al. (46,47) for industrial factory work of presumably less intensity than sugar cane cutting. Their subjects were nutritionally normal workers engaged in the production of detonator fuses, which could be measured in terms of the number of fuses produced per day. They found that body weight, height, and LBM were significantly correlated with productivity and that after partialing out the effect of height, weight and LBM were still significantly correlated with productivity. That is, the total daily work output was significantly higher in those with higher body weight and LBM.

STUDIES IN CHILDREN

With the recognition that the reduced work capacity found in malnourished adults was largely the result of reduced muscle mass, the next question to be addressed was the effect of chronic marginal malnutrition, which is so prevalent in the poorer segments of developing countries, on the growth of work capacity in school-aged children. There are few studies of exercise and work capacity in malnourished children, and most of these have been carried out using submaximal exercise testing. Areskog et al. (48) determined the physical work capacity at a heart rate of 170 (PWC_{170}) in 10- and 13-year-old Ethiopian boys from public and private schools with the aim of including both poorly nourished (public schools) and well-nourished (private schools) subjects. The older public school boys were shorter, weighed less, and had smaller skinfolds and midarm circumferences than their private school counterparts. The performance of the public school boys was somewhat better than the private school children in the tests of PWC_{170}. Davies

(49) predicted $\dot{V}O_2$ max from submaximal bicycle ergometry, demonstrating that malnourished (underweight) children had low values for $\dot{V}O_2$ max but that maximal aerobic power in terms of body weight, LBM, or leg volume was well within the normal range. Satyanarayana et al. (50) have also reported the results of measurements of PWC_{170} in boys 14–17 years of age categorized according to their nutritional status at age 5 years. They found that about 64% of the variation in PWC_{170} could be explained by the subjects' body weight at the time of the testing, and another 10% by their habitual physical activity levels. But even severe malnutrition at age 5 had no effect on work performance when PWC_{170} was expressed in terms of body weight. However, the undernourished subjects had higher values for f_H at the same submaximal work load, i.e., were working at a higher percentage of $\dot{V}O_2$ max than normal children.

In the work to be described from our laboratory, all subjects were boys and had to present their official birth certificates as a first condition for inclusion in the study. They were grouped into five age groups at 2-year intervals from 6 to 16 years of age. According to the Colombian standards established by Rueda-Williamson et al. (51), children were selected who had weight for age and weight for height >95% (but <110%) of predicted as being nutritionally normal (N) and without a history of undernutrition. Those with both weight for age and weight for height <95% of the standard were considered to be undernourished at the time of study. The choice of 95% as the cut-off point was entirely arbitrary, and the expectation was that the group averages would be considerably below this point (52). The details of the selection process and the methodology employed in the anthropometric and maturation (52), $\dot{V}O_2$ max (53), body composition (54), and work efficiency measurements (55) have been described previously.

Anthropometry, Sexual Maturation, and Body Composition in Boys

The average heights and weights of the five age groups of nutritionally normal and undernourished boys are plotted on the NCHS percentile grids in Fig. 5. The number of subjects in each group varied from 24 to 60. The nutritionally normal boys followed the 50th percentile in the younger age groups and deviated towards the 25th percentile in the older groups (Fig. 5) for both height and weight. The tendency towards shorter stature in these boys is probably the result of the high percentage of mestizos (74%), who have shorter stature than other children (56,57). Both height for age and weight for age of the undernourished boys were on or below the fifth percentile during this period of growth. The weight for height of the normal subjects fell slightly above the 50th percentile throughout this period, whereas the undernourished boys followed approximately the 10th percentile (52). In addition to the depressed growth pattern seen in Fig. 5, the undernourished subjects had significantly lower values for skinfolds, significantly delayed growth spurt and sexual maturation (52), and, in a subgroup, increased fasting levels of circulating growth hormone *(unpublished)*. Consequently, the selection process resulted in the separation of undernourished boys, who were smaller and

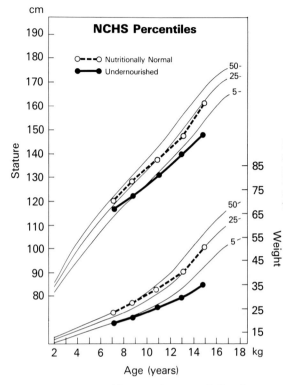

FIG. 5. Average values of height and weight of control and undernourished school-aged Colombian boys plotted as a function of average group ages on NCHS percentiles. (Spurr *et al.*, ref. 52.)

thinner than normal boys, who were following essentially normal growth development compared to either national or international (NCHS) norms. However, the physiologic data (slowed growth velocity, delayed sexual maturation, and high circulating growth hormone concentrations) make it clear that the reason for their smallness and thinness is that they were undergoing a process of chronic malnutrition, which is no doubt "marginal" in nature but nevertheless real. Furthermore, the fact, that there is a progressive deviation from predicted values of height and weight for age from younger to older boys (Fig. 5) (52) indicates that the process is cumulative with age.

We have demonstrated (54) that the empirical equations developed by Pařízková (58) for estimating body fat from skinfolds in children also apply to our subjects. The results of average estimates of LBM derived from these equations are plotted in Fig. 6 (panel C) together with values for height and weight for the 6 to 8, 10 to 12, and 14 to 16-year-old boys (panels A and B) to compare with similar values for the four groups of adult Colombian men discussed previously (C, M, I, and S) and a group of 10 nutritionally normal North American men. The LBM of the C group was calculated from the skinfold equations of Pascale et al. (59), and that of the American men from those of Durnin and Womersley (60). The LBM of the three groups of malnourished Colombian men (M, I, and S) were obtained from measurements of total body water (24).

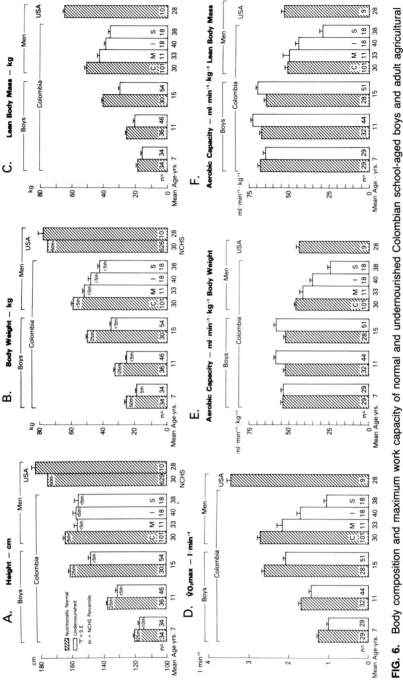

FIG. 6. Body composition and maximum work capacity of normal and undernourished Colombian school-aged boys and adult agricultural workers classified as nutritionally normal control subjects (C) or as mild (M), intermediate (I), and severe (S) in the degree of their nutritional deprivation. Also shown are the values for a group of North American men and the NCHS 50th-percentile values of weight and height for adult men.

It can be seen (Fig. 6C) that the development of LBM of the undernourished boys is significantly attenuated during growth (54). When expressed as percentage of body weight, the undernourished boys had significantly higher values of LBM than well-nourished subjects because of lower fat values in the former (54).

Growth of Work Capacity

The growth of $\dot{V}O_2$ max in the youngest, oldest, and intermediate age groups of boys presented in Fig. 5 is shown in Fig. 6D. The $\dot{V}O_2$ max of the nutritionally deprived boys was significantly lower ($\sim 85\%$) than the normal subjects throughout the age range studied (53). When expressed as per kilogram of body weight, with the exception of the youngest age group, the undernourished boys had higher aerobic capacities than the normal boys (Fig. 6E), which was thought to be because of differences in body composition (53). Subsequent studies (54) demonstrated that even when expressed in terms of LBM, the aerobic capacity of the undernourished subjects, at least in the older age groups, was significantly higher (Fig. 6F). That is, the undernourished boys show evidence of better physical condition (61). In a similar study on rural Colombian boys, although the difference in aerobic capacity between nutritionally normal and undernourished subjects expressed per kilogram of body weight was similar to that found for urban subjects (Fig. 6E) (53), the difference disappeared when aerobic capacity was calculated in terms of LBM (Fig. 6F); i.e., the rural boys did not exhibit a training effect (54). These results may be caused by a relative increase in the daily physical activity of the undernourished boys (in relation to their lower total $\dot{V}O_2$ max) (62,63) or result from greater access of urban children to sports training facilities than rural boys (53,54,64).

These results make it clear that the lower values of $\dot{V}O_2$ max for the nutritionally deprived children are related to their lower body weights. This is essentially the same conclusion reached by Davies (49) and Satyanarayana et al. (50). As mentioned earlier for adults, there does not appear to be any basic deficit in muscle function in marginally malnourished children, only in the quantity of muscle available for maximal work. We have deliberately avoided analyzing these data on the basis of so-called "developmental" age because such an analysis would tend to obscure the differences seen in Fig. 6D; the responsibilities of adulthood occur with chronological, not developmental age.

BODY SIZE, COMPOSITION, AND $\dot{V}O_2$ max IN MEN AND BOYS

Persons of larger size in general appear to function better than those with smaller stature (65) in relation to reproduction (66), disease (67), cognition (68), and work performance (13,14). Because physical work capacity is a function of body size (10), i.e., the mass of muscle tissue involved in the maximum effort, and muscle constitutes about 40% of the body weight and 50% of the LBM

(69,70), it is interesting to note the correlations between the three components of body size and $\dot{V}O_2$ max presented in Table 2. The correlations in boys are higher than those in men, probably because of a threefold greater range in values, but in either case it is clear that in nonobese subjects there are significant correlations between parameters of body size and PWC as measured by $\dot{V}O_2$ max. Taller individuals have more LBM and higher $\dot{V}O_2$ max values (Fig. 6). Similar relationships exist for adult women, but the correlation coefficients are lower (71).

All of the data presented in Fig. 6 are from various studies in our laboratory (22–26,44,52–54,63) and permit a comparison between Colombian boys and men and between the latter and a small group of North American adult males. The differences in height between adults of developing and developed countries is well known (12). The average value of the C group of men in Fig. 6 is very close to that published for low-income Colombian men (12) and probably reflects some period(s) of undernutrition during the period of growth. The heights of the three groups of malnourished (M, I, S) men were not significantly different from each other but were lower than the C group. This is probably a result of more severe nutritional deprivation in groups M, I, and S during growth than occurred in group C. It is difficult to predict the adult height of the oldest boys, but it is likely that the nutritionally normal children will be taller (Fig. 6A) and perhaps have a higher $\dot{V}O_2$ max than group C (Fig. 6D), whereas the undernourished group of boys in adulthood will most likely resemble more closely group M.

The lower values of aerobic capacity per kilogram of body weight and of LBM in adults than in boys are also well known and at least in part probably reflects the progressive decline in these measurements with age from the youngest ages (72). The differences also may reflect differences in the states of physical training in the boys and men.

ENERGY COST OF LOAD CARRYING

The smaller size of nutritionally at-risk populations has been considered an advantage when resources are limited, since energy expenditure for the maintenance

TABLE 2. *Correlation coefficients of weight, height, lean body mass, and maximal oxygen consumption in nutritionally normal boys 6 to 16 years of age and adult males*[a]

	Boys (n = 406)			Men (n = 35)		
	Weight (kg)	Height (cm)	Lean body mass (kg)	Weight (kg)	Height (cm)	Lean body mass (kg)
Height	0.970	—	—	0.758	—	—
LBM	0.986	0.965	—	0.875	0.702	—
$\dot{V}O_2$ max	0.931	0.911	0.932	0.562	0.489	0.724

[a]Data on boys from Spurr et al. (53) and Barac-Nieto et al. (54); data on men from von Dobeln (71). All are statistically significant ($p < 0.01$).

of a small body would be less than that for a larger one, and the energy cost of movement would also be less.

The manual transportation of loads in developing countries persists as a major occupation of the adult work force (5,73), and although there have been a number of studies on the energy cost of load carrying (73,74), there seem to be none that compare this activity in nutritionally normal and malnourished subjects. Because the relationship between body size and energy expenditure in carrying out work tasks is incompletely understood, we have recently done some experiments on load carrying in nutritionally normal and malnourished boys and well-nourished men (63). The latter were included to give a wider range of body weights as well as a different environmental background. Three age groups of boys (6–8, 10–12, and 14–16 years of age) were studied while walking on a treadmill (3 miles per hour) at 0, 4, 8 and 12% grade without and with a 3-, 6-, or 9-kg backpack load in the youngest to oldest age groups, respectively. The adults also carried a 9-kg load. The results are summarized in Fig. 7, where the energy expended at each work load (grade) is expressed as a function of the body weight (without load) or body weight plus load.

Two conclusions are immediately evident from these results. First, the energy expended in treadmill walking without and with loads is a function of the body weight and the weight carried and not of nutritional status, since the two nutritional groups fall on the same line. Furthermore, age per se does not seem to influence the relationship except as it influences body size (weight). Similar results were also obtained by Mahadeva et al. (75) for nutritionally normal subjects. They concluded that no significant increase in precision was obtained by also taking into account height or age. The linear regression values for walking at 0% grade in our experiments (Fig. 7) are very similar to those obtained by these authors (75). Sec-

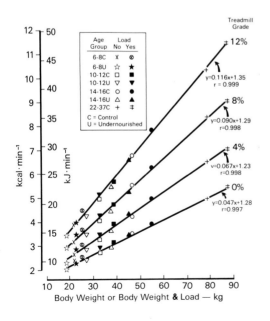

FIG. 7. Mean energy expenditure as a function of treadmill grade, body weight, and body weight plus weight of load carried in nutritionally undernourished boys walking at 3 miles per hour. Boys 6 to 8, 10 to 12, and 14 to 16 years old carried 3, 6, and 9 kg, respectively, and adults also carried 9 kg. (From Spurr and Reina, ref. 63.)

ondly, the energy cost of carrying a given load (i.e., in excess of that required to move the body weight) is the same regardless of nutritional status or body size, since the slope and intercepts are constants and at a given body weight, only the change in weight carried will increase energy expenditure. A third conclusion can be deduced indirectly from the results in Fig. 7; since $\dot{V}o_2$ max (Fig. 6D) is less in the smaller (younger and malnourished) subjects, the O_2 cost of carrying a given load will be relatively higher (percentage $\dot{V}o_2$ max) in these subjects than in bigger ones. This is borne out by direct calculations (63). Finally, the divergence of subjects (normal and malnourished Colombian boys and North American adults) gives the expectation that the relationships seen in Fig. 7 may apply to other groups (racial, sexual, etc.) as well (63,75).

Hypothetical Work Task

A task is contrived in Fig. 8 to approximate a possible work situation to which we might apply the equation from the 0% grade in Fig. 7. The figures in Fig. 8 are unloading a truck carrying sacks a distance that, at 3 miles per hour, takes 1 min and returning at the same speed for the next load. The calculations of energy expenditure are also shown.

Using the average values of body weight and $\dot{V}o_2$ max for the five groups of adults presented in Fig. 6, it is possible to make estimates of the rate of energy expenditure, relative effort, and total energy expenditure during the 7.5-hr work day for men carrying loads of 20 or 50 kg, which are presented in Fig. 9. The rate (kcal/min) and total (kcal/7.5 hr of work) energy expenditure of the largest (North American) men (Fig. 6) were the highest, and there is a progressive decline proportional to the body weight in the other subjects (Fig. 6). The difference between 20 and 50 kg of weight carried is constant, so that the smallest men have

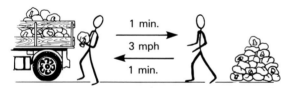

Rate of Transfer = 30 Sacks/hr.

Work Day:	8:00 A.M. — 12 Noon; 15 min. rest
	12:30 P.M. — 4:30 P.M.; 15 min. rest
Total =	7.5 hrs.
Productivity =	225 sacks/day

FIG. 8. Hypothetical work task based on 0° grade load carrying (presented in Fig. 7) and calculated energy expenditure (presented in Fig. 9).

Energy Expenditure (EE; kcal/min)

$$EE = [(0.047 \times wt. + 1.28) + (0.047 \times (wt + Load) + 1.28)]/2$$
$$\dot{V}O_2 = EE/4.9 = l/min$$
$$\text{Relative Effort} = \% \dot{V}O_2 max = (\dot{V}O_2/\dot{V}O_2 max) \times 100$$

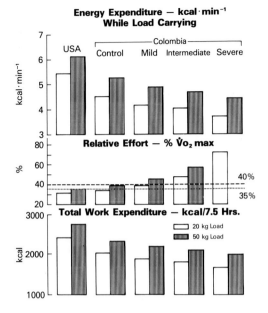

FIG. 9. Theoretical energy expenditure and relative effort of work load described in Fig. 8 in nutritionally normal North American and Colombian men and in three groups of undernourished Colombian men classified as mild, intermediate, and severe in the degree of their nutritional deprivation. Estimated data while carrying 20- and 50-kg loads are shown.

to increase their energy output by the same amount as the largest when changing from the 20- to the 50-kg load (Figs. 7 and 9).

The most interesting estimates in Fig. 9 are those based on relative effort. Lines at 40% and 35% of $\dot{V}o_2$ max have been drawn for easy reference. For the moment, we assume that those who work below this level can sustain this work for 8 hr, whereas those who have to work above 40% $\dot{V}o_2$ max would become fatigued and unable to continue some time before the end of an 8-hr workday. With only this as a criterion, the U.S. and Colombian nutritionally normal subjects could sustain both work loads, whereas the mildly malnourished group M could carry out only the 20-kg task. The intermediate and severely malnourished groups could not sustain either work load; indeed, the percentage $\dot{V}o_2$ max of group S during carriage of the 50-kg load (Fig. 8) was calculated to be greater than 100%, and so no value for this situation is plotted in Fig. 9.

Rarely, particularly in physiology, is anything as absolute as the above discussion would imply. Michael et al.'s (33) estimate of the maximum percentage $\dot{V}o_2$ max substainable for 8 hr of treadmill work in the laboratory was 35%, as was our own in sugar cane cutters in the field (26). However, of the 54 cutters studied, 16 sustained estimated efforts greater than 40%, one as high as 56%, during 8 hr of work (76). Although Åstrand's (34) estimate was about 40% of $\dot{V}o_2$ max, Jørgensen (77) has recently suggested that individual tasks must be adjusted to metabolic levels not to exceed 30 to 35% $\dot{V}o_2$ max.

What this points to is that there has been an attempt to estimate upper limits of daily work and, consequently, of effects on productivity from too few data (13,14), particularly concerning undernourished subjects. There is little information on sustained work efforts (percentage $\dot{V}O_2$ max) in undernourished subjects (21–23). Furthermore, the question arises about whether energy expenditure measurements are appropriate indicators for fatigue and productivity. There is some indication that strain and fatigue of back muscles (Fig. 8) can occur in long-term work even when metabolic rates are below so-called acceptable levels (77).

In any event, more detailed studies are needed of relative efforts sustainable for long periods in individuals of small stature as well as those with poor nutritional intakes. Anecdotal information abounds of small men, perhaps poorly nourished, who seem to perform superhuman work tasks. However, data are scarce.

EFFICIENCY OF SUBMAXIMAL WORK IN MALNUTRITION

It has been suggested that adults from developing countries are mechanically more efficient than their taller counterparts from the developed nations (78). The arguments on which this contention was made have been contested (13,55).

Edmundson (79,80) has presented data on basal metabolic rate (BMR) and mechanical work efficiency of men in East Java together with a review of related literature and attempted to make a case for metabolic adaptation to "undernutrition" as judged by the well-known reduction in BMR that occurs in undernourished subjects (81) and an increase in mechanical work efficiency in subjects on a chronic low energy intake. We consider only the mechanical work efficiency measurements made on two groups of his subjects who were selected from a group of 54 subjects studied. One group of five subjects was composed of high-energy-intake individuals (mean 2,754 kcal/day, 11.5 MJ/day) who were nearly identical in average height and weight to a group of six low-energy-intake subjects (mean 1,770 kcal/day, 7.4 MJ/day). It seems, therefore, that the subjects were selected for differences in their existing "metabolic efficiency." The BMR of the high-energy-intake group was almost twice that of the low-energy-intake subjects, and, perhaps not surprisingly, the gross calculated efficiency at 600 kpm/min on a bicycle ergometer was significantly higher in the latter group than in the former, although the difference at 300 kpm/min was not statistically significant. The Δ efficiencies calculated from Edmundson's (79,80) data were $16.1 \pm 6.48\%$ (range 7.6–23.0%) in the high-intake subjects and $23.6 \pm 5.26\%$ (range 16.8–31.0%) in the low-intake group and were not significantly different ($t = 2.07$; $p = 0.07$). It may be that a larger number of subjects would show a statistically significant difference in Δ efficiency since the range of efficiencies is large. Also, the values are somewhat lower than those reported by others (16).

We have also reported on the efficiency of submaximal treadmill walking in the normal and marginally malnourished school-aged children described above (55). The submaximal $\dot{V}O_2$ of treadmill walking at 3.5 miles per hour and 15% grade increased with age (body size) and was lower in malnourished boys than in their nutritionally normal counterparts. The gross economy (efficiency) followed the same pattern (55). However, when efficiency was expressed in terms of O_2 cost per kilogram of body weight, the opposite was true, i.e., higher $\dot{V}O_2$/kg body weight in younger (smaller) than older (bigger) subjects and in undernourished (smaller) than control (larger) boys.

The observation that the O_2 cost of treadmill walking or bicycle ergometry increases with age in children and decreases with age when expressed in terms of body weight is an old one (82,83) that has been repeatedly confirmed (84–86). The increase in $\dot{V}O_2$ with age is an expected result, since $\dot{V}O_2$ is related to body mass, and older and heavier boys are performing more work at the same treadmill speed and grade. This effect of body weight also seems to be a reasonable explanation for the fact that the smaller undernourished children follow a similar pattern with age but at lower $\dot{V}O_2$s than their nutritionally normal counterparts.

It has been implied that the fall in submaximal $\dot{V}O_2$, expressed in terms of body weight, with age represents an improved "efficiency" (86), perhaps as a result of the fact that younger, shorter individuals need to take more steps at the same speed than older, taller subjects (83,85). When Pate (85) analyzed his data on boys and men using stepping frequency as a covariate, the difference in submaximal $\dot{V}O_2$ between men and boys persisted. However, using only body weight as the covariate, the statistically significant difference disappeared, suggesting that the difference between men and boys may be accounted for by variation in body weight. This would also explain the results reported here, i.e., lower O_2 cost per kilogram of body weight in the heavier (older or nutritionally more adequate) boys. The possible reasons for this apparent "inefficiency" in smaller individuals have been discussed (62,63,87).

When Δ efficiencies were calculated for the normal and undernourished Colombian boys, there were no significant differences with age or between nutritional groups. The lack of age effects in Δ efficiency have been confirmed by Cooper et al. (88). Consequently, marginal malnutrition in school-aged Colombian boys does not appear to have any effect on the Δ efficiency of muscular work. Claims for increased work efficiency in populations of underdeveloped countries (78–80) are unconvincing.

WORK PERFORMANCE IN LARGE AND SMALL INDIVIDUALS

The data presented in Table 2 and Fig. 6 demonstrate that larger individuals have higher values for $\dot{V}O_2$ max. But when expressed per kilogram of body weight or LBM (Fig. 6E,F), larger individuals may have similar (North American versus Colombian groups C and M) or lower values (men versus boys) than smaller ones. The lower values for aerobic power of men compared to boys does not mean that the latter are capable of more work than the former. Rather, the higher values of $\dot{V}O_2$ max indicate greater work capacity, since they result from greater muscle mass performing maximally. The values of $\dot{V}O_2$ max per kilogram of mass (weight or LBM) are not indicators of quantity of work the individuals can perform, as has been suggested (3), but rather of O_2 consumption per kilogram of tissue at maximum effort, i.e., the physical condition. Furthermore, one can draw no conclusions from such data about work efficiency, as has also been suggested (3).

SUMMARY

Studies in nutritionally normal and malnourished men have shown that the physical work capacity, as measured by the $\dot{V}o_2$ max, is dependent on nutritional status such that, relative to the degree of malnutrition, undernourished subjects have depressed work capacities largely because of decreased muscle mass. Since productivity in hard physical work is also directly related to physical work capacity, by implication the productivity of undernourished individuals would also be depressed in heavy physical work.

During the growth of school children, even marginal malnutrition results in growth retardation, slowing of sexual maturation, delay of the growth spurt, and reduction in physical work capaqcity ($\dot{V}o_2$ max) because of the smaller body size. There are implications that in adulthood these smaller boys will be unable to produce as well in heavy physical work as their nutritionally normal counterparts. Studies of load carrying in men and boys indicate that only the body size (weight) and weight of the load carried influence the energy expended independently of nutritional status. Although bigger men have more lean body mass and higher values for maximum physical work capacity, they also expend more energy on body movement during work, but at lower relative effort (percentage $\dot{V}o_2$ max) than smaller nutritionally normal or undernourished men. The limits of effort that can be sustained for an 8-hr work day are about 35 to 40% $\dot{V}o_2$ max, but more studies are needed of small individuals working at heavy tasks in developing countries. There are no indications that smaller or undernourished people are more efficient in physical work.

Small children may have higher $\dot{V}o_2$ max values per kilogram of body weight or LBM than adults, but their total $\dot{V}o_2$ max is related to their body size and therefore is very much lower than that of adults. Consequently, the proper expression of the physical work capacity of individuals, children or adults, is in terms of total $\dot{V}o_2$ max.

ACKNOWLEDGMENTS

Various aspects of the work described from our laboratory have been supported by USAID contracts AID/CSD2943 and AID/TA-C 1424, NIH grant HD10814, Nestlé Research Grants Programme, United Nations University, Zablocki VA Medical Center, and the Fundación para la Educación Superior, Cali.

REFERENCES

1. Seckler D. "Small but healthy": a basic hypothesis in the theory, measurement and policy of malnutrition. In: Sukhatme PV, ed. *Newer concepts in nutrition and their implications for policy.* Pune, India: Maharashtra Association for the Cultivation of Science Research Institute, 1982: 127–37.
2. Gopalan C. "Small is healthy?" For the poor, not for the rich! *Bull Nutr Found India* 1983: October.

3. Margen S. Energy–protein malnutrition: the web of causes and consequences. In: Brožek J, Schürch B, eds. *Malnutrition and behavior: critical assessment of key issues*. Bern: Hans Huber, 1984:20–31. (Nestlé Foundation Publication Series; vol 4).
4. Smil V. Energy flows in the developing world. *Am Sci* 1979;67:522–31.
5. Department of International Economy and Social Affairs. *United Nations demographic year book* (1979). 32nd ed. New York: United Nations, 1980.
6. Arteaga LA. The nutritional status of Latin American adults. *Basic Life Sci* 1976;7:67–76.
7. Berg A. *The nutrition factor: its role in national development*. Washington: The Brookings Institution, 1973.
8. Shephard RJ. *Human physiologic work capacity*. New York: Cambridge University Press, 1978.
9. Andersen KL, Shephard RJ, Denolin H, Vernauskas E, Masironi R. *Fundamentals of exercise testing*. Geneva: WHO, 1971.
10. Åstrand P-O, Rodahl K. *Textbook of work physiology*. New York: McGraw-Hill, 1977.
11. Viteri FE, Torún B, Immink MDC, Flores R. Marginal malnutrition and working capacity. In: Harper AE, Davis GK, eds. *Nutrition in health and disease and international development*. New York: Alan R Liss, 1981:277–83.
12. Spurr GB, Barac-Nieto M, Maksud MG. Childhood undernutrition: implications for adult work capacity and productivity. In: Folinsbee LJ, Wagner JA, Borgia JF, Drinkwater BL, Gliner JA, Bedi JF, eds. *Environmental stress: individual human adaptations*. New York: Academic Press, 1978:165–81.
13. Spurr GB. Nutritional status and physical work capacity. *Am J Phys Anthropol* 1983;26(suppl 4):1–35.
14. Spurr GB. Physical activity, nutritional status and physical work capacity in relation to agricultural productivity. In: Pollitt E, Amante P, eds. *Energy intake and activity*. New York: Alan R. Liss, 1984:207–61.
15. Whipp BJ, Wasserman K. Efficiency of muscular work. *J Appl Physiol* 1969;26:644–8.
16. Gaessar GA, Brooks GA. Muscular efficiency during steady-state exercise: effects of speed and work rate. *J Appl Physiol* 1975;38:1132–9.
17. Donovan CM, Brooks GA. Muscular efficiency during steady-state exercise. II. Effects of walking speed and work rate. *J Appl Physiol* 1977;43:431–9.
18. Stainsby WN, Gladden LB, Barclay JK, Wilson BA. Exercise efficiency: validity of base-line subtractions. *J Appl Physiol* 1980;48:518–22.
19. Cavanagh PR, Kram R. The efficiency of human movement—a statement of the problem. *Med Sci Sports Exerc* 1985;17:304–8.
20. Viteri FE. Considerations on the effect of nutrition on the body composition and physical working capacity of young Guatemalan adults. In: Scrimshaw NS, Altshull AM, eds. *Amino acid fortification of protein foods*. Cambridge, MA: MIT Press, 1971:350–75.
21. Viteri FE, Torún B. Ingestión calórica y trabajo fisico de obreros agrícolas en Guatemala. Efecto de la suplentación alimentaria y su lugar en los programas de salud. *Bol Of Sanit Panam* 1975;78:58–74.
22. Barac-Nieto M, Spurr, GB, Maksud MG, Lotero H. Aerobic work capacity in chronically undernourished adult males. *J Appl Physiol* 1978;44:209–15.
23. Barac-Nieto M, Spurr GB, Dahners HW, Maksud MG. Aerobic work capacity and endurance during nutritional repletion of severely undernourished men. *Am J Clin Nutr* 1980;33:2268–75.
24. Barac-Nieto M, Spurr GB, Lotero H, Maksud MG. Body composition in chronic undernutrition. *Am J Clin Nutr* 1978;31:23–40.
25. Barac-Nietro M. Spurr GB, Lotero H, Maksud MG, Dahners HW. Body composition during nutritional repletion of severely undernourished men. *Am J Clin Nutr* 1979;32:981–91.
26. Spurr GB, Barac-Nieto M, Maksud MG. Energy expenditure cutting sugar cane. *J. Appl Physiol* 1975;39:990–6.
27. Spurr GB, Maksud MG, Barac-Nieto M. Energy expenditure, productivity, and physical work capacity of sugar cane loaders. *Am J Clin Nutr* 1977;30:1740–6.
28. Maksud MG, Spurr GB, Barac-Nieto M. The aerobic power of several groups of laborers in Colombia and the United States. *Eur J Appl Physiol* 1976;35:173–82.
29. Tasker K, Tulpule PG. Influence of protein and calorie deficiencies in the rat on the energy-transfer reactions of the striated muscle. *Biochem J* 1964;92:391–8.
30. Raju N V. Effect of early malnutrition on muscle function and metabolism in rats. *Life Sci* 1974;15: 949–60.
31. Lopes J, Russell DM, Whitwell J, Jeejeebhoy KN. Skeletal muscle function in malnutrition. *Am J Clin Nutr* 1982;36:602–10.

32. Heymsfield SB, Stevens V, Noel R, McManus C, Smith J, Nixon D. Biochemical composition of muscle in normal and semistarved human subjects: relevance to anthropometric measurements. *Am J Clin Nutr* 1982;36:131–42.
33. Michael ED, Hutton KE, Horvath SM. Cardiorespiratory responses during prolonged exercise. *J Appl Physiol* 1961;16:997–1000.
34. Åstrand I. Degree of strain during building work as related to individual aerobic capacity. *Ergonomics* 1967;10:293–303.
35. Barac-Nieto M. Body composition and physical work capacity in undernutrition. In: White PL, Selvey N, eds. *Malnutrition: determinants and consequences.* New York: Alan R Liss, 1984: 165–8.
36. Hanson-Smith FM, Maksud MG, Van Horn DL. Influence of chronic undernutrition on oxygen consumption of rats during exercise. *Growth* 1977;41:115–21.
37. Bergstrom J, Hermansen L. Hultman E, Saltin B. Diet, muscle glycogen and physical performance. *Acta Physiol Scand* 1967;71:140–50.
38. Gollnick PD, Piehl K, Saubert CW, Armstrong RB, Saltin B. Diet, exercise and glycogen changes in human muscle fibers. *J Appl Physiol* 1972;33:421–5.
39. Durnin JVGA. Muscle in sports and medicine—nutrition and muscular performance. *Int J Sports Med* 1982;3:52–57.
40. Durnin JVGA, Passmore R. *Energy, work and leisure.* London: Heinemann, 1967.
41. Hansson JE. *The relationship between individual characteristics of the worker and output of logging operations.* Stockholm: Skogshogskolan, 1965:68–77. (Studia Forestalia Suecia; no. 29).
42. Davies CTM. Relationship of maximum aerobic power output to productivity and absenteeism of East African sugar cane workers. *Br J Ind Med* 1973;30:146–54.
43. Davies CTM, Brotherhood JR, Collins KJ, et al. Energy expenditure and physiological performance of Sudanese cane cutters. *Br J Ind Med* 1976;33:181–6.
44. Spurr GB, Barac-Nieto M, Maksud MG. Productivity and maximal oxygen consumption in sugar cane cutters. *Am J Clin Nutr* 1977;30:316–21.
45. Thomson AM. The later results in man of malnutrition early in life. In: McCance RA, Widdowson EM, eds. *Calorie deficiencies and protein deficiencies.* Boston: Little Brown, 1968:289–99.
46. Satyanarayana K, Nadamuni Naidu A, Chatterjee B, Narasinga Rao BS. Body size and work output. *Am J Clin Nutr* 1977;30:322–5.
47. Satyanarayana K, Nadamuni Naidu A, Narasinga Rao BS. Nutrition, physical work capacity and work output. *Indian J Med Res* 1978;68(suppl):88–93.
48. Areskog N-H, Selinus R, Vahlquist B. Physical work capacity and nutritional status in Ethopian male children and young adults. *Am J Clin Nutr* 1969;22:471–9.
49. Davies CTM. Physiological responses to exercise in East African children II. The effects of shistosomiasis, anaemia and malnutrition. *J Trop Pediatr Environ Child Health* 1973;19:115–9.
50. Satayanarayana K, Nadamuni Naidu A, Narasinga Rao BS. Nutritional deprivation in childhood and the body size, activity and physical work capacity of young boys. *Am J Clin Nutr* 1979;32:1769–75.
51. Rueda-Williamson R, Luna-Jaspe H, Ariza J, Pardo F, Mora JO. Estudio seccional de crecimento, desarrollo y nutrición en 12,138 niños de Bogotá, Colombia. *Pediatria* 1969;10:337–49.
52. Spurr GB, Reina JC, Barac-Nieto M. Marginal malnutrition in school-aged Colombian boys: anthropometry and maturation. *Am J Clin Nutr* 1983;37:119–32.
53. Spurr GB, Reina JC, Dahners HW, Barac-Nieto M. Marginal malnutrition in school-aged Colombian boys: functional consequences in maximum exercise. *Am J Clin Nutr* 1983;37:834–47.
54. Barac-Nieto M, Spurr GB, Reina JC. Marginal malnutrition in school-aged Colombian boys: body composition and maximal O_2 consumption. *Am J Clin Nutr* 1984;39:830–9.
55. Spurr GB, Barac-Nieto M, Reina JC, Ramirez R. Marginal malnutrition in school-aged Colombian boys: efficiency of treadmill walking in submaximal exercise. *Am J Clin Nutr* 1984;39:452–9.
56. Malina RM. Ethnic and cultural factors in the development of motor abilities and strength in American children. In: Raric GL, ed. *Physical activity, human growth and development.* New York: Academic Press, 1973:333–64.
57. Zavaleta AN, Malina RM. Growth, fatness and leanness in Mexican-American children. *Am J Clin Nutr* 1980;33:2008–20.
58. Pařízková J. Total body fat and skinfolds in children. *Metabolism* 1961;10:794–807.
59. Pascale LR, Grossman MI, Sloane HS, Frankel T. Correlations between thickness of skinfolds and body density in 88 soldiers. *Hum Biol* 1956;28:165–75.

60. Durnin JVGA, Womersley J. Body fat assessed from total body density and its estimation from skinfold thickness: measurements on 481 men and women aged from 16 to 72 years. *Br J Nutr* 1974;32:77–97.
61. Halloszy JO. Biochemical adaptations in muscle. Effects of exercise on mitochondrial O_2 uptake and respiratory enzyme activity in skeletal muscle. *J. Biol Chem* 1967;242:2278–82.
62. Spurr GB, Reina JC, Barac-Nieto M. Marginal malnutrition in school-aged Colombian boys: metabolic rate and estimated daily energy expenditure. *Am J Clin Nutr* 1986;44:113–26.
63. Spurr GB, Reina JC. Marginal malnutrition in school-aged Colombian boys: body size and energy costs of walking and light load carrying. *Hum Nutr Clin Nutr* 1986;40:409–19.
64. Shephard RJ, Lavallee H, Larivière G, et al. La capacité physique des enfants canadiens: une comparaison entre les enfants canadiens-français, canadiens-anglais et esquimaux. I. Consommation maximale d'oxygène et débit cardiaque. *Union Med Can* 1974;103:1767–77.
65. Calloway DH. Functional consequences of malnutrition. *Rev Infect Dis* 1982;4:736–45.
66. Thomson AM. The importance of being tall. *Hum Ecol Forum* 1980;10:4–10.
67. Reddy V, Jagadeesan V, Ragharamulu N, Bharkaram S, Srikantia SG. Functional significance of growth retardation in malnutrition. *Am J Clin Nutr* 1976;29:3–7.
68. Klein RE, Breeman HE, Kagan J, Yarbrough C. Is big smart? The relation of growth to cognition. *J Health Soc Behav* 1972;13:219–25.
69. Clarys JB, Martin AD, Drinkwater DT. Gross tissue weights in the human body by cadaver dissection. *Hum Biol* 1984;56:459–73.
70. Buskirk ER, Mendez J. Lean-body-tissue assessment, with emphasis on skeletal-muscle mass. In: Roche AF, ed. *Body-composition assessments in youth and adults.* Report of the 6th Ross Conference on Medical Research. Columbus, OH: Ross Laboratories, 1985:59–65.
71. von Dobeln W. Human standard and maximal metabolic rate in relation to fat free mass. *Acta Physiol Scand [suppl]* 1956;126:1–79.
72. Dehn MM, Bruce RA. Longitudinal variations in maximal oxygen intake with age and activity. *J. Appl Physiol* 1972;33:805–7.
73. Datta SS, Chatterjee BB, Roy BM. The relationship between energy expenditure and pulse rates with body weight and the load carried during load carrying on the level. *Ergonomics* 1973;16:506–13.
74. Givoni B, Goldman RF. Predicting metabolic energy cost. *J Appl Physiol* 1971;30:429–33.
75. Mahadeva K, Passmore R, Woolf B. Individual variations in the metabolic cost of standardized exercises: the effects of food, age, sex and race. *J Physiol* 1953;121:225–31.
76. Spurr GB, Barac-Nieto M, Maksud MG. Efficiency and daily work effort in sugar cane cutters. *Br J Ind Med* 1977;34:137–41.
77. Jørgensen K. Permissible loads based on energy expenditure measurements. *Ergonomics* 1985;28:365–9.
78. Martorell R, Lechtig A, Yarbrough C, Delgado H, Klein RE. Small stature in developing nations: its causes and implications. In: Margen S, Ogar RA, eds. *Progress in human nutrition; vol 2.* Westport, CT: Avi Publishing Co, 1978:142–56.
79. Edmundson W. Individual variations in basal metabolic rate and mechanical work efficiency in East Java. *Ecol Food Nutr* 1979;8:189–95.
80. Edmundson W. Adaptation to undernutrition: how much food does man need? *Soc Sci Med* 1980;14D:119–26.
81. Keys A, Brožek J, Henschel A, Mickelsen O, Taylor HL. *The biology of human starvation.* Minneapolis: University of Minnesota Press, 1950.
82. Robinson S. Experimental study of physical fitness in relation to age. *Arbeitsphysiologie* 1938;10:251–333.
83. Åstrand P-O. *Experimental studies of physical working capacity in relation to sex and age.* Copenhagen: Ejnar Munksgaard, 1952.
84. Daniels J, Oldridge N, Nagle F, White B. Differences and changes in Vo_2 among young runners 10 to 18 years of age. *Med Sci Sports* 1978;10:200–3.
85. Pate RR. Oxygen cost of walking, running and cycling in boys and men. [Abstract]. *Med Sci Sports Exerc* 1981;13:123–4.
86. Montoye JH. Age and oxygen utilization during submaximal treadmill exercise in males. *J Gerontol* 1982;37:396–402.
87. Kleiber M. *The fire of life. An introduction to animal energetics.* Huntington, NY: Krieger, 1975.
88. Cooper DM, Weiler-Ravell D, Whipp BJ, Wasserman K. Aerobic parameters of exercise as a function of body size during growth in children. *J Appl Physiol* 1984;56:628–34.

DISCUSSION

Dr. Waterlow: You made a very convincing case, but I am not completely convinced. At the very end you almost let yourself off the hook by saying that you are dealing with heavy physical work. I would like to refine that a little and suggest that what we need to do for different activities and occupations or for different types of work is to separate out quantitatively, if possible, the component that depends on moving the body and the component that depends on doing some other kind of work such as cutting cane or carrying loads. Your conclusions are crucially dependent on this. If the main part of the work requires moving the body, then being small does not matter because the cost is proportional to the body weight. This comes out in the FAO/WHO report on energy requirements for walking on a treadmill without loads but with different body weights. Ann Ashworth (1), in Jamaica, gave people the task of carrying bricks from point A to point B. She made them carry either the number of bricks that was most convenient to them or fewer or more bricks and measured the energy cost. The energy cost of transferring these bricks was actually lower if they carried more at a time because the distance element was greater than the load element. I would therefore suggest that there is a continuum of situations from those in which a great deal of external work is done to those, as in farmers walking to distant fields, in which virtually all the work is moving the body. We then have to be very careful in generalizing, and we should try to pinpoint where we are on that continuum when referring to physical work.

Dr. Spurr: There is not enough information on this topic. I wasn't aware of Ashworth's work on the brick carrying, but it sounds as if it would fit in with some of our hypotheses. I contrived a work situation (Figs. 8 and 9) in order to separate the effect of body size, but we clearly need more measurements in real work situations. It is possible with the data obtained on the load-carrying experiments (Fig. 7) to estimate energy expenditure under varying percentage contributions of load carrying versus non-load-carrying work, i.e., the "load" versus "distance" components you mention. These estimates lead to the same conclusion. What I am trying to do with the information we have is to make people question some of the statements that occur in the literature, that if you are small, it really doesn't make any difference because you are going to expend less energy but are still able to do the same amount of work. I simply don't think that this is so, even with the information at our disposal.

Dr. Keller: I always thought that the daily energy expenditure for work in tropical countries was considerably less than 1,500 to 2,000 kcal. Is that really common? I think it was at Dr. Gopalan's institute that they measured the energy expenditure of farmers in South India, and, if I remember correctly, they came out with about 500 work kilocalories per day. The reason is possibly that there are circulatory limitations to getting rid of the heat. What do you think is the daily workload that can be reasonably expected?

Dr. Spurr: Sugar cane cutting is extremely heavy physical work. We estimated (2) for the sugar cane cutters who were working in a hot environment that their total daily energy expenditure was about 3,600 kcal and that their maintenance estimate would be somewhere around 1,800, so you are getting pretty close to 2,000 kcal daily energy expenditure for work.

Dr. Davies: Have you looked at work capacity in normal small people as opposed to abnormal small people? Is it a function of muscle mass or of the composition of muscle mass?

Dr. Spurr: These Colombian agricultural workers, who included sugar cane cutters, loaders, and general farm laborers, are small, but they are nutritionally normal. From all the data that we have and that have been derived from Viteri and Torún's studies (3,4) at INCAP, it is not the quality of muscle but the quantity that is important. We do not have any data to indicate that chronic malnutrition affects the ability of the muscle that is there to do work; it is rather the quantity of muscle that is available.

Dr. Milner: Could I ask you to expand on the technology of measuring $\dot{V}o_2$ in children? The physiological maximum heart rate increases as age decreases; if you take a child to a heart rate of 190, he may not have achieved a plateau. I also noticed that you used 3-min time intervals when you were measuring $\dot{V}o_2$ max in the children. Did you use a Bruce protocol? We found that 3-min intervals are quite long for children to tolerate. The third problem that we found most difficult is tolerance to the mouthpiece. That led us to switch to having the children working to a heart rate maximum and voluntary cessation of the work whether they had achieved a $\dot{V}o_2$ max or whether they were on a heart rate plateau (5).

Dr. Spurr: Performance of the $\dot{V}o_2$ max test is difficult and has to be done with a great deal of care, particularly with children. The 3-min protocol that you saw was for a submaximal test. We routinely use 2-min intervals, and we start them after a 3-min warm-up at 5% grade. Then we increase by 2.5% grade increments until maximum is reached.

Dr. Millner: With constant speed?

Dr. Spurr: Yes, we choose a constant speed and maintain it there. We use either 3, 3.5, or 4.2 miles per hour, depending on the heart rate response during the warm-up. The average maximum heart rates of our children are somewhere around 207 or 208. We have had children going up to 230. That is unusual, but it happens. We do not accept a $\dot{V}o_2$ max measurement unless the heart rate is above 200 and unless the heart rate as well as the oxygen consumption are plateauing or at supramaximal values. We are very careful about accepting a measurement as a true $\dot{V}o_2$ max. In the studies that we have performed, we did $\dot{V}o_2$ max measurements on over 1,100 boys, and we got acceptable values in about 92% of the subjects (6).

Dr. Milner: How did you get them to accept the mouthpiece?

Dr. Spurr: The smaller children in particular cannot get the mouthpiece in, but we can make it smaller. We have mouthpieces of various sizes. We put the children through a preliminary test a day or so before the real test in which we explain what it is we want, what the mouthpiece is going to feel like; we teach them how to walk on the treadmill, etc.

Dr. Waterlow: I would find it a little easier to assess what you mean by "mild, moderate, and severe malnutrition" if you expressed the results as body mass index, at least for the adults. Nobody really knows what the lower limit of acceptable body mass index is; not many people in industrialized countries are lower than about 19 or 18. Shetty's laborers in India (7) were around 15 to 16 and apparently very fit. So for comparative purposes, it would be very helpful. I am not at all happy with Colombian standards because I have no idea what the standards are.

Dr. Spurr: We did not use body mass index. In adults, the classification "mild, intermediate, and severe malnutrition" was based on a point system derived from three parameters: weight-for-height ratio, serum albumin level, and 24-hr creatinine excretion (8). We set up a point system. Table 1 in the chapter gives the values that we used to make that decision. The Colombian norms that we used to classify the children were established in Bogotá in the upper socioeconomic group. The results that I presented here were all on children from lower socioeconomic classes. We did not include the studies that we made in the upper socioeconomic group (6,9). Within the lower socioeconomic group, it is possible to find children with a relatively normal growth curve. I don't really think it makes any difference what norm is used, a local one or an international one, as long as some decision is made about cut-off points. We have artificially established our own cut-off points for marginal malnutrition at less than 95% of the Colombian standards, with the expectation that the average group values would be much lower than that. And they were (9).

Dr. Waterlow: It doesn't make any difference to you because you are comparing groups in the same population, but it makes a lot of difference to me if I want to compare your data with, say, Indian data. Regardless of the physiological validity of the international reference, as more and more people are performing similar studies to yours, it is important to use the same reference.

Dr. Spurr: One ought to be able to compare our children with Indian children or any other group. Ours grow on or below the fifth centile of the NCHS data (10), and our published work (Fig. 5) has been in reference to these standards (9).

Dr. Nnanyelugo: Was the food intake of the subjects standardized? Could the type of food consumed not affect work capacity?

Dr. Spurr: We were unable to control the dietary intake in these subjects; our children were recruited from the public schools in Cali. We have attempted time and time again to get some reasonable information on dietary intake without much success, because we could not send technicians into the homes for weighing. As far as the dietary recall method is concerned, it is absolutely unacceptable.

Dr. Kraisid: Do you analyze your $\dot{V}o_2$ max and heart rate data in relation to hematocrit or hemoglobin levels?

Dr. Spurr: In a sense, yes. We measure hemoglobin and hematocrit in all our subjects. In children, when we compute $\dot{V}o_2$ max as a function of body weight, to remove the effect of body size, and plot that against hemoglobin concentration, we get an absolutely flat curve: the correlation was 0.03 in children. Between 9 and 16 g/dl of hemoglobin, in children, there does not seem to be any relationship with oxygen-carrying capacity (6). That means that there have to be some other physiological adaptations in children that perhaps do not exist in adults, in which Viteri and Torún's work (11) has shown that there is a very close relationship between $\dot{V}o_2$ max and oxygen-carrying capacity of the blood. Earlier studies by Parsons and Wright (12) and Vellar and Hermansen (13) also indicated that in children there is some other adaptation, perhaps in blood flow or increased oxygen extraction across the capillary bed. These mechanisms have not yet been studied.

Dr. Golden: I am impressed by the psychological effects of malnutrition. Could you comment on the influence of nutritional status on the training effect and also on effort? You used the term "whining." Do malnourished children put less voluntary effort into the task that you have set them than well-nourished children?

Dr. Spurr: As far as I know, there is no information on the influence of nutritional status on training and training effect. I would like to be able to carry out some studies, particularly during recuperation from malnourished states, on the effect of exercise on recuperation, for example. One of the things that we saw in severely malnourished adults during dietary repletion was a reduction in endurance time, defined as the time during which a subject is able to work at about 80% of $\dot{V}o_2$ max. Endurance studies are very difficult to perform; very few have been performed, even in adults. We did these measurements, comparing the three nutritional groups, and did not observe any statistically significant difference except in the severely malnourished subjects during dietary repletion, when there was a progressive and finally statistically significant decrease in endurance (14). We have never been able to go back and repeat it, and we have never been able to explain it. Is it the muscle that is reconstituted during the 3- or 3.5-month repletion period that is different, or is it because these subjects were sedentary during the whole period of repletion? Would it be different if they were undergoing exercise training? I don't know, but here I am talking about the effect of nutritional status on effort in terms of percentage $\dot{V}o_2$ max, whereas you are talking about a psychological effect. We have no measures of that. All I can say, subjectively, is that the marginally malnourished children do not behave differently as far as their willingness to perform work is concerned.

Dr. Gopalan: I think you made a very important comment when you said that these laboratory studies must be supported by observations in real-life conditions. There is a need for more work of that kind, which unfortunately, up to now, seems to be largely done by observational social scientists and economists rather than by health and nutrition scientists. That would be great support to the type of work that you are doing in the laboratory.

Dr. Spurr: The measurement of energy expenditure in heavy physical work under field conditions is difficult. The use of the double-labeled water technique could be interesting. Even the minute-by-minute heart rate recording method might be used if done under appropriate conditions.

Dr. Waterlow: In relation to this last point, many years ago in Jamaica a study was done of the output of sugar cane cutters in relation to food intake. The men who ate the most food had the biggest output, but the relationship wasn't as simple as it appeared because the men who ate the most food were those who were married and had good food provided. In Jamaica, you only marry if you are a steady, hard-working, productive person; otherwise you don't marry. At least, that, I believe, used to be the case. This illustrates that sociologists do have something to contribute.

REFERENCES

1. Ashworth A. An investigation of very low calorie intakes reported in Jamaica. *Br J Nutr* 1968;22:341–55.
2. Spurr GB, Barac-Nieto M, Maksud MG. Energy expenditure cutting sugar cane. *J Appl Physiol* 1975;39:990–6.
3. Viteri FE. Considerations on the effect of nutrition on the body composition and physical working capacity of young Guatemalan adults. In: Scrimshaw NS, Altshull AM, eds. *Amino acid fortification of protein foods*. Cambridge, MA: MIT Press, 1971:350–75.
4. Viteri FE, Torún B, Ingestión calórica y trabajo fisico de obreros agrícolas en Guatemala. Efecto de la suplementación alimentaria y su lugar en los programas de salud. *Bol Of Sanit Panam* 1975;78:58–74.
5. Houlsby WT. Functional aerobic capacity and body size. *Arch Dis Child* 1986;61:388–93.
6. Spurr GB, Reina JC, Dahners HW, Barac-Nieto M. Marginal malnutrition in school-aged Colombian boys: functional consequences in maximum exercise. *Am J Clin Nutr* 1983;37:834–47.
7. Shetty PS. Adaptive changes in basal metabolic rate and lean body mass in chronic undernutrition. *Hum Nutr Clin Nutr* 1984;38C:443–52.
8. Barac-Nieto M, Spurr GB, Lotero H, Maksud MG. Body composition in chronic undernutrition. *Am J Clin Nutr* 1978;31:23–40.
9. Spurr GB, Reina JC, Barac-Nieto M. Marginal malnutrition in school-aged Colombian boys: anthropometry and maturation. *Am J Clin Nutr* 1983;37:119–32.
10. Hamill PVV, Drizd TA, Johnson CL, Reed RB, Roche AF, Moore WM. Physical growth: National Center for Health Statistics percentiles. *Am J Clin Nutr* 1979;32:607–29.
11. Viteri FE, Torún B. Anaemia and physical work capacity. *Clin Haematol* 1974;3:609–26.
12. Parsons CG, Wright FH. Circulatory function in the anemias of children. I. Effect of anemia on exercise tolerance and vital capacity. *Am J Dis Child* 1939;57:15–23.
13. Vellar OD, Hermansen L. Physical performance and hematological parameters. *Acta Med Scand [Suppl]* 1971;522:1–40.
14. Barac-Nieto M, Spurr GB, Dahners HW, Maksud MG. Aerobic work capacity and endurance during nutritional repletion of severely undernourished men. *Am J Clin Nutr* 1980;33:2268–75.

Linear Growth Retardation in Less Developed Countries, edited by John C. Waterlow. Nestlé Nutrition Workshop Series, Vol. 14. Nestec Ltd., Vevey/Raven Press, Ltd., New York © 1988.

Linear Growth Retardation and Mortality

W. Van Lerberghe

ENOV-URESP Unit for Research and Training in Public Health, Institute for Tropical Medicine, B-2000 Antwerp, Belgium

When discussing the relationship between stunting and mortality in developing countries, one has to distinguish two separate issues. (a) Does being stunted, i.e., presenting with retarded linear growth, carry an additional risk of dying? (b) Does stunting, i.e., presenting with deceleration of linear growth, carry an additional risk of dying? Very little is known on either subject.

The data gathered by Keller and Fillmore on the prevalence of protein–energy malnutrition throughout the world (1) show that countries with high juvenile and infantile mortality rates also invariably have high prevalences of stunted children, and those with low prevalences invariably have low mortality rates (Fig. 1). There are, nevertheless, a number of countries such as Yugoslavia, Sri Lanka, Costa Rica, or Panama where low juvenile mortality rates coexist with high prevalences of stunted children.

Thus, poor countries that tend to have high mortality rates also tend to have high prevalences of stunted children.

Very little data are available from a small number of community-based longitudinal studies that can be used to evaluate the relationship between anthropometric indicators and mortality (Table 1).

Only the two more recent studies from Bangladesh (4,6) question the relationship between being stunted and risk of dying, and only Bairagi (6) also addresses the importance of stunting. In this chapter, these observations will be confronted with some of the data from the Kasongo (Zaire) study.

The Kasongo study was a multiround survey whose principal objective was to assess the influence of measles vaccination on the survival pattern of under-5s. More than 32,500 weight, height, and arm-circumference measurements were taken in over 7,000 children. A detailed description of the study population and the way in which the survey was conducted may be found elsewhere (8).

The growth curves[1] of the Kasongo children show a fairly typical pattern for

---

[1]Unless it is specifically mentioned that local or other reference data were used, the NCHS data (9) were used as "reference." Between 24 and 36 months, when length and stature reference data overlap, these were averaged, as were their corresponding standard deviations.

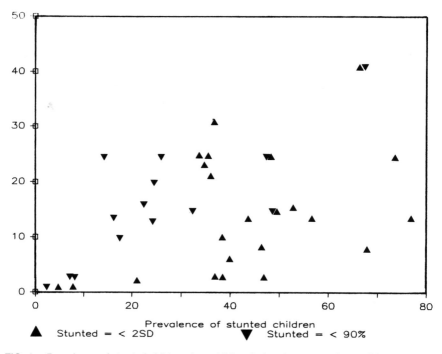

FIG. 1. Prevalence of stunted children, i.e., children below the mean minus 2 SD of the reference height for age (23 countries) or less than 90% of the reference height for age (14 countries) at the age of 1 year, and child mortality rate. (From Keller and Fillmore, ref. 1.)

TABLE 1. *Anthropometric indicators whose relationship with mortality has been investigated in nonhospitalized populations*[a]

	Single measurements						
Reference	W/A	W/H	H/A	AC/A	AC/H	WtQ	HtQ
Sommer and Lowenstein, 1975, Bangladesh (2)					*		
Kielmann and McCord, 1978, India (3)	*						
Chen et al., 1980, Bangladesh (4)	*	*	*	*	*	*	*
Kasongo Project Team, 1983, Zaire (5)	*	*		*	*		
Bairagi et al., 1985, Bangladesh (6)	*	*	*				

	Measurements of velocity or loss				
	W/A	H/A	W/H	AC/A	AC/H
Bairagi et al., 1985, Bangladesh (6)	*	*			
Kasongo Project Team, 1986, Zaire (7) (7)	*		*	*	*

[a]W/A, weight for age; W/H, weight for height; H/A, height for age; AC/A, arm circumference for age; AC/H, arm circumference for height; WtQ, weight quotient; HtQ, height quotient (WtQ and HtQ are the ratios of the weight-age or height-age, i.e., the age at which the weight or height of the child is at the 50th percentile of the Harvard standard, divided by the child's chronological age).

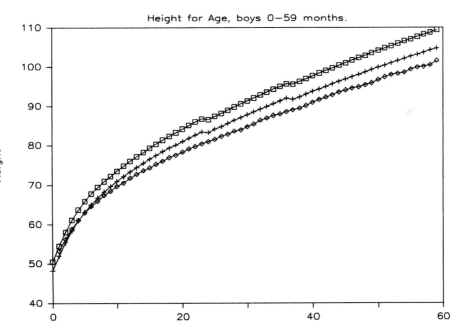

FIG. 2. Height for age of boys in Kasongo (◇) and median (□) and median minus 1 SD (+) of the NCHS reference. Reference data for length and stature at ages 24 to 35 months are averages. (From Kasongo Project Team, ref. 8.)

African under-5s, with a deficit in weight for age that becomes evident from 5 to 6 months on. The deficit in height for age starts earlier and is already noticeable at the age of 2 months (Fig. 2). Figure 3 shows that the whole distribution is shifted to the left when compared to the NCHS distribution; the whole population is affected by growth retardation. However, as is evidenced by the weight-for-height curve, which is quasiidentical to the NCHS reference, longitudinal growth deficit and weight deficit in this population are quite proportional; wasting is relatively rare. Figures 4 and 5 show the prevalence of stunted children by age according to the classical Waterlow classification (10) or using the median minus 2 SD of the NCHS reference as criterion: the prevalence increases progressively and peaks during the third year of life; it stabilizes at a slightly lower level after 36 months.

OBSERVATIONS ON THE ASSOCIATION BETWEEN BEING STUNTED AND SUBSEQUENT MORTALITY

The first study providing evidence for an association between being stunted and subsequent mortality was published by Chen et al. in 1980 (4) on the basis of a 2-year follow-up of 2,019 children in Bangladesh. For any given level of weight-for-height deficit at ages 12 to 23 months, a deficit in height for age was associated

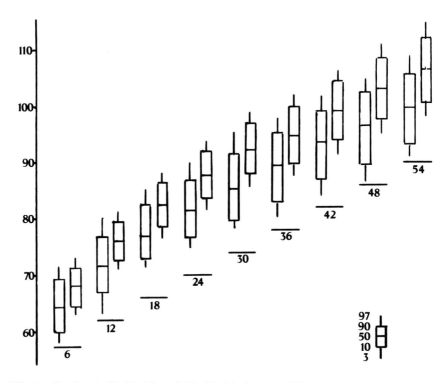

FIG. 3. Centiles 3, 10, 50, 90, and 97 of height for age of Kasongo boys **(left)** and of the NCHS reference **(right)** at selected ages (months).

with high mortality rates during the two subsequent years. Children who died were 1.2 times as likely to be less than 90% and 2.0 times less than 85% of the Harvard median height for age than the overall study population. Risk of dying increased sharply below a threshold situated around 85% of the reference values.

Table 2 shows the ratio of the risk of dying during the two subsequent years for children below and above 85% of height for age. A height for age below 85% was associated with increased risk of dying whether the weight for height was above or below 80%, independently of indicators of maternal nutrition and housing size.

Poor height or weight of the mother was not associated with an increased risk of dying for children above 85% (risk ratios of 0.99 and 0.92), whereas it was for children below 85% (risk ratios of 1.58 and 1.25); small housing size was associated with a higher risk for both stunted and other children, but more so for the stunted children, with a risk ratio of 2.29 instead of 1.24. This supports the hypothesis that stunted children are more vulnerable than others to whatever ultimately will be the direct "cause" of death.

Bairagi et al. (6), who studied children in the same population as Chen et al. (4) (actually, about 40 children were included in both studies), confirmed the association of low height for age with subsequent mortality, but without finding Chen's threshold phenomenon.

In principle, the most convincing evidence for the hypothetical association

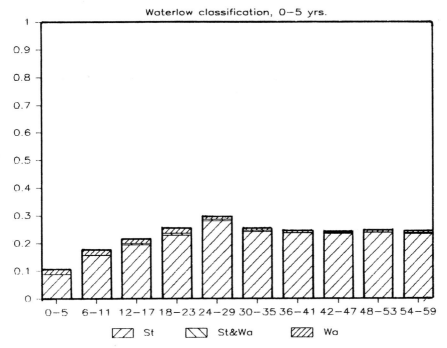

FIG. 4. Prevalence by age of stunted, stunted and wasted, and wasted children, according to the Waterlow classification.

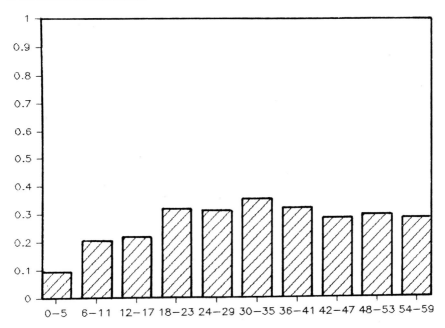

FIG. 5. Prevalence by age of stunted children using the NCHS median minus 2 SD of height for age as cutoff.

TABLE 2. *Ratios of risk of dying within 2 years for children above and below 85% of the Harvard standard height for age*

All children	2.98
Wt/Ht $\geq$ 80%	2.88
Wt/Ht $<$ 80%	1.54
Shorter mother	3.45
Taller mother	2.16
Lighter mother	3.35
Heavier mother	2.48
Small housing size	2.29
Large housing size	4.23

From Chen et al. (4).

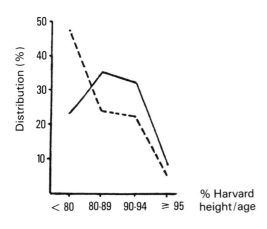

FIG. 6. Height distribution of the Matlab study population (*solid line*) and of subsequently dying children (*dashed line*). (From Chen et al., ref. 4.)

would be provided by a comparison of the height distribution of the subsequently dying children and the overall population. Such a comparison of distributions is preferable to one of "prevalences" (11). One would expect subsequently dying children to be shorter than the other children of the same age in the population: the height distribution of subsequently dying children should be different—shifted to the left of that of the overall population.

Chen and his co-workers (4) observed this shift to the left (Fig. 6). However, in Kasongo the pattern is different.

Methods

Anthropometric information is available for 137 children who died at the age of 6 months or older (including three deaths at the age of 61 months). Z scores of height for age at the last measurement before death (the average interval between measurement and death being 2.3 months) were calculated for each of these children, using the local mean and standard deviation of height for age. This provides an age-independent distribution that can easily be compared with that of the population, assuming that at any age the latter is a normal distribution (the mean $= 0$ and 1 SD $= 1$). The statistical significance of differences between the distribution of subsequently dying children and that of the overall population was tested using a Kolmogorov–Smirnov one-sample test.

Results

The distribution of the Z scores of height for age at the last measurement made on each child (Fig. 7) is not significantly different from the overall distribution of the population (Kolmogorov–Smirnov $Z = 0.910$; $p = 0.380$). This is further confirmed by Table 3, which shows that the average Z scores do not differ significantly from the population average of 0.

Thus, the distribution of the Z scores does not corroborate the hypothesis of an association between being stunted and subsequent mortality. The corollary of this distribution is that risk of dying is fairly homogeneously distributed among the Kasongo children of a given age, whatever their attained height.

OBSERVATIONS ON THE ASSOCIATION BETWEEN THE STUNTING PROCESS AND MORTALITY

If an association between the stunting process and subsequent mortality exists, then children who die should have experienced periods of less intensive linear

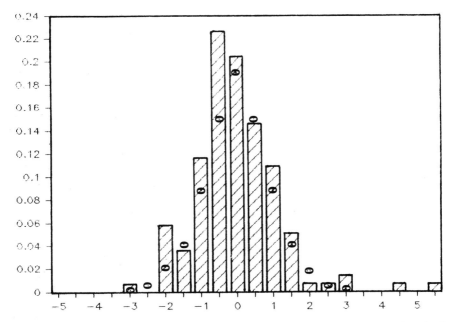

FIG. 7. Distribution of the Z scores of height for age at the last measurement before death, using the local mean and SD as reference; $n = 137$. Average interval between measurement and death was 2.3 months; *circles,* overall distribution for all children.

TABLE 3. *Mean Z score of height for age (using the local mean and SD as reference) at the last measurement before death*

	Age at death (months)					
	6–11	12–17	18–23	24–35	36–61	6–61
Z score	0.17	0.06	0.02	− 0.34	− 0.09	− 0.02
SD	1.63	1.09	0.90	1.14	0.89	1.19
N	30	30	27	25	25	137

growth than one would expect in the overall population.

Bairagi et al. (6) examined the association between mortality and growth velocities (g or cm/month over periods of 2 months) in 1- to 4-year-old children from Matlab. They did find an association between mortality and weight velocity, but not with height velocity. However, for a number of reasons their results are difficult to interpret. The small number of deceased children on whom previous anthropometric information was available[2] did not make it possible to control for age, which should affect height velocities measured in that fashion. The survey was conducted in the aftermath of a famine: catch-up growth was observed, as evidenced by a U-shaped relationship between weight velocity and mortality. There were also important seasonal variations in growth. With that background, the fact that height velocities were not significantly lower for subsequently dying children does not provide a formal argument against the hypothesis of an association; it merely provides no formal argument for it.

Material and Methods

In order to test for such an association in Kasongo, the process of growth faltering had to be measured in some way that makes it possible to compare the growth of the subsequently dying children and that of the overall population by taking age into account. The difference between the Z scores of two measurements, divided by the time interval between those measurements, provides a convenient standardized expression of the growth increment during this interval as a number of SD units of change per month. If this "standardized monthly velocity" is negative; i.e., if the Z score at the second measurement is lower than the first, there is growth deceleration (as compared to the average monthly increment of the reference population, which by definition is equal to zero); if it is positive, there is growth acceleration. If height for age is being measured, a deceleration can be called stunting.

For 78 children who died at the age of 6 months or older, information is available for 238 time intervals. It was thus possible to calculate standardized monthly

---

[2]Apparently height measurements less than 5 months preceding death were available for only 14 children; growth velocity in these children was less than 0.40 cm/month in the period preceding death, compared to velocities ranging from 0.60 to 0.68 cm/month for surviving children.

TABLE 4. *Average standardized monthly growth velocities at different ages in Kasongo (measured in SD score units per month)[a]*

	Age group				
	0–5 months	6–11 months	1 year	2 years	3–4 years
H/A	− 0.014	− 0.025	− 0.040	− 0.025	− 0.004
W/A	− 0.050	− 0.125	− 0.008	0.012	− 0.008
W/H[b]		− 0.040	− 0.050	< 0.004	

[a]H/A, height for age; W/A, weight for age; W/H, weight for height.
[b]Approximation from the average Z scores of weight-for-height curves for ages 0–5, 6–11, 12–23, and 24–59 months.

TABLE 5. *Average standardized monthly height-for-age velocities (SD units/month) of subsequently dying children[a]*

	Age group (months)				
	0–5	6–11	12–23	24–35	36–59
a. All intervals:	− 0.575	− 0.082	− 0.061	− 0.059	− 0.002**
b. Velocities measured < 12 months before death	− 0.217	− 0.099	− 0.075	− 0.061	− 0.008*
c. Velocities measured during intervals ending ≤ 3 months before death	− 0.268	− 0.066	− 0.099	− 0.090	− 0.019

[a]Significance: *$p < 0.05$; **NS; all others $p < 0.01$. All children died between 6 and 61 months. Number of months of observation for the calculation in each age group: (a) 70, 288, 457.5, 228, 158; (b) 44, 118, 116 (two outliers removed), 118, 99; (c) 20, 81, 48 (two outliers removed), 74, 47.

growth velocities of height for age, weight for age, or weight for height at different ages. These standardized monthly velocities were averaged for each of the following age groups: 0 to 5, 6 to 11, 12 to 24, 24 to 35, and 36 to 59 months. (If any interval overlapped with one of these age groups, the total standardized growth change was accordingly divided between the different age groups for calculation of the monthly standardized velocities.) This was done (a) using all the available information on subsequently dying children, which totaled just over 100 child-years of observation, (b) for the year preceding the death of each child (a total of 495 months of observation), and (c) for time intervals ending not more than 3 months before death; the average duration of time interval was 2.7 months (a total of 270 months of observation).

For each age group, these averages were compared with the average standardized monthly growth increments of the whole population (Table 4). Statistical significance of differences from the standardized monthly growth increment of the whole population in the same age group was assessed with a one-sided Z test.

The average standardized monthly height velocities of subsequently dying children (Table 5) are negative and significantly more so than those of the overall population (Table 4). This is true at all ages; from the age of 1 year the difference is most marked when only growth increments in the months immediately preceding death are taken into consideration (Table 5, c).

The difference between the standardized monthly height-for-age velocity during the period preceding death and that of the overall population is graphically represented in Fig. 8. Monthly height-for-age velocity of children who will die within the coming months (average 1.7 months after the last measurement) is 19 times slower (i.e., actual stunting) than expected at ages 0 to 5 months, 2.6 times slower at ages 6 to 11 months, and 2.5, 3.6, and 4.7 times larger at ages 1, 2, and 3 through 4 years, respectively.

As shown in Table 6, the decelerations of linear growth during the last months preceding death were also accompanied by larger than expected decelerations of weight for age and weight for height, i.e., actual wasting. In fact, 47.4% of 190 child-months with negative standardized monthly height-for-age velocity also showed a negative figure for weight for height; in 6.3%, this exceeded 0.5 SD units per month, indicating marked wasting. Wasting was much more frequent for those child-months without stunting: 84.8% of 106 child-months; 22.6% with a wasting of more than 0.5 SD units of weight for height per month.

Nevertheless, Table 7 shows that stunting during the period preceding death was more intense than in the general population, even for those children who did not show growth deceleration in terms of weight for height, i.e., who were not wasting, and even for children who presented little or no deceleration in terms of weight for age.

THE IMPLICATIONS

The discussion of the implications of the findings focuses on three aspects: (a) the apparent contradiction between the lack of association between mortality and

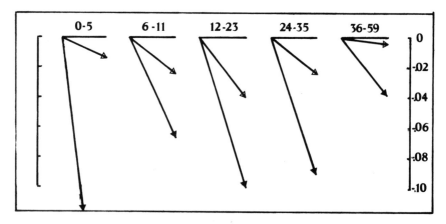

FIG. 8. Standardized monthly height-for-age velocities (SD units/month) at different ages; base line, reference population (zero by definition); *open arrows,* average for all children; *solid arrows,* average for subsequently dying children.

TABLE 6. *Average standardized monthly velocities of weight for age and weight for height of subsequently dying children[a]*

	Age group (months)				
	0–5	6–11	12–23	24–35	36–59
Weight for age	− 0.171	− 0.190	− 0.115	− 0.186	− 0.075
Weight for height	− 0.056	− 0.087	− 0.163	− 0.124	− 0.066

[a]Averages based only on intervals ending ≤ 3 months before death.

TABLE 7. *Average standardized monthly height-for-age velocity of subsequently dying children (a) without weight for height deceleration, (b) with decelerations of less than 0.25 SD units of weight for age per month, and (c) without weight-for-age decelerations[a]*

	Age group (months)				
	0–5	6–11	12–23	24–35	36–59
No W/H deceleration	− 0.632	− 0.328	− 0.270	− 0.147	− 0.078
W/A deceleration of less than 0.25 SD units	− 0.218	− 0.193	− 0.169	− 0.094	− 0.046
No W/A deceleration	0.018	− 0.354	− 0.147	− 0.123	− 0.048

[a]Velocities measured during intervals ending ≤ 3 months before death. All children died between 6 and 61 months of age. Number of children observed: 29, 31, and 21.

being stunted and the association with the process of stunting, as well as the discrepancies between the Matlab and Kasongo findings; (b) the causal nature of the association between stunting and mortality; (c) finally, some remarks on the implications of the results and their interpretation for the monitoring and evaluation of the health status of young children.

Being Stunted, Stunting, and Dying

Apparently the association between being stunted and increased subsequent risk of dying is found in Matlab but not in Kasongo. This contrast is even more impressive if one considers that the association in Matlab was demonstrated for risk of dying during the two subsequent years, whereas in Kasongo the interval between measurement and death was much shorter, an average of 2.3 months. One would expect the association to be stronger for short-term than for long-term mortality.

On the other hand, there is definitely an association between the stunting process and subsequent mortality in Kasongo. This association is most marked if one considers the period immediately preceding death (subgroup c in Table 5). It is present even in the absence of growth decelerations in terms of weight for height and weight for age. Those children who did not experience stunting in the months preceding death often experienced wasting.

The lack of association between mortality and attained height in Kasongo is not really surprising. Similar observations have been made for weight for age and height and, to a lesser extent, for arm circumference measurements (5). This lack of association could be explained by the specificity of the socioeconomic and cultural situation in Kasongo, where all children are basically exposed to a similar physical and nutritional environment. This would be responsible for a shift to the left of the growth curve of the entire population. Thus, a child on the upper fringe of the local distribution presents a growth retardation (with associated increased mortality risk), just as a child on the lower fringe does. Consequently, anthropometric measurement will not discriminate between children with greater or smaller environment- or nutritional-status-associated mortality risk.

An environment that causes a shift to the left for the entire population would also explain the apparent contradiction with the Matlab data. Whereas Kasongo children, on both the upper and lower fringes of the distribution, would be exposed to the same environment and the same risk of dying, the Bangladeshi child on the upper fringe of the height distribution for a certain age would probably be exposed to a different environment than a child on the lower fringe and would therefore be less exposed to the risk of dying. For the Matlab children this is certainly true to a certain extent: attained height and weight not only reflect the recent famines but also are correlated with indicators of socioeconomic status (6). The association between attained height and mortality in the Matlab studies, and especially Chen's demonstration of a cut-off point with increasing risk (4), is possibly related to a more important social stratification with nutritional corollaries than in Kasongo and to the fact that the overall nutritional situation appears to be considerably worse and disequilibrated in the Matlab study population.

Within this explanatory framework, the lack of association between being stunted and mortality does not preclude an association between mortality and stunting. If the stunting process is associated with mortality but is not restricted to a subgroup of the population and affects all children, then an associated excess mortality is plausible even in the absence of discriminatory power of attained height. On the other hand, in situations where attained height permits discrimination, such as in Matlab, the absence of association between mortality and stunting is unlikely.

In any case, the scarcity of available evidence should make us very cautious about extrapolating results of nutritional screening from one population to the other and making causal inferences from them.

The Causal Nature of the Association Between Stunting and Mortality

The association between stunting and mortality in Kasongo satisfies a number of the criteria required to call the stunting process a risk factor[3] for subsequent death. In order for the evidence to support a causal interpretation, however, a

---

[3] It is better to speak of "risk factor" rather than of "necessary" or "contributory cause": the death of young children in developing countries has a multifactorial etiology. Together with our limited ability to understand and observe the causal process, this makes it difficult to work with a purely deterministic framework (15).

plausible and intelligible biological mechanism has to be available (12,13). One should thus be able to formulate at least a tentative answer to the question of why a stunting child would be more at risk of dying.

Within this context it is useful to mention what was observed during a study of the influence of measles on the growth pattern of the children in Kasongo (14). Measles appears initially to cause weight loss and reduction of arm circumference. Four to 5 months after the onset of measles, the arm circumference regains its former level, but some deficit of weight for age, as compared to the NCHS reference, persists, and a statistically significant decrease of height for age starts to appear.

These phenomena could possibly be explained as follows. The height retardation would be the delayed effect of the nutritional stress caused by measles as a result of an incomplete recuperation during which recovery of an acceptable weight for height is privileged over ongoing linear growth. Stunting would become measurable in the aftermath of a serious stress. If a child is exposed to another infectious or nutritional stress while still recuperating from the previous one, it makes sense that he/she would be more vulnerable than the average child.

The nature of the association between stunting and subsequent mortality may be explained as follows: the final and direct cause of death in a stunting child would operate on a child still recuperating from recent stress, stunting being essentially a marker of the general vulnerability of the child to a new aggression. In such an explanatory framework, the frequency of infectious aggressions to which a child is exposed in a developing country (16) becomes extremely important and makes the association between stunting and mortality possible.

Unless a biological mechanism can be suggested through which the stunting process—or being stunted—per se would operate to make the child more vulnerable, the available evidence does not point towards an interpretation of stunting as a direct contributory cause of excess mortality. Rather, the association between stunting and mortality appears to be through their common cause, poverty, and its corollary of frequent nutritional and infectious stresses that do not allow for complete recuperation.

If poverty operates in conjunction with social stratification, as it appears to do in Matlab, attained height will reflect this stratification and therefore show an association with the poverty-linked increased risk of dying. If it operates in a less stratified way, as in Kasongo, attained height will not differentiate, within the population, groups more or less exposed to the poverty-linked increased risk of dying. Stresses affecting the child's health may be differently distributed within these populations, but in both situations, basic mechanisms are similar: a common effect of stress on a child's health is stunting; a less common effect is death, the latter occurring particularly when stresses occur in rapid succession and health care behavior at the microlevel does not enable the child to recuperate rapidly.

Linear Growth as a Monitor of Health Status of Children

Whatever its causal nature, the association between stunting and mortality makes it tempting to use it for evaluation purposes. A full discussion on the selection of indicators for monitoring health status of children goes beyond the scope of this chapter. Some remarks can nevertheless be made, keeping in mind that one has to distinguish (as for the evaluation of the nutritional status) (17) between the value of stunting as a tool to monitor the health status of individual children or to monitor and evaluate the health status of populations of children.

A statistically significant association can be demonstrated between stunting and the individual child's risk of dying. This, however, does not necessarily provide a practical screening instrument for the identification of children at risk. Do static (as in Bangladesh) or dynamic (as in Kasongo) height-for-age measurements provide a significant marginal benefit over screening on the basis of weight or weight-for-height measurements?

In the population studied by Chen et al. (4), a cut-off point at 80% of the reference weight for height permits selecting a group with a mortality risk 1.15 times higher than in the whole group. Cross classifying with height for age (cut-off point 90% of the reference) improves the ratio to 1.78, with a much higher sensitivity, but at the cost of an important loss of specificity. Only 28% of the children are not considered at risk, and a selected child has a probability of dying during the next 2 years of 0.06; this is a higher risk indeed but remains low from a statistical or operational point of view. There is not enough information available to assess the potential improvement gained from, as well as the cost entailed by, the introduction of velocity measurements (height or weight) as a screening tool in that population.

In Kasongo, standardized growth decelerations of weight for age of a magnitude of -1 SD unit or more over a period of 3 months are fairly frequent—about 6% above 24 months, more than 20% between 6 and 11 months—and robust to either errors in measurement or determination of age. They are more promising than static measurements as a tool for the identification of children at risk (7). Looking for linear growth decelerations among children who do not present decelerations in weight growth does not increase sensitivity (for detection of death within the next 100 days) if the measurements are made after the age of 24 months, whereas it does reduce specificity. Between the ages of 6 and 24 months, an increase in sensitivity can be obtained, from 56 to 77%, but again with a reduction of specificity, from 54 to 38%.

The formulation of concrete recommendations in this regard requires additional research on the characteristics of the screening criteria (sensitivity, specificity, predictive value at various cut-off points, etc.) in different situations, on the possibilities of operationalizing velocity measurements in community settings, and on the possibilities of intervention on children identified as at risk. However, the actual choice of an indicator of faltering or faltered growth is probably less important than whether it is used in conjunction with information on the child's recent or present morbidity and its socioeconomic environment. This might enable us to discriminate those episodes of growth faltering for which an intervention could be implemented, aiming at diminishing exposure and increasing resistance to nutritional or infectious stresses when the child is particularly vulnerable.

What is the value of the prevalence of stunted children as a tool for the evaluation or monitoring of the health of a population of children? The data presented do not permit more than speculation; still, the measurement of height deficits seems to be useful.

If both stunting and mortality are different outcomes—often successive but without direct causal relationship—of a succession of stresses on the children's health, then the measurement of the height of children in a community is an even more valuable tool for evaluation. Indeed, the measurement of the prevalence of stunted children then becomes an operationally fairly feasible, be it indirect, measurement of poverty-related disease frequency and of the inability of rapid recuperation. Stunting may not be a "disease" per se or a "cause of death"; it probably only results from the adaptation of the body to an incomplete recuperation after exposure to various stresses in an unfavorable environment. The measurement of the prevalence of stunted children in a community does not tell us whether this adaptation was obtained with a high or low cost of human lives; we need other indicators for that. However, it provides us with a tell-tale sign that such an adaptation was necessary, because aggressions were not avoided and/or the children were not able to overcome their debilitating effect.

The prevalence of stunted children appears to be a good overall indicator of the health status of a community of children, as are mortality levels. Both have similar limitations and certainly may not be substituted for socioeconomic or health service functioning indicators, which may be more directly relevant for decision making. But measurement of prevalence of stunted children does have some advantages: it is a cheap measurement, and in situations in which a number of frequent "biological" causes of mortality such as malaria or tetanus are under control, it might be a sensitive indicator showing that the effects of poverty on the child's health have not been completely overcome.

ACKNOWLEDGMENTS

This work was supported in part by grants 3.4541.85 of the F.N.R.S. and 22.363 of the N.F.W.O., Belgium.

REFERENCES

1. Keller W, Fillmore CM. Prevalence of protein–energy malnutrition. *World Health Stat Q* 1983;36:168–200.
2. Sommer A, Lowenstein MS. Nutritional status and mortality: a prospective validation of the QUAC stick. *Am J Clin Nutr* 1975;28:287–92.
3. Kielmann AA, McCord CW. Weight for age as an index of risk of death in children. *Lancet* 1978;2:1247–50.
4. Chen LC, Alauddin Chodhury AKM, Huffman SL. Anthropometric assessment of energy–protein malnutrition and subsequent risk of mortality among preschool aged children. *Am J Clin Nutr* 1980;33:1836–45.
5. Kasongo Project Team. Anthropometric assessment of young children's nutritional status as an indicator of subsequent risk of dying. *J Trop Pediatr* 1983;29:69–75.

6. Bairagi R, Chowdhury MK, Kim YJ, Curlin GT. Alternative anthropometric indicators of mortality. *Am J Clin Nutr* 1985;42:296–306.
7. Kasongo Project Team. Growth decelerations among under-5-year-old children in Kasongo (Zaire). Part 2. Relationship with subsequent risk of dying, and operational consequences. *Bull WHO* 1986;64:703–9.
8. Kasongo Project Team. Weight, height and arm circumference in 0 to 5 year-old children from Kasongo (Zaire). *Ecol Food Nutr* 1982;12:19–28.
9. National Center for Health Statistics. *NCHS growth charts, 1976*. Rockville, MD: National Center for Health Statistics, 1976; DHEW publication no. (HRA) 76-1120 [Monthly vital statistics report; series 25; no 3 (suppl)].
10. Waterlow JC. Classification and definition of protein–energy malnutrition. In: Beaton GH, Bengoa JM, eds. *Nutrition in preventive medicine. The major deficiency syndromes, epidemiology, and approaches to control.* WHO Monograph Series 62. Geneva: WHO, 1976:530–55.
11. Keller W. Choice of indicators of nutritional status. In: Schürch B, ed. *Evaluation of nutrition education in third world communities.* Bern, Stuttgart, Vienna: Hans Huber, 1983:101–13 (Nestlé Foundation Publication Series; vol 3).
12. Bradford Hill A. *Principles of medical statistics.* Oxford: Oxford University Press, 1971.
13. Van Parijs P. *Explication et modèles en sciences humaines. Essais d'épistémologie concrète.* Louvain la Neuve, Belgium: Diffusion Universitaire Ciaco, 1981.
14. Kasongo Project Team. Growth decelerations among under-5-year-old children in Kasongo (Zaire). Part 1. Occurrence of decelerations and impact of measles on growth. *Bull WHO* 1986;64:695–701.
15. Kleinbaum DG, Kupper LL, Morgenstern H. *Epidemiologic research. Principles and quantitative methods.* London: Lifetime Learning Publications, 1982.
16. Mata LJ, Kromal RA, Urrutia JJ, Garcia B. Effect of infection on food intake and the nutritional state: perspectives as viewed from the village. *Am J Clin Nutr* 1977;30:1215–27.
17. Tanner JM. Growth as a monitor of nutritional status. *Proc Nutr Soc* 1976;35:315–22.

DISCUSSION

Dr. Tanner: I feel rather bad that it rests with me to make some methodological or technological criticism, particularly in respect to this extremely interesting and important paper with which I agree almost entirely, apart from this technical point, which is nonetheless an important one. If you consider the change in Z score with age as a measure of the probability of velocity in terms of distribution (that is, the velocity centile as usually understood), it is biased and therefore inaccurate. It is a very easy one to get wrong. A lot of people have fallen into this trap, but it is perfectly well known and is in the auxology textbooks (1). So you must look at it in terms of velocity itself.

Dr. Van Lerberghe: I am not familiar with velocity measurements, and I was uneasy about the way in which to express them. To me, this was an operational measure enabling us to see whether there was a difference between the overall population and the children who died. I agree that it may be a biased measure of the probability of velocity, but I was only looking for something different occurring in the children who died, in the period before they died, compared to the overall population. It is this difference that is important.

Dr. Tanner: I agree with you, but if you start comparing the differences between the dying and the nondying between ages, you might draw the conclusion that certain ages are worse than others; then you are in trouble.

Dr. Martorell: Dr. Van Lerberghe, in relation to mortality, there is a third study you may want to include, by Peter Heywood in New Guinea (2). He performed anthropometric measurements in over 1,000 children with a follow-up of 18 months. When the initial status in terms of weight for height was adequate, being stunted did not seem to make a difference in terms of mortality. There was, however, a strong interaction between stunting and wasting: the group with the highest mortality was the one that was stunted and wasted.

You mentioned the influence of maternal size and maternal height on child mortality. I think that is another area we might want to look at to get a full picture of what stunting means in terms of mortality. We studied maternal height and child survival in about 400 Mayan women in Guatemala (3). Maternal height was strongly related to infant mortality. When we divided these women into terciles of height, the infant mortality for the tallest was about 200 per 1,000; for the midtercile, it was about 150 per 1,000; and for the shortest, it was about 100 per 1,000. So there is a strong relationship between maternal height and infant mortality. Could you comment on this?

Dr. Van Lerberghe: Both maternal height and weight have been used by Chen as indicators of maternal nutrition. It is interesting to see that this indicator of maternal nutrition does not make any difference to the child's risk of dying if the child is not severely stunted. The risk ratios for children above 85% of the reference are 0.99 for height and 0.92 for weight, whereas if you look at children below 85% of the reference, then the risk ratios are 1.58 and 1.25. So there seems to be an association, but again this should really be analyzed in the context of the social stratification within the population. I am not familiar with the Matlab population, but I wonder whether it really is one homogeneous population or whether it is composed of a number of subpopulations in which the environmental associated risk is different. In the Zaire situation, the physical and nutritional environments of all the children in the population appear to be identical; there are no gross differences. We do not have any data on maternal nutritional status, but my guess is that it would not be an indicator of differences in the environment of the child and that it would not interfere very much with child mortality. However, this is totally speculative.

Dr. Tomkins: I should like to hear your opinion on the duration of follow-up. What worries me about the interpretation of these studies is that the Matlab study by Chen (4) was over a 24-month period; the analysis by Bairagi (5) was over a 12-month period. Chen showed a stepwise threshold; Bairagi showed a linear relationship, at least for two of the seasons. Your study was over 100 days, I believe. Is this difference in duration of follow-up important if we are going to make recommendations for the future? I wonder if you could comment on what bias might be introduced by looking at children over different periods of time?

Dr. Van Lerberghe: The choice of length of follow-up depends on a number of things. One of the reasons we chose a relatively short follow-up period is that we were looking for an operational tool to identify the children for whom we could do something on a short-term basis. I have very incomplete data on long-term risk evaluation; you will find some in the chapter. It seems that the association in Kasongo, at least, is no different for long- and short-term follow-up. As far as velocity is concerned, the mixed long- and short-term follow up (in Chen's paper the long- and short-term follow-ups are also mixed) shows significant differences, but the differences are smaller than for the short-term follow up. That means that the nearer the measurements are to death, the bigger is the difference compared to what was expected.

Dr. Tomkins: I think that this is a real problem, and I am glad that you differentiated between different communities. Another question is whether there could be a bias between these studies because of the different causes of death? If I understand correctly, 54% of the children in your study died from measles. It is very interesting to realize that nutrition itself may not be a particularly severe risk factor in urban-type measles: work from Guinea Bissau (6) and from South Africa (7) emphasized that it might be a severe problem in relatively well-nourished children. I wonder if you had an opportunity to look at the difference between height for age and subsequent risk for nonmeasles death, as opposed to measles death, because I do not think that 54% of the children in Matlab died from measles. What do you feel about the potential bias introduced by different causes of death?

Dr. Van Lerberghe: I cannot answer your question as far as height is concerned, but for weight, weight for height, arm circumference, and arm circumference for height, we did see the same pattern in measles and nonmeasles deaths. It might be different for height.

Dr. Gopalan: Don't you think that the level of health care could influence the relationship between stunting and mortality? Of course, it is to be expected that in many of the poor population groups where there is a great deal of stunting, access to health care is also poor, but even in the most extreme cases of kwashiorkor, we now know that fatalities are not inevitable. Even in kwashiorkor, with proper treatment the mortality rate is now very low. The effort that is needed to reduce mortality is clearly very different from the effort needed to reverse stunting. Many developing countries may be able to afford the first but not the second. The pool of stunted children may actually increase because of the reduction in child mortality. It could very well be that health care in one location was inadequate with, as a consequence, stunting and mortality going together, and this may not apply in another location. Could you comment on the level of health care in the area where you were working?

Dr. Van Lerberghe: There are a number of questions involved. One could speculate that the level of stunting is a good indicator of whether there is integrated health care or not. When health care is restricted to a few single actions such as vaccination and oral rehydration and maybe two or three other simple things, I don't think that the health care system will thoroughly influence the level of stunting because it will not consider a number of minor aggressions that end up debilitating the health of the child. That is why the prevalence of stunted children is probably a good indicator of dysfunctioning of the health system. On the other hand, the efficiency of the use of anthropometric data within the context of an integrated primary health care system (curative care, preventive care, promotive care, and so on) is bound to increase very considerably for purely mathematical reasons. The predictive value of a screening test, if you use anthropometry as a screening instrument, increases if the prevalence of what you want to predict increases. If the screening is conducted within the context of general curative care, then the chance is high that anthropometry will be related to a pathological situation that requires intervention; this automatically increases the efficiency of the screening instrument. If you have got a good health system, the prevalence of stunted children should go down, and the usefulness of anthropometry should rise.

Dr. Gopalan: I don't want to continue this discussion, but I think the statement that the level of stunting is a reflection of the efficiency of the health system may be an oversimplification; it may be a reflection of socioeconomic deprivation; I wish it were that simple. Stunting is not a disease like goiter or keratomalacia; there is no vaccine against stunting. On the other hand, the reduction of mortality may be much more closely related to the efficiency of the health care system.

Dr. Van Lerberghe: This is true in extreme situations with very high levels of mortality and very high levels of stunted children. I don't believe that this remains true in an intermediary situation, when single causes of death have been eliminated—I mean those causes of death for which very simple technological measures exist. For instance, if there is a high mortality from tetanus and the health system starts vaccinating pregnant women, then the best indicator for the functioning of the health system will be the reduction in mortality level and not the reduction in stunting. If such causes of death have been eliminated, the causal structure of mortality changes and becomes more diffuse, the causes of death being a number of different conditions such as respiratory diseases, chronic diarrhea, and so on, as in Latin America or some parts of Africa. At that point, the prevalence of stunted children becomes an indicator of health system functioning and of socioeconomic status, which are also interrelated. It doesn't, however, really identify what goes wrong. It just shows that something is wrong, and one should start looking for the causes.

Dr. Valyasevi: The main causes of mortality, especially in young children in rural areas in developing countries, are probably diarrhea and infection of the respiratory tract. These are thoroughly influenced by the availability of health care, as has been observed in Thailand. Before infant health care systems were implemented about 10 or 15 years ago, the infant mortality rate was very high, about 70 or 80 per 1,000. Up to 3 or 4 years ago, the preventive and promotive aspects of health care were really not emphasized. Nevertheless, the infant mortality dropped to below 50. This was mainly because of the availability of health care in the villages, primarily focusing on curative aspects. This seems to support Dr. Gopalan's remark that mortality is rather an index of the availability of health care, whereas stunting probably reflects the socioeconomic situation. At least, this is my experience.

Dr. Nabarro: I am concerned that we appear to be making international generalizations about processes whose nature will vary from location to location. Chen and his colleagues reported the relationship between children's anthropometric indices and subsequent mortality in 1980 (4). Their data have been used by a number of writers to explain the nature of the relationship and its implications for those making decisions about the allocation of resources to undernourished children. However, workers in Papua New Guinea (8) and your group in Zaire (9) found quite different anthropometry–mortality relationships. There appears to be considerable variety in these relationships, depending both on the interval over which children's mortality risks are studied and the location in which the study took place. I would suggest that both the socioeconomic status of the population and the infections that are experienced by children are important determinants of the relationship. I consider it premature to suggest that the prevalence of stunting can be used as a universal index of health service performance or of the impact of development programs.

Dr. Van Lerberghe: Stunting is only a single measure, and as such it has the same limitations as other single measures. It can certainly not be substituted either for socioeconomic indicators or for indicators of health service functioning. In my opinion, health service functioning indicators are much more important because they help us to make decisions adapted to the local situation. Some indicators might be applicable everywhere; however, one should avoid claiming that single indicators explain everything, because it is evident that one cannot evaluate a complex situation just by looking at one single measurement.

Dr. Martorell: Knowing the mechanism is helpful for generalizing. For instance, wasting may be related to mortality partly through biological mechanisms, impaired immunocompetence and so on, in which case generalization is easier. In the case of stunting, I would agree with you that it probably reflects many aspects of the socioeconomic environment, and it is difficult to isolate the mechanisms involved; these need to be investigated in each location. As a result, one cannot generalize easily concerning the meaning of stunting in different places.

Dr. Van Lerberghe: If such a mechanism could be suggested for stunting, then I would certainly speak of a risk factor and of some degree of causal association. In the case of stunting there are so far no such biological explanations available.

Dr. Golden: I would like to reemphasize the importance, in analyzing this type of data, of breaking it down in terms of cause-specific mortality. In her study of mental stimulation of malnourished children in Jamaica, Sally McGregor was horrified to find that children who were stimulated were dying from increased numbers of accidents, such as traffic injury, burns, etc. If we don't break mortality down to cause-specific mortality, we might end by reaching quite wrong conclusions. Measles deaths are different from diarrheal deaths and from accidents. We must clean the data in terms of the cause of death.

Dr. Van Lerberghe: It is already very hard to find studies where a reasonable number of deaths are analyzed. In the Bairagi study (5), fewer than 20 children have had height measurements in the months preceding death; we cannot start breaking down 20 deaths by cause and analyzing those different categories. In our study, we had 137 deaths that we could analyze in children between 6 and 61 months. That is still a very small group. Now we can break it down into measles and nonmeasles, or maybe into measles, diarrhea, and "nonmeasles–nondiarrhea," but with 3-monthly visits you cannot get reasonable morbidity data, and you start having difficulties in identifying the causes of death. If we want to identify the causes of death on a prospective basis, we need a multiround survey with visits every 15 days, but then we get an extremely biased study. There is really no way out unless we use sophisticated designs combining prospective cohort studies with case control.

REFERENCES

1. Tanner JM. Use and abuse of growth standards. In: Falkner F, Tanner JM, eds. *Human growth.* 2nd ed, vol 3. New York: Plenum Press, 1986:95–112.
2. Heywood PF. Growth and nutrition in Papua New Guinea. *J Hum Evol* 1983;12:133–43.
3. Martorell R, Delgado H, Valverde V, Klein RE. Maternal stature, fertility and infant mortality. *Hum Biol* 1981;53:303–12.
4. Chen LC, Chowdhury AKMA, Huffman SL. Anthropometric assessment of energy–protein malnutrition and subsequent risk of mortality among pre-school aged children. *Am J Clin Nutr* 1980;33:1836–45.
5. Bairagi R, Chowdhury MK, Kim YJ, Curlin GT. Alternative anthropometric indicators of mortality. *Am J Clin Nutr* 1985;42:296–306.
6. Aaby P, Bukha J, Lisse IM, Smits AJ. Measles mortality, state of nutrition and family structure. A community study from Guinea-Bissau. *J. Infect Dis* 1983;147:693–701.
7. Coovadia HM, Wesley A, Brain P, Henderson LG, Hallet AF, Vos GH. Immunoparesis and outcome in measles. *Lancet* 1977;1:619–21.
8. Heywood P. The functional significance of malnutrition—growth and prospective risk of death in the highlands of Papua New Guinea. *J Food Nutr* 1982;39:13–9.
9. The Kasongo Project Team. Anthropometric assessment of young children's nutritional status as an indicator of subsequent risk of dying. *J Trop Pediatr* 1983;29:69–75.

Linear Growth Retardation in Less Developed Countries, edited by John C. Waterlow. Nestlé Nutrition Workshop Series, Vol. 14. Nestec Ltd., Vevey/Raven Press, Ltd., New York © 1988.

Stunting: Significance and Implications for Public Health Policy

C. Gopalan

The Nutrition Foundation of India, New Delhi 110049, India

Available anthropometric data on different communities around the world broadly indicate a close relationship between the heights of children (and, for that matter, of adults) in a community and the level of its socioeconomic development. The greater the socioeconomic deprivation in a community, the greater, generally, are the extent and degree of stunting in it.

Socioeconomic underdevelopment (poverty) generally signifies the following: (a) low levels of income, (b) inadequate diets, (c) low-paid unskilled and semi-skilled manual occupations of adults, (d) poor levels of education, (e) poor environmental sanitation and housing conditions, (f) large family size, and (g) high prevalence of morbidity and clinical signs of undernutrition (other than growth retardation), especially among children. Among communities subject to socioeconomic deprivations, these attributes of the "poverty syndrome" invariably coexist and tend mutually to reinforce their respective ill effects. Children and adults caught up in this situation cannot but be stunted.

All these factors of the poverty scenario listed above, however, must ultimately act through a final common pathway to bring about stunting, the ultimate determinant being the lack of availability at the cellular level, in adequate amounts, in proper combinations, and at appropriate times, of all the essential nutrients required for growth, development, maintenance, repair, and normal functions of the organism. Stunting associated with poverty is, therefore, in the final analysis, a direct reflection of the undernutrition induced by it. It is the most convenient and practical quantifiable index of undernutrition available to the health scientist.

There may be academic debates as to what stunting per se does or does not do, but there can be no two opinions about the need for eradication of poverty, which automatically implies the eradication of stunting as well.

Physical stunting in poverty-stricken cases is invariably associated with varying degrees of impairment of mental development as well, as is ably pointed out by Dr. Colombo in this volume, though these two attributes may not always be directly causally related. In the same way as physical stunting is not a reflection of low genetic potential for growth, mental stunting is not a reflection of low intellectual potential but presumably results from environmentally induced learning disabilities and lack of adequate opportunities for cultivation of such potential in poverty situations.

A community in which a very high proportion of children and adults are stunted is most likely to be a community whose human resources are of poor quality.

RECENT INDIAN STUDIES

Three recent Indian studies throw light on the context and real-life setting in which stunting is generally seen.

An extensive longitudinal study on growth and development of children of different socioeconomic groups, followed from birth for periods extending now to nearly 15 years, has been ongoing in Delhi in India since 1969. These unique studies originally initiated by Ghosh and colleagues (1) are now being continued by S. K. Bhargava and V. Kapani. The observations presented here are based on an as-yet unpublished report of S. K. Bhargava and V. Kapani.

Nearly 8,200 children have been covered in this study. The communities investigated ranged from the poorest (less than Rs 50/- per person per month, 1969

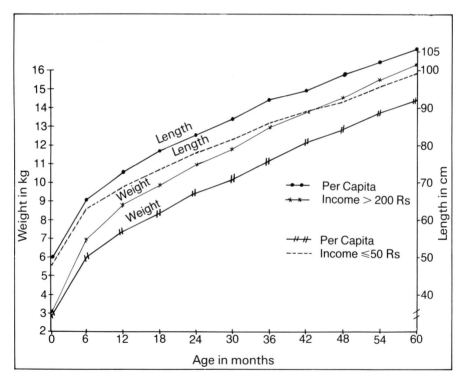

FIG. 1. Weight and lengths/standing heights of girls by *per capita* income and age. (From S.K. Bhargava and V. Kapani, *unpublished data.*)

level) to the fairly well-to-do upper middle class (more than Rs 200/- per person per month, 1969 level). The longitudinal data from children belonging to these two income groups (Fig. 1) show the clear relationship between socioeconomic status and heights and weights of children.

K. Satyanarayana and colleagues (2) at the National Institute of Nutrition, Hyderabad, have assembled data from longitudinal observations on the heights and weights of children of different socioeconomic groups in rural Hyderabad observed over a 15-year period (5 to 20 years). The children belonging to their group I, with heights between the mean and the mean minus 2 SD of the Boston Standard, mostly came from families of affluent landlords owning more than 5 acres of fertile land; those of their group III were from the poorest rural households owning no land of their own, with adults being illiterate and eking out their living from seasonal agricultural wage labor. Some of their observations have been set out in Table 1. The same table also shows data on heights and weights of children of the most affluent Indian communities as observed and reported by D. Hanumantha Rao and Gowrinath Sastry (3) of the same institute on the basis of their cross-sectional studies. The striking difference between the different socioeconomic groups is again obvious.

The National Nutrition Monitoring Bureau in Hyderabad, India, has recently completed a study of the dietary, nutritional, and anthropometric status of 32,332 subjects (12,925 adults and 19,407 children) drawn from 15 major cities of India (4). The sample households were classified into five major socioeconomic categories.

The high-income group (HIG) and the slum laborers (SL) represented the two extreme ends of the economic spectrum, with the other three groups lying in between. The SL was the group subject to the greatest socioeconomic deprivation— poor, largely illiterate or semiliterate, living in highly overcrowded and unhygienic

TABLE 1. *Longitudinal studies of growth of Indian children of different socioeconomic groups*

Group	Initial (5 years of age)		Final (20 years of age)	
	Height (cm)	Weight (kg)	Height (cm)	Weight (kg)
Mostly from families of well-to-do landlords (owning about 5 acres of fertile land) (mean ± SD)[a]	104.7 ± 2.90	15.3 ± 1.4	167.8 ± 6.26	51.5 ± 6.6
Mostly from families of agricultural laborers on seasonal daily wages (mean ± SD)[a]	89.2 ± 4.02	11.5 ± 1.08	157.8 ± 6.09	44.0 ± 3.91
Highly affluent[b]	108.0	18.3	171.8	59.6

[a]Satyanarayana et al. (2).
[b]Hanumantha Rao and Gowrinath Sastry (3).

conditions and having to depend mostly on unskilled manual labor to eke out a precarious livelihood. Their diets were decidedly lower in energy content, and their children showed a higher prevalence of signs of vitamin deficiencies.

The heights and weights of children and adults faithfully reflected the socioeconomic gradient, with the HIG at one end and SL at the other and the other groups falling in between. For the sake of convenience, only part of the data from the two groups at the extreme ends (HIG and SL) are shown in Tables 2 and 3.

THE POVERTY TRAP

The outstanding finding in all three studies cited above is the striking relationship between income and occupational status on the one hand and physical stature on the other. It appears that the more lowly (using the expression for the sake of convenience) the job that a community is engaged in, the greater is the degree of stunting in its children and adults. The cart pullers, scavengers, manual laborers

TABLE 2. *Heights and weights of children from the highest (HIG) and lowest (SL) socioeconomic groups in 15 major cities of India*

Age (years)	Sex	Height (cm)		Weight (kg)	
		HIG	SL	HIG	SL
5	Boys	110.4	99.8	18.2	13.9
	Girls	107.6	98.7	16.2	13.6
12	Boys	144.2	132.6	30.8	25.1
	Girls	140.4	133.7	29.9	26.8
16	Boys	164.5	154.7	46.2	38.6
	Girls	156.2	148.6	43.1	39.1

From the National Nutrition Monitoring Bureau (4).

TABLE 3. *Heights and weights of adults from the highest (HIG) and lowest (SL) socioeconomic groups in 15 major cities in India*

Age group	Heights (cm)		Weights (kg)	
	HIG	SL	HIG	SL
20–25 years, M	166.4	161.4 (161.0–164)[a]	50.4	46.6 (47.2–49.8)
20–25 years, F	154.6	150.1 (149.4–151.9)	46.8	41.7 (41.0–44.2)
40–45 years, M	166.8	161.2	66.3	48.1
40–45 years, F	153.1	149.6	56.0	41.6

[a]Figures within parentheses in columns 3 and 5 are measurements of the corresponding rural group.
From the National Nutrition Monitoring Bureau (4).

(including those engaged in strenuous work), stone cutters, porters having to carry heavy loads, and agricultural laborers are apparently the ones who are most stunted and have the lowest body weights; unfortunately, these are precisely the occupation groups who stand in greatest need of a sturdy body build for optimal productivity and output and for earning a reasonable wage from their occupation.

In developed countries, it is most unlikely that one sees such a striking relationship between the occupation a community is engaged in and its physical stature. For instance, it should be surprising if the Canadian lumbermen, Norwegian fishermen, or Swedish farm workers of today were significantly shorter and lighter than people engaged in intellectual activities in those countries. If anything, they may be expected to be far sturdier. It may also be similarly expected that the children of Canadian lumbermen and Swedish farm workers will not be stunted from lack of adequate food and end up as stunted adults only fit for unskilled manual labor with low levels of productivity and earning capacity. Even the lowest jobs in those countries fetch incomes adequate for at least the basic minimal diet.

It may be reasonable to argue that in the developed countries of today (whatever the position might have been in the early part of this century), the occupation an individual takes on is largely (though not entirely) determined by his innate talents, interests, and abilities. In short, it is the genetic endowment, and not the accident of birth, that largely determines the occupation. Those with "more brawn than brain" may be moving into occupations involving strenuous labor. In developing countries, on the other hand, where communities are caught up in the poverty trap, neither the genetic potential for physical growth nor that for intellectual activity is able to find adequate expression, and a considerable part of the human resources of the state run to waste and are forced to drift to jobs calling mostly for unskilled or semiskilled manual labor.

Stunting is the outstanding feature of this poverty trap. In fact, it appears to be the feature that ensures that not this generation only but the next as well does not escape from the poverty trap. Stunted children with impaired learning abilities and schooling end up as stunted adults with low levels of productivity, educational attainment, and resourcefulness, earning low incomes and thus continuing to be enmeshed in the poverty trap and so unable to feed their children adequately. Stunted women beget offspring with low birth weight who thus start their lives with an initial handicap, which compounds the effects of superimposed undernutrition in their infancy and childhood. Thus, stunting and the poverty with which it is invariably associated continue from one generation to another.

THE COST OF STUNTING

In most discussions of the significance of stunting, the enormous "cost" that stunting implies to the society and to the state seems to be hardly appreciated. On the basis of cross-sectional data obtained from communities of growth-retarded children, "synthetic" growth curves have been constructed projecting the illusion that the growth of poverty-stricken children follows a well-ordered, well-regulated, uneventful, smooth trajectory, no doubt running well below the "normal" curve, somewhat akin to what is observed in rats reared in laboratories on deficient diets. In an earlier publication (5), I pointed out the fallacy of this concept. In actual fact, many "apparently adapted" older children and adults are those who had just managed to scrape through the "valley of death" in their early preschool years.

A community in which a considerable part of the population is stunted is usually a community with high infant and child mortality, high levels of morbidity in children, and a high rate of dropouts from schools. This is also a community in which children have lost valuable time for learning skills, mothers have lost a considerable part of their daily wages, and health services are so overburdened with a heavy load of curative work to the point that preventive and promotive health programs are relegated to the background.

Even if, for argument's sake, we accept the position that those who have arrived at adulthood in a stunted state with body weights appropriate to their heights and currently with no obvious sign of nutritional deficiency are "functionally normal" and, therefore, do not need to be bothered about—a position that I do not accept—we cannot ignore the enormous cost to the community that this stunting process had been associated with. There can, therefore, be no equivocation over the position that stunting is undesirable and needs to be prevented irrespective of the question of whether stunting in adulthood is consistent with normal function or not.

Does Stunting per se Really Matter?

It is argued that a stunted subject with a weight appropriate to his height, currently showing no obvious signs of nutritional deficiency, and going about his job with no obvious disability could be considered "normal" or "adapted." We may concede that a number of people showing marginal degrees of stunting do not exhibit obvious functional disability, even as a large number of people with hemoglobin levels of 8 g/dl go about their jobs apparently normally. The term "adaptation" is unfortunately being used, in this connection, loosely as almost equivalent to normality.

The factual position is that large sections of stunted subjects in developing countries, including those who are moderately and severely stunted, have "adapted" themselves to function within the poverty trap. To call this "normal functioning" would be cruel irony. It must also be remembered that (a) many of these stunted (seemingly adapted) subjects might not, in the first place, be doing the jobs they are currently doing if they had access to adequate nutrition, schooling, and health care in their childhood, in which case they would not have been stunted at all, and (b) even in the jobs they are currently engaged in (particularly heavy manual labor), they might have been able to earn more and to escape dire poverty if they had better physical stamina.

It is not necessary to go over the ground so ably covered by Dr. Spurr *(this volume)*, nor need I expand on the work of Satyanarayana and colleagues (6), which showed a direct correlation between productivity and body weight in industrial workers drawn from the poor socioeconomic groups even with respect to operations in which body weight may not be expected to make a difference. It is meaningless and cynical to argue that per kilogram of body weight the output of these workers was not significantly lower; unfortunately, workers are paid their wages on the basis of their individual output and not on the basis of output per kilogram body weight.

Indeed, it is hardly necessary to resort to functional tests in laboratories to show that the productivity of stunted subjects, especially in strenuous manual occupations, is impaired. Observations in the field under real-life conditions provide indubitable evidence. The stunted rickshaw puller from the slums of Calcutta plies his rickshaw just for a few hours of the day until he has made his 50 cents to a dollar, which will just help him and his family to escape starvation for the next day. He has neither the physical stamina nor the will to ply his vehicle for longer hours to earn a larger daily income. One does not need functional laboratory tests to guess that the work that one Canadian lumberman can do in the course of the day will probably require at least three stunted Indian workers. The fact that stunted Indian laborers are still managing to work and survive in a marginal state of poverty is no argument in support of the sweeping conclusion that the stunted state is quite compatible with "normal" function. Stunting can at best help to "preserve" them in a state of poverty and underdevelopment.

In a longitudinal study on undernourished boys in India by Satyanarayana and colleagues (7,8), it was found that the wages earned by adolescent boys employed by farmers in rural areas were significantly related to body weight and height.

> Better nourished boys were sought after by the farmers and were assigned the more demanding jobs and were paid higher wages that went with those jobs. . . . Poorly nourished young men could never compete with normally nourished matched counterparts either with respect to work capacity or wages earned. Men and women with better nutritional anthropometry earned 30% to 50% additional incentive money (over and above the uniform basic pay) in factories where an individual incentive system based on work output was in operation. (8)

Maternal Stunting and Low Birth Weights

An important aspect that has largely been ignored in discussions on the public health significance and implications of stunting is in the effect of stunting in the mother on the birth weight of her infant. In India, as in many other developing countries, more than one-third of all infants born alive have a birth weight below 2,500 g. Bhargava and colleagues (9) in India have carried out extensive studies in this area.

The follow-up studies of Bhargava and Kapani had been referred to earlier. In

TABLE 4. *Height measurements from birth to 14 years of premature, appropriate for gestational age (AGA), full-term, small for gestational age (SGA), and full-term, AGA infants in India*

Age	Preterm AGA (cm)	Full-term SGA (cm)	Full-term AGA (cm)
Birth	44.6	43.4	49.3
1 year	69.3	67.9	73.7
2 years	79.3	77.5	83.0
3 years	87.0	85.4	90.7
4 years	94.3	92.6	96.5
5 years	100.5	96.9	102.3
6 years	106.6	100.3	107.4
7 years	112.9	109.6	115.8
8 years	121.0	114.5	121.5
9 years	126.4	119.7	124.3
10 years	131.6	125.3	126.4
11 years	136.6	131.6	131.7
12 years	142.6	137.0	140.0
13 years	148.4	145.0	146.9
14 years	154.5	147.0	156.4

From S.K. Bhargava and V. Kapani (*unpublished observations*).

TABLE 5. *Weight measurements from birth to 14 years of premature, appropriate for gestational age (AGA), full-term, small for gestational age (SGA), and full-term, AGA infants in India*

Age	Preterm AGA (kg)	Full-term SGA (kg)	Full-term AGA (kg)
Birth	1.8	1.7	3.0
1 year	7.3	6.7	8.8
2 years	9.4	8.7	10.7
3 years	11.4	10.5	12.4
4 years	12.9	12.0	13.7
5 years	14.3	13.1	15.2
6 years	15.8	15.1	16.5
7 years	18.6	16.2	19.1
8 years	20.6	17.6	21.5
9 years	23.2	19.8	23.8
10 years	24.1	22.0	26.9
11 years	26.4	24.9	28.4
12 years	27.2	28.9	30.5
13 years	33.3	34.0	35.9
14 years	42.0	35.6	43.6

From S.K. Bhargava and V. Kapani (*unpublished observations*).

Tables 4 and 5, the results of their longitudinal studies of three categories of infants have been indicated:

1. Premature infants with low birth weights (weights appropriate for their gestational age, AGA).

2. Full-term infants with birth weights less than 2,500 g (small for gestational age, SGA).
3. Full-term infants with birth weights above 2,500 g.

With respect to both height and weight, infants who start with the initial handicap of low birth weight in spite of their being full term (SGA) apparently never fully recover from their initial handicap, unlike infants of the AGA group. Thus, low birth weights in full-term infants make a lasting contribution to stunting.

It may, however, be argued that since a great majority of SGA infants may be expected to come from poor households, unlike the "normal controls" with birth weights above 2,500 g, their poorer growth performance may be caused by their substandard postnatal nutrition and not necessarily be a reflection of their initial handicap of low birth weight.

In order to be able to answer this question, Bhargava and Kapani's data on the growth performance of SGA infants in both the poor (less than Rs 50/- per person per month) and the well-to-do groups (more than Rs 200/- per person per month) was compared to that of infants in both groups who started with normal birth weights are also shown (Figs. 2 and 3). In each income group, the growth performance of SGA infants was poorer than that of infants with normal birth weights in the same income group. The worst growth performance was seen in infants who belonged to the poor group and who also had the additional handicap of low birth weight to start with.

There is apparently a direct relationship between stunting in the mothers and the occurrence of low birth weights in their offspring (Table 6). According to the recommendation of international agencies, maternal heights below 145 cm may be considered to be indicative of risk of obstetric complications and low birth weight. It can be seen in Table 6 that a distinctly higher proportion of offspring of mothers with heights less than 145 cm were of low birth weight (SGA).

Here is direct evidence that stunting in the mother contributes to stunting in the infant; thus, the effect of stunting is not confined to the present generation alone. If reproduction of a healthy child who can grow normally is an important physiological function, here we have evidence that stunting in the mother does compromise this basic function of immense significance not just to this generation but to the next as well.

POLICY AND PROGRAMS

It is thus clear that stunting, now seen widely among poor communities around the world, cannot be viewed approvingly as an acceptable form of so-called "adaptation," as has been loosely suggested in some quarters. Acceptance of this hypothesis will only help perpetuate the current state of their underdevelopment. It is true that in a number of developing countries including India, a majority of children are stunted to varying degrees. This staggering vastness of the numbers of stunted itself provides the psychological temptation to raise the question

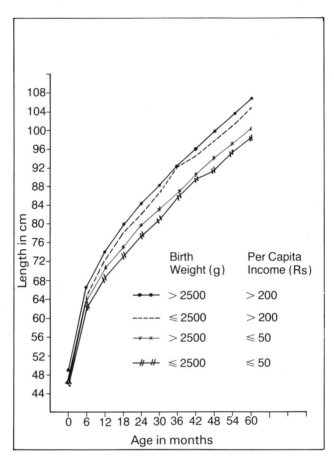

FIG. 2. Mean length/standing height by *per capita* income, birth weight, and age. (From S.K. Bhargava and V. Kapani, *unpublished data.*)

whether we should call such subjects abnormal at all and whether we should not accept stunting in these populations of developing countries as a feature of no consequence for them. Even according to the highly conservative estimate of India's Planning Commission, more than 40% of India's population is below the poverty line, and this so-called "poverty line" is based on very rigid criteria that signify only the most extreme degrees of economic deprivation and dire poverty by the standards of most developed countries of the world. Not more than 15% of India's population can be considered affluent according to the average standards of developed countries of Europe and North America. If, as has been pointed out above, stunting is a concomitant feature of poverty, it is inevitable that it must be as widespread as poverty itself.

The removal of factors in the socioeconomic and health scene that prevent children from attaining their genetic potential for growth and development must

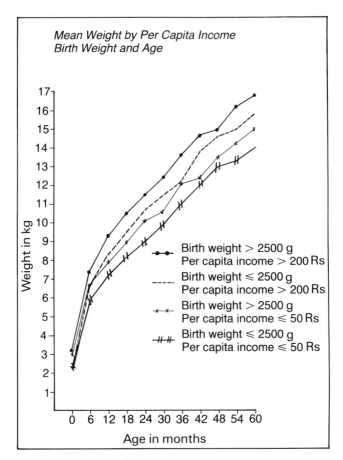

FIG. 3. Mean weight by *per capita* income, birth weight, and age. (From S.K. Bhargava and V. Kapani, *unpublished data.*)

TABLE 6. *Maternal height and incidence of low birth weight (LBW) in offspring*

Maternal height (cm)	Income group	Incidence of LBW
Less than 145 cm	Less than Rs 50/- per person per month	35.5%
More than 145 cm	Less than Rs 50/- per person per month	24.2%
More than 145 cm	More than Rs 200/- per person per month	15.0%

From S.K. Bhargava and V. Kapani (*unpublished observations*).

clearly be the central objective of any national health policy devoted to the improvement of the quality of a country's human resources.

Antipoverty Programs

Such a public health policy will imply not just narrow vertical programs confined to the health sector alone but broad-based programs of social and economic uplift that address the social and economic determinants of poverty and undernutrition. In the formulation and implementation of such integrated programs, health scientists and nutrition scientists must play a crucial role in order to ensure that health and nutrition aspects receive adequate focus and that the appropriate target groups are addressed.

Among populations of most developing countries, we may expect an almost continuous socioeconomic gradient between the affluent groups at the top and the abjectly poor at the bottom. Poverty will be found to deepen progressively and stunting to increase in severity as we descend the socioeconomic scale. Because of their severe resource constraints, it is most unlikely that developing countries will be able to eradicate their massive problem of poverty and its accompaniments (including stunting) within the next decade. Hard realities will demand that they settle for gradual elimination of these problems in a phased manner. For this purpose, they will have to set for themselves, from time to time, during various stages of their development, targets that fall far short of the eventual goal of total eradication of these problems. This is perfectly understandable. The level of poverty and the level of stunting that are to be chosen as a cut-off point for identifying target groups for action programs at a given stage of development have to be decided by each country depending on its resources, its perception of priorities, and its value systems. It will be wrong to attempt to invest such practical arbitrary decisions with scientific validity. In particular, it will be unscientific to ''adjust'' standards of normality to suit the actual scale of problems within the country. Standards are expected to determine the magnitude of a problem; it would be perverse to let the magnitude of a problem determine the standard.

Long-range integrated antipoverty programs will naturally take time to show results. In the immediate short run, intensive programs in the health and social welfare sectors will be necessary. Where resources are limited, it will be prudent to direct such resources to the early phases of growth and development, namely, the intrauterine phase (pregnancy), infancy, and early childhood. It could be inferred from the studies of Satyanarayana et al. (2) that if stunting can be averted until the fifth year, normal growth thereafter may be possible even at current levels of socioeconomic development.

Maternal Nutrition

Through intensive antenatal care, nutrition education of pregnant women directed to improving their diets during the second and third trimesters of pregnancy, and correction of anemia, it may be possible to bring about a significant reduction in the incidence of low birth weights. This program must be given high priority. The great majority of pregnant women in many developing countries currently receive no health care.

Breast Feeding

For most developing countries, the remarkable ability of even their poorest women to successfully breast feed their infants for prolonged periods has been the most valuable national asset in an otherwise bleak child nutrition scene. This salutary practice, which now faces the threat of progressive erosion, must be preserved and protected.

It has been suggested that since in some studies growth faltering in breast-fed infants is detectable even by the end of the second month after delivery, supplements to breast milk may have to be introduced even by that period. In the first place, this growth faltering by the second month is apparently by no means a universal phenomenon. Cowan (10) has actually demonstrated that infants can be reared successfully through exclusive breast feeding for 6 months. Growth faltering in early infancy in breast-fed infants, where it is seen, may also well be related to faulty breast-feeding practices (offering water to the infant in between feeds, not putting the infant to the breast as often as may be necessary, etc.) and not to inadequacy in breast milk as such. What may be needed, then, is education with respect to improving beast-feeding practices and not early supplementation.

Even if there is some faltering of growth by the end of the second month, it will be prudent in the case of mothers belonging to the poorest communities living in highly unsanitary surroundings to advise them to continue with exclusive breast feeding of their infants until at least the end of the fourth month if not the sixth month (11). This is because in such situations, the marginal nutritional advantage of earlier supplementation (if any) will be more than offset by the definite disadvantage of earlier supervention of diarrheal episodes. In fact, a study carried out by the Nutrition Foundation of India among poor communities has shown that infants who had received supplements before the fourth month arrived at their ninth month with a poorer anthropometric status than those who had been exclusively breast fed for 4 to 6 months (12).

Supplements

Supplements to breast milk to be introduced after at least 4 months of exclusive breast feeding must be based on inexpensive, locally available foods within the economic reach of the poor. There is a great need for educating mothers and children (and health workers) as to how such locally available foods can best be successfully used for infant feeding. Efforts in this area are at present woefully inadequate, and much of the undernutrition and stunting in children of developing countries may be traced to poor education and training in this regard.

Misuse of Commercial Baby Foods

Among poor communities living in highly unhygienic conditions, the use of commercial baby foods as supplements must be actively discouraged. The poor have neither the means to buy these foods in adequate amounts for feeding their infants nor the facilities to feed them hygienically. Unfortunately, these foods are currently being widely misused much to the detriment of infant nutrition in many developing countries. A study by the Nutrition Foundation of India (13) showed that in the urban slums and periurban rural areas of Bombay, Calcutta, and Madras, 22% to 30% of mothers belonging to the poorest income group were currently misusing these foods with results that could only be described as disastrous.

Outreach of Health Care

Infections (respiratory and gastrointestinal) account for much of the undernutrition (and stunting) in children in poor communities. The present poor outreach of health services in many developing countries precludes efforts at effective prevention and treatment of such infections. Perhaps even more important than the extension of government health services to villages is the need to develop programs within the villages to improve self-reliance and health/nutrition awareness of the community (especially the women) and to involve the community in its own health-care operations. It is gratifying that many developing countries have now launched programs for raising women's clubs and health volunteer forces in villages so that health care becomes a people's (and not the government's) movement. In the long run, it is through such means that real social transformation can come about in the villages and the basic factors that underlie their present poverty will be addressed.

Monitoring and Surveillance

Any meaningful health policy must rest on a proper information system and data base. Currently, few developing countries have adequate facilities for nutrition monitoring and surveillance. With few exceptions, such data on the prevalence of stunting in children as are available are based on *ad hoc* surveys; and since such surveys have not often been based on standardized methodology and sampling design, results obtained at different times and in different locations are often not comparable; it has also not been possible, under the circumstances, to evaluate the impact of action programs. The setting up of national systems for continuous nutrition monitoring should not be considered a luxury that developing countries can ill afford; indeed, it would help them to utilize their meager resources to maximal advantage and enable them to inject timely midcourse corrections in their action programs.

Research

There are still major gaps in our knowledge of the pathogenesis and significance of growth retardation. We do not know, for example, if the environmental constraints on growth in childhood that eventually lead to stunting and those that lead to wasting are necessarily always identical, or whether in certain situations, some factors in the environment (deficiencies of specific nutrients such as zinc) may preferentially contribute to stunting as opposed to wasting. We still do not know whether, given the same order of stunting, previous growth experience (the growth route the child took to arrive at the present stunted state) makes a difference with respect to functional performance. Clearly, answers to these and other questions can only come from extensive and careful studies conducted in developing countries. The need for continuing research in this area must not, therefore, be underestimated.

REFERENCES

1. Ghosh S, Sudershan K, Bhargava SK, Bhargava V. Growth and development of infants with severe intrauterine growth retardation. *Proc Nutr Soc* 1972;11:1–5.
2. Satyanarayana K, Nadamuni Naidu A, Narasinga Rao BS. Adolescent growth spurt among rural Indian boys in relation to their nutritional status in early childhood. *Ann Hum Biol* 1980;7: 359–65.
3. Hanumantha Rao D, Gowrinath Sastry J. Growth pattern of well-to-do Indian adolescents and young adults. *Indian J Med Res* 1977;66:950–6.
4. National Nutrition Monitoring Bureau. *Report on urban populations, 1975–79*. Hyderabad: National Institute of Nutrition, 1985.
5. Gopalan C. "Small is healthy?" For the poor, not for the rich. *Bull Nutr Found India* 1980;4 (Oct):4–8.
6. Satyanarayana K, Nadamuni Naidu A, Chatterjee B, Narasinga Rao BS. Body size and work output. *Am J Clin Nutr* 1977;30:322–5.
7. Satyanarayana K, Nadamuni Naidu A, Narasinga Rao BS. Nutritional deprivation in childhood, and the body size, activity, and physical work capacity of young boys. *Am J Clin Nutr* 1979;32:1769–75.
8. Satyanarayana K, Nadamuni Naidu A, Narasinga Rao BS. Agricultural employment, wage earnings and nutritional status of teenage rural Hyderabad boys. *Indian J Nutr Diet* 1980;17:281–6.
9. Bhargava SK, Ghosh S, Lall VB. A study of low birth weight infants in an urban community. *Health Popul Perspect Issues* 1979;2:54–65.
10. Das D, Dhanoa J, Cowan B. Exclusive breast-feeding for six months—an attainable goal for poor communities. *Bull Nutr Found India* 1982;3:2–5.
11. Gopalan C. Appropriate supplementation of breast milk. *Bull Nutr Found India* 1981;2:4–5.
12. Gopujkar PV, Chaudhuri SN, Ramaswami MA, Gore MS, Gopalan C. Infant feeding practices with special reference to the use of commercial infant foods. In: *Nutrition Foundation of India, Scientific Report, 1984*. New Delhi: Nutrition Foundaiton of India, 1985:90–5.
13. Gopujkar PV, Chaudhuri SN, Ramaswami MA, Gore MS, Gopalan C. Infant feeding practices with special reference to the use of commercial infant foods. In: *Nutrition Foundation of India, Scientific Report, 1984*. New Delhi: Nutrition Foundation of India, 1985:59–77.

DISCUSSION

Dr. Waterlow: Dr. Gopalan, you used the phrase, "the problem of undernutrition and stunting." Is stunting a problem? I get the impression, for example, from Dr. Van Lerberghe, that it isn't a problem but a kind of index.

Dr. Van Lerberghe: That is exactly what I wanted to say. I think it is dangerous to talk about the "problem of stunting." Is "stunting" a problem, or is "poverty" a problem for which stunting could be an indicator? If we go on using the term "stunting problem," we might be formulating "stunting control programs," which could create the illusion that we can solve the "stunting problem." But why should we solve a so-called "stunting problem" as such and let the problem of poverty remain? Such "stunting control programs" would divert attention from looking at the real solutions, which conceptually are much more difficult to develop and will certainly go far beyond what is considered to be the territory of the nutritionist.

Dr. Gopalan: I totally agree with you. I am not talking about "stunting control," and I do not look at "stunting" as an isolated problem. I look at it in its full context, in a real-life situation, as a manifestation of poverty and undernutrition, as an index. I do not think that there is any conflict at all. I am talking of eradication of poverty and undernutrition.

Dr. Martorell: This is an important point. I think all of us agree that growth retardation is an indicator, and I liked Dr. Gopalan's emphasis at the end that we should try to pinpoint when the process of stunting really takes place. This is important because it allows us to identify the real problems. I think it is clear that stunting surfaces during the preschool period, particularly during the first 3 years. We know that stunting is associated with problems that arise during the weaning process. It is precisely in the area of child feeding and health practices that we need to work, and all the evidence we have today indicates that height retardation is our best indicator of how successful our programs, whatever specific policies we implement, will be. We can also use stunting as an indicator of the quality of life, as an indicator of social inequalities; we can map countries and talk about areas of high and low prevalence and infer that there are social inequalities that have to be corrected. I totally agree that stunting is best viewed as an indicator. From the policy point of view, I think that it is the wrong approach to emphasize the implications of stunting; let's rather talk about the causes and use stunting as an indicator of those causes.

Dr. Gopalan: I agree that stunting is a good indicator, but there is more to it than that. Stunting by itself, as pointed out by Dr. Spurr, has its deleterious repercussions. It helps to perpetuate poverty. For example, to what extent is low birth weight related to stunting in women? To what extent does stunting reduce productivity? Does stunting perpetuate poverty over the generations? Stunting is not just an indicator but an undesirable feature that has got to be corrected. But I am not talking of stunting in isolation; it can only be corrected as part of an overall attack on the problem of poverty and undernutrition. When I spoke about the implications of stunting, I did not mean that these flow out of stunting per se; I said: "the community in which you see a lot of stunting is a community that is afflicted by a number of other things that go with stunting." That is what I meant by "the cost of stunting and its implications." It is not a relationship of cause and effect.

Dr. Martorell: I agree that there are some areas we talked about, infant mortality, for instance, where you can argue in that way. But it is much more difficult in other areas, productivity, for example. I think we stand a better chance of improving the situation if we emphasize that stunting is an indicator of social inequalities.

Dr. Kraisid: About 6 years ago, the National Economic and Social Development Board sponsored a study in Thailand on the use of malnutrition in terms of wasting and stunting as a social indicator. We have a so-called poverty eradication program, the concept of which was just as you mentioned. I think it is important to emphasize, for all countries who initiate similar programs, that they need to be supported from the top; many processes are involved, and the approach needs to be a holistic one.

Dr. Golden: I would like to ask how you reconcile the data presented earlier by Dr. Keller, in which no change in the distribution of stunting was seen in Jordan from 1974 until 1985 and yet, during that time, they had all sorts of public health programs, such as improving the literacy of the mothers, introducing oral rehydration, etc. No change at all was observed in the profile of stunting, but quite marked changes in the profile of wasting. We have contradictory data that we have to reconcile, and I would like your comments.

Dr. Gopalan: As I mentioned, I don't think that intensive health care alone can solve the problem of stunting. You can have a very efficient health service but a great deal of poverty, and if you haven't addressed the question of poverty, you are not going to solve the problem of stunting. This is what I mean by integrated development: income generation programs, which go hand in hand with health care, education of women, etc. There must be a comprehensive attack on the problem of poverty; otherwise, you may reduce deaths and that is all.

Dr. Waterlow: In other words, you are assuming that in Jordan there was no change in the degree of poverty in the refugee camps.

Dr. Gopalan: I don't know the Jordan situation, but I wouldn't be surprised if the emphasis were all on intensive health care and not on overall economic improvement.

Dr. Van Lerberghe: We still seem to get stuck with stunting either as a problem or as an indicator. Stunting is not a problem, but it is also certainly not the only indicator. I am not surprised by data like those from Jordan, where you do not find significant associations between the prevalence of stunting and the implementation of public health programs. This indicator does not work everywhere; it is one of the indicators one can use in order to obtain effective decision making, but it is not the only one.

Dr. Valyasevi: I agree almost totally with what Dr. Gopalan has said. It is the overall development that is important. Our government in Thailand is heading this way. But children are born every day, and we cannot wait until the total socioeconomic situation has improved, because this may take 10 to 20 years. I thus have three practical questions. If resources are limited:

1. What are the at-risk groups? Dr. Gopalan mentioned the fetus *in utero* and young children up to 5 years of age; this seems acceptable to me.
2. Which indicators should be used? These need to be reasonably sensitive, specific, and applicable in the existing social structure. At present, the public health authority in Thailand uses weight by age, but it has been criticized for that; what else should be recommended?
3. When should intervention programs start and stop? Here, of course, since resources are limited, we need to think in terms of cost effectiveness.

Dr. Gopalan: Questions as to what the mix in the intervention package should be, when it should start, and within which target groups are matters for local governments to decide. In a country like India, this cannot be legislated from New Delhi. There is a need for studying the problems locally. I am not able to say what has to be done in all developing countries. An important question, when we are talking of intervention, is "what is the intervention we are talking about?" If we are referring to education, for example, educating mothers on how to feed their children, then that should go on continuously as part of the health care program; in fact, it should start even before a girl becomes a mother. I would put great emphasis on that. Supplementation, giving nutrient supplements, is very expensive—it involves a lot of investment—and there, of course, we run into political pressures.

Dr. Aponso: Dr. Gopalan, you have given the right perspective of the situation in Third World countries. You mentioned seven different factors that converge to a common pathway and produce chronic undernutrition, stunting, and deterioration of child health in our countries. You called the common pathway the "poverty syndrome." This is true, but I know you will agree that it is not merely a question of poverty, but it is a triad of (a) poverty; (b) ignorance; and (c) customs, beliefs, and tradition.

Most of our villages are bound by some of these customs, beliefs, and traditions: some are very good; some are harmful. Our resources are limited; we need time and money. Some resources are available in our countries. You mentioned nutrition education; this is excellent, but we should make use not only of health professionals but of social scientists as well. With the resources we have, we can increase our productivity if we accept the use of the community itself and if we accept community participation. Our community is today made up of people who are used to doing things as they are told. We should educate them to do things not merely because they are asked to do so but as an expression of their own self-will; in other words, as active acceptors.

Dr. Gopalan: The extensive use of health volunteers, as in Sri Lanka and Indonesia, is a very good thing. I wish it could happen on a large scale in India also.

Dr. Mukerhjee: In developing countries, the poverty syndrome—poor food, housing, education, and employment opportunity, frequent illness, and inadequate health care—represents a formidable problem. To meet the challenge we should make a sincere effort in prevention: early screening of cases, improvement of weaning practices, education in general as well as health and nutrition education, application of knowledge in practice, and teaching and training of parents and paramedical and medical personnel in health and nutrition of children.

Dr. Nabarro: Most of the interventions that have been suggested are likely to have only a limited impact. The association between stunting and socioeconomic deprivation implies that reducing the incidence of stunting requires broad development strategies and not just public health interventions. The implementation of poverty-focused development programs is both difficult and costly. I would predict that the average cost of preventing Nepalese children from becoming stunted would be at least U.S.$100 per child per year; it would certainly be much more than the present figure for health care expenditure (U.S.$1 to 2 per year).

Dr. Gopalan: I am not discouraged by prophecies of gloom. I challenge this calculation of over U.S.$100 per child per year. It may be correct under the American scale, but not under the Nepalese scale.

Dr. Tomkins: There is an increasing tendency for people to perceive nutrition and stunting as things that could be changed by vertical programs. I wonder what advice you would give for the next 10 to 20 years as to how we are going to avoid being obsessed with vertical programs within the health sector as opposed to the more integrated approaches that you have suggested.

Dr. Gopalan: Except for interventions for eliminating conditions such as goiter or to a certain extent keratomalacia, I don't think that vertical programs are the answer. Primary health care as it is now being conceived, which is an integrated effort, is the way to go about it. That is what I am pushing for.

Dr. Davies: This meeting has been very helpful, but it does share one thing in common with many others of its kind in involving those who are already convinced. Since strategies that are supposed to improve matters are so much in the hands of politicians and social scientists, I sometimes feel that to have a political presence in these meetings would be helpful, so that at least we could have the opportunity of putting questions and points of view to people who are primarily responsible for making and implementing decisions. I would value comments from others on whether or not these symposia would be more meaningful and strategies for improvement more relevant had we also a political presence?

Dr. Gopalan: I agree.

Dr. Waterlow: As a physiologist, I am disappointed that nobody seems to be interested in the biology of stunting, in what actually causes it eventually. We know that this is a preventable phenomenon, so there must be a metabolic nutritional biological cause. I don't think we know these causal factors. Can we do anything useful without really knowing the causal factors? I am not proposing an antistunting program, but it somehow seems wrong, and I rather agree with Professor Davies, to turn our back on ignorance and simply talk to each other as if we knew all the answers.

Dr. Tanner: Although, intellectually, I agree with Professor Waterlow, I think that that train of thought is extremely dangerous, because I think we may have the answer to his question in the not too distant future (in terms of the physiology of IGF I). We might then be tempted to do a kind of phenylketonuria program, what I believe you call a vertical intervention program, and then what will happen? You will still have massive poverty, but the people will not be short. So what have you achieved? I am thus absolutely at one with all the last few speakers. Height is only important as a proxy for social deprivation (as between groups).

Dr. Guesry: Nestlé Nutrition Workshops are supposed to be scientific workshops. We are not here to make decisions in the name of any government. I was also disappointed that the biological aspect has not been touched on.

Dr. Waterlow: To repeat what Dr. Golden said, we can't apply knowledge we don't have. Coming back to the political dimension, surely you would agree, Dr. Gopalan, that it has been extremely useful to know, if we are convinced by Dr. Colombo, that failure of physical growth has no direct relationship to failure of mental growth. The data of Dr. Spurr are very important. I am not suggesting, when looking at the biological implications, that, as a result, we should try to prevent stunting. I am trying to put it in its proper perspective, that's all.

Dr. Valysevi: I agree with Dr. Waterlow; we all like to understand what is happening. However, in Japan, for example, in the past 30 years, the final length has remarkably increased; in Thailand too, although we still don't know the causes of stunting, the height of school children has now increased by at least 2 inches compared to 20 years ago. Therefore, I think that both the physiological and political aspects of the problem need to be addressed together.

Dr. Golden: Undoubtedly there must be a biological reason, quite apart from poverty. If we look at many of the populations in Africa, we find populations living quite close to each other, in one of which the staple is sorghum and in the other plantain; both populations have equal body weights, but the cereal-eating population is much taller and thinner than the plantain-eating population, which is short and fat. In West Africa, where we have yam- and grain-eating people, we find exactly the same thing, although if we look at the level of poverty in these villages, we really find very little difference in terms of disposable income. There must be biological reasons that we have to tackle and not just put them all down to poverty.

Dr. Waterlow: I would like to suggest that two points of practical application have come out of the "biological" part of our discussion. One is that the data have emphasized, more than we knew before, that this growth failure starts very early in life and that it therefore has some application to the question of "where should we concentrate our resources?" The precise determination will depend on local conditions, but this would bring us to concentrate our efforts on the first year of life rather than on the fifth.

The second important point that has emerged, again at the technical level, is the great sensitivity of velocity measurements as opposed to distance measurements and, as Professor Tanner and Dr. van Lerberghe have said, the value these may have for decision making. Perhaps we could agree that we don't have two completely distinct points of view on this?

Dr. Nabarro: Is it really appropriate to propose that interventions be concentrated on the first year of life just because this is the period when linear growth retardation is more prominent? Do we know enough about the functional consequences of this growth retardation to be able to make such prescriptions? I would suggest that we do not yet have sufficient information at our disposal to make such recommendations.

Dr. Gopalan: I think that we should take the whole period of intrauterine development, infancy, and the preschool period as a continuum if only because some of the effects that you see in infancy could still be corrected in the preschool period. I would rather suggest that we treat this as one unit.

Dr. Waterlow: I do not agree with Dr. Nabarro, and I do not much care for the so-called "holistic," antianalytical point of view, which seems to me just a reiteration of received and obvious doctrine. However, disagreement among scientists is perhaps a sign that the subject is in a healthy state. It would be interesting to repeat this symposium in 5 years' time to see whether the disagreements persist in the light of whatever new information we may have succeeded in getting by then.

SUBJECT INDEX

Subject Index